Ostheimer's Manual of

OBSTETRIC
ANESTHESIA

D1021006

Ostheimer's Manual of
OBSTETRIC ANESTHESIA

THIRD EDITION

David J. Birnbach, M.D.

Associate Professor, Departments of Anesthesiology and
Obstetrics and Gynecology
College of Physicians and Surgeons
Columbia University;
Director, Obstetric Anesthesiology
St. Luke's–Roosevelt Hospital Center
New York, New York

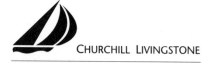

CHURCHILL LIVINGSTONE

A Harcourt Health Sciences Company
New York Edinburgh London Philadelphia

Churchill Livingstone
A Harcourt Health Sciences Company

The Curtis Center
Independence Square West
Philadelphia, Pennsylvania 19106

Library of Congress Cataloging-in-Publication Data

Ostheimer's manual of obstetric anesthesia / [edited by] David J. Birnbach.—3rd ed.

p.   cm.

Rev. ed. of: Manual of obstetric anesthesia / edited by Gerard W. Ostheimer. 2nd ed. 1992.
Includes bibliographical references and index.

ISBN 0–443–06554–3

1. Anesthesia in obstetrics—Handbooks, manuals, etc.   I. Birnbach, David J.   II. Ostheimer, Gerard W.

[DNLM: 1. Anesthesia, Obstetrical—methods. WO 450 085 2000]
RG732 .M36 2000
617.9′682 21—dc21   99–035204

Acquisitions Editor: Allan Ross
Developmental Editor: Melissa Dudlick
Production Editor: Evelyn Adler
Production Manager: Norman Stellander
Illustration Specialist: Francis Moriarty
Book Designer: Jonel Sofian

OSTHEIMER'S MANUAL OF
OBSTETRIC ANESTHESIA   ISBN 0–443–06554–3

Printed in the United States of America.

Last digit is the print number: 9   8   7   6   5   4   3   2   1

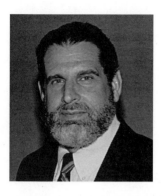

We dedicate this third edition of Ostheimer's Manual of Obstetric Anesthesia *to the memory of Gerard W. Ostheimer, M.D. As our teacher, friend, and mentor, he inspired the contributors to this book, each of whom trained under his guidance at the Brigham and Women's Hospital or its predecessor, the Boston Lying-In. We have now come together to revise and sustain his* Manual of Obsetric Anesthesia *because we believe that a manual for residents and fellows who are learning obstetric anesthesia is just as indispensable today as it was when it was first published 16 years ago. In addition, we, his fellows, know how important this book was to Gerry. In dedicating this book to his memory, we acknowledge Dr. Ostheimer's numerous contributions to obstetric anesthesia and his commitment to the training of residents and fellows in this field. His vision changed the practice of obstetric anesthesia and our lives.*

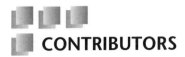
CONTRIBUTORS

Angela M. Bader, M.D.
Associate Professor of Anaesthesia, Harvard Medical School; Director, PreAdmitting Test Center, Brigham and Women's Hospital, Boston, Massachusetts
Neonatal Resuscitation

David J. Birnbach, M.D.
Associate Professor, Departments of Anesthesiology and Obstetrics and Gynecology, Columbia University College of Physicians and Surgeons; Director, Obstetric Anesthesiology, St. Luke's–Roosevelt Hospital Center, New York, New York
Academic Goals for the Obstetric Anesthesiology Rotation; Techniques of Neuraxial Analgesia for Labor

Corey A. Burchman, B.A., M.D.
Attending Anesthesiologist, York Hospital, York, Pennsylvania
Anesthetic Management of the Pregnant Surgical Patient

Gerald A. Burger, M.D.
Staff Anesthesiologist, Wyoming Medical Center, Casper, Wyoming
Principles of Perinatal Pharmacology

William R. Camann, M.D.
Associate Professor of Anesthesia, Harvard Medical School; Director of Obstetric Anesthesia Education, Brigham and Women's Hospital, Boston, Massachusetts
Physiologic Adaptations During Pregnancy

Barry Corke, M.B., Ch.B., F.R.C.A.
Attending Anesthesiologist, Christiana Health Care System, Wilmington, Delaware
Maternal Mortality

Regina Fragneto, M.D.
Associate Professor and Director, Obstetric Anesthesia, University of Kentucky College of Medicine, Lexington, Kentucky
Obstetric Complications

Stephen P. Gatt, M.D., F.A.N.Z.C.A., F.F.I.C.A.N.Z.C.A.
Senior Lecturer in Anaesthesia, University of New South Wales, Sydney, Australia; Head of Division of Anaesthesia and Intensive Care, Programme Director, Acute Services Programme, Head of Division, Anaesthesia and Intensive Care, The Prince of Wales, Sydney Children's, and Prince Henry Hospitals, Sydney, Australia
Preeclampsia and Eclampsia

Ronald Hurley, M.D.
Assistant Professor of Anesthesia, Harvard Medical School; Associate Director of Obstetric Anesthesia, Brigham and Women's Hospital, Boston, Massachusetts
The High-Risk Parturient

Kathleen Leavitt, M.D.
Assistant Professor, Department of Anesthesiology; Director, Division of Obstetric Anesthesiology, George Washington University, Washington, DC
Techniques of Neuraxial Analgesia for Labor

Andrew M. Malinow, M.D.
Associate Professor of Anesthesiology and Obstetrics, Gynecology and Reproductive

Sciences, University of Maryland School of Medicine; Director of Obstetric Anesthesiology, Associate Vice-Chair, Department of Anesthesiology, University of Maryland Medical Center, Baltimore, Maryland
  Embolic Disease

Ramon Martin, M.D., Ph.D.
Instructor, Harvard Medical School; Staff Anesthesiologist, Brigham and Women's Hospital, Boston, Massachusetts
  Antepartum Fetal Assessment

Timothy B. McDonald, M.D., J.D.
Assistant Professor, Anesthesiology; Assistant Professor, Pediatrics, University of Illinois at Chicago College of Medicine, Chicago, Illinois
  Legal and Ethical Issues in Obstetric Anesthesia

Norah Naughton, M.D.
Clinical Assistant Professor, University of Michigan Medical School; Clinical Assistant Professor, University of Michigan Health System, Ann Arbor, Michigan
  Regional Anesthesia for Cesarean Section

Lee S. Perrin, M.D.
Associate Clinical Professor of Anesthesia, Tufts University School of Medicine; Vice Chairman, Department of

Anesthesiology, St. Elizabeth's Medical Center, Boston, Massachusetts
  Guidelines for Obstetric Anesthesia

Ferne B. Sevarino, M.D.
Associate Professor of Anesthesiology; Chief, Section of Obstetrical Anesthesiology; Associate Director, Acute Pain Service, Yale University School of Medicine, New Haven, Connecticut
  Postoperative Pain Management After Cesarean Delivery

Glenn Shopper, M.D.
Assistant Professor, Jefferson Medical College, Thomas Jefferson University; Director of Obstetric Anesthesia, Albert Einstein Medical Center, Philadelphia, Pennsylvania
  General Anesthesia for Cesarean Section

Maya S. Suresh, M.D.
Professor, Department of Anesthesiology, Baylor College of Medicine; Director, Service Chief of Anesthesiology, Baylor College of Medicine, Houston, Texas
  Obstetric Hemorrhage

Esther M. Yun, M.D.
Chief of Obstetric Anesthesia, Lenox Hill Hospital, New York, New York
  Pharmacology of Local Anesthetics

PREFACE TO THE THIRD EDITION

The *Manual of Obstetric Anesthesia* is the outgrowth of physiologic and pharmacologic approaches to pain relief the obstetric patient developed and practiced at the Brigham and Women's Hospital, Harvard Medical School. The approach to clinical care that is presented in this *Manual* is the result of more than 30 years of obstetric anesthesia research, teaching, and clinical experience at the Brigham and Women's Hospital and its predecessor institutions (the Boston Lying-In Hospital and the Boston Hospital for Women) and is a testament to the institution and those who have tirelessly worked to improve the practice of obstetric anesthesiology.

Each of the 19 authors completed their training in obstetric anesthesiology under the nurturing, dedicated, and demanding guardianship of the late Gerard W. Ostheimer, M.D., who inspired not only us but an entire generation of anesthesiologists. He believed in the importance of a clear and concise manual for the resident learning obstetric anesthesiology, and it is our hope that this third edition will keep his dream alive and continue to help the next generation of anesthesiologists.

The goal of this book is not to produce another encyclopedic textbook, as there are several excellent obstetric anesthesiology textbooks already available. As the title suggests, this is a manual geared to residents and fellows. However, as in the first two editions of the Ostheimer manual, I hope that it will also be useful to practicing anesthesiologists, obstetricians, and nurses who want concise up-to-date and clinically oriented information on obstetric anesthesia, and also that it will find a place as a reference in Labor and Delivery suites.

Eight years and numerous changes in the field of obstetric anesthesiology have occurred since the publication of the second edition. The third edition of the *Manual* is in many ways a completely new book. Most chapters have been completely rewritten to include current practice. The description of old techniques has been revised, and new areas of interest such as combined spinal epidural anesthesia and the new amide local anesthetics have been added. The biggest change, however, is that the format of this book more closely resembles that of the first edition so that it can be more easily carried and therefore be more readily accessible to the clinician on the labor floor. As in any book with multiple authors, a small amount of duplication is found. However, as in previous editions, this is intentional so that the reader can learn all the necessary information on each topic in one chapter.

Special thanks to Michael Houston and his colleagues at

ngstone, who believed that the Ostheimer Man-
continue despite the untimely death of its first
lissa Dudlick of W.B. Saunders who kept the
om getting too loose; and to Daniel M. Thys,
irman, mentor, and friend, without whose sup-
ouragement this book would never have been

DAVID J. BIRNBACH, M.D.

CONTENTS

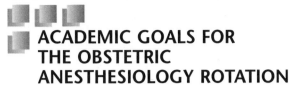

ACADEMIC GOALS FOR THE OBSTETRIC ANESTHESIOLOGY ROTATION

David J. Birnbach, MD

The checklist below represents the subjects that should be learned during your obstetric anesthesiology rotation. Each item should be checked off when it is fully understood.

I. Physiologic changes of pregnancy
1. Cardiovascular
☐ a. Changes to cardiac output and blood volume in each trimester
☐ b. Changes occurring during labor
☐ c. Changes in the postpartum period
2. Pulmonary, respiratory, and airway
☐ a. Changes in upper airway
☐ b. Changes in respiratory mechanics
☐ c. Changes in gas exchange
3. Gastrointestinal
☐ a. Hormonal changes
☐ b. Anatomic changes
4. Renal
☐ a. Normal values of blood urea nitrogen, creatinine, and glomerular filtration rate in pregnancy
☐ b. Changes in renal function due to disease states
5. Hematologic
☐ a. Anemia of pregnancy
☐ b. Changes in coagulation factors
6. Central nervous system
☐ a. Effect of pregnancy on minimal alveolar concentration
☐ b. Pressure and volume changes within the epidural space

II. Perinatal pharmacology
☐ 1. Anatomy of the placental-fetal unit
☐ 2. Regulation of umbilical–placental circulation
☐ 3. Uteroplacental circulation and its determinants
☐ 4. Measurement of uteroplacental blood flow
☐ 5. Placental transfer of anesthetics
☐ 6. Fetal adaptations to hypoxia

III. Fetal and neonatal assessment
- [ ] 1. Intrapartum fetal heart rate tracings
  - [ ] a. Early decelerations
  - [ ] b. Late decelerations
  - [ ] c. Variable decelerations
- [ ] 2. Apgar scores
- [ ] 3. Nonstress testing, contraction stress testing
- [ ] 4. Fetal blood sampling
- [ ] 5. Definition of perinatal mortality

IV. Neonatal physiology
- [ ] 1. Intrapartum resuscitation
- [ ] 2. Neonatal adaptations to extrauterine life
- [ ] 3. Newborn resuscitation

V. Labor analgesia
- [ ] 1. Stages of labor and pain pathways
- [ ] 2. Effect of analgesia on labor and delivery
- [ ] 3. Options available for maternal analgesia
- [ ] 4. Epidural analgesia technique
- [ ] 5. Complications of neuraxial analgesia for labor
- [ ] 6. Combined spinal-epidural technique
- [ ] 7. Continuous spinal techniques

VI. Cesarean section
- [ ] 1. Obstetric indications for abdominal delivery
- [ ] 2. Indications for emergency cesarean section
- [ ] 3. Anesthetic options for elective/emergency cesarean sections
- [ ] 4. Management of the patient with antepartum hemorrhage for cesarean section
- [ ] 5. Treatment of postpartum uterine atony
- [ ] 6. Anesthesia for multiple pregnancies
- [ ] 7. Anesthesia for breech position
- [ ] 8. General anesthesia for cesarean section
  - [ ] a. Indications for use of general anesthesia
  - [ ] b. Induction agents and doses
  - [ ] c. Maintenance of general anesthesia
  - [ ] d. Recognition and management of the "difficult airway"
  - [ ] e. Algorithm for failed intubation in the parturient
  - [ ] f. Prevention, recognition, and treatment of pulmonary aspiration
- [ ] 9. Regional anesthesia for cesarean section
  - [ ] a. Spinal needles, drugs, and dosage
  - [ ] b. Epidural anesthesia for emergency and elective cesarean section
  - [ ] c. Contraindications to regional anesthesia
  - [ ] d. Spinal anesthesia for cesarean section
  - [ ] e. Continuous spinal anesthesia

☐   f. Combined spinal-epidural techniques for cesarean section
☐   g. Complications of regional anesthesia and their treatment
☐ 10. Postoperative pain management after cesarean delivery
    ☐ a. Patient-controlled analgesia
    ☐ b. Subarachnoid opioids
    ☐ c. Epidural infusions
    ☐ d. Oral treatments: Nonsteroidal anti-inflammatory drugs and oral opioids

VII. Local anesthetics
  ☐ 1. Pharmacology of local anesthetics
  ☐ 2. Treatment of local anesthetic toxicity
  ☐ 3. Diagnosis and treatment of total spinal
  ☐ 4. Effects of anesthetics on the fetus
  ☐ 5. Effects of vasoconstrictors and other local anesthetic additives

VIII. Neuraxial opioids
  ☐ 1. Pharmacology of neuraxial opioids
    ☐ a. Sufentanil
    ☐ b. Fentanyl
    ☐ c. Meperidine
    ☐ d. Morphine
  ☐ 2. Side effects of neuroaxial opioids
    ☐ a. Respiratory depression/arrest
    ☐ b. Pruritis
    ☐ c. Hypotension
    ☐ d. Fetal bradycardia
  ☐ 3. Fetal effects of neuraxial opioids
  ☐ 4. Interaction between neuraxial opioids and local anesthetics

IX. Obstetric complications and their anesthetic management
  ☐ 1. Obstetric hemorrhage
    ☐ a. Abruptio placenta
    ☐ b. Placenta previa
    ☐ c. Placenta accreta
    ☐ d. Retained placenta
  ☐ 2. Uterine inversion
  ☐ 3. Uterine rupture
  ☐ 4. Amniotic fluid embolism
  ☐ 5. Preterm labor
  ☐ 6. Multiple gestation
  ☐ 7. Multiparity

X. Hypertensive disorders of pregnancy
  ☐ 1. Pathophysiology
  ☐ 2. Definition of severe preeclampsia

☐ 3. Antihypertensive options for pregnancy-induced hypertension
☐ 4. Magnesium sulfate
☐ 5. Management of oliguria
☐ 6. Indications for invasive monitoring
☐ 7. Anesthetic options for cesarean section
☐ 8. HELLP syndrome

XI. The high-risk paturient
  ☐ 1. Morbid obesity
  ☐ 2. Asthma
  ☐ 3. Diabetes
  ☐ 4. Cardiac disease
  ☐ 5. Diabetes
  ☐ 6. Renal disease
  ☐ 7. Neurologic disease
  ☐ 8. Substance abuse
  ☐ 9. Human immunodeficiency virus infection
  ☐ 10. Cardiac arrest

XII. Anesthesia for nonobstetric surgery during pregnancy
  ☐ 1. Teratogenicity of anesthetic agents
  ☐ 2. Maternal considerations
  ☐ 3. Fetal considerations
  ☐ 4. Fetal surgery
  ☐ 5. Postpartum surgery

XIII. Guidelines for obstetric anesthesia
  ☐ 1. Definitions
     ☐ a. Practice parameters
     ☐ b. Standards
     ☐ c. Guidelines
  ☐ 2. Guidelines for regional anesthesia in obstetrics
  ☐ 3. Standards for basic anesthesia monitoring
  ☐ 4. Standards for postanesthesia care
  ☐ 5. Practice guidelines—ASA Task Force on obstetrical anesthesia

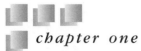

chapter one

PHYSIOLOGIC ADAPTATIONS DURING PREGNANCY

William R. Camann, MD

The transition from the nonpregnant to the pregnant state is heralded by the growth and development of the fetoplacental unit within a constantly enlarging uterus. Profound physiologic and anatomic changes due to this gravid state result in maternal adaptations in all organ systems. The anesthesiologist caring for the pregnant patient must understand these physiologic changes to provide safe analgesia and anesthesia to mother and safe deliverance to the fetus.

CARDIOVASCULAR SYSTEM

Cardiac Output

Oxygen consumption is increased in pregnancy and maternal cardiac output rises to meet these demands. The rise in cardiac output is a result of increased heart rate, increased stroke volume, and decreased afterload (Table 1-1). Cardiac output rises most rapidly during the second trimester (Fig. 1-1) and then remains steady until term when labor and uteroplacental transfusion of blood into the intravascular system result in additional increases in cardiac output. Central filling pressures (CVP, PA, pulmonary capillary wedge pressure) do not change during normal pregnancy. Although left ventricular diastolic volume is increased, hypertrophy and dilation can allow for this increased volume without an increase in pressure.

■ Table 1–1
MATERNAL CARDIOVASCULAR ALTERATIONS AT TERM

Variable	Change	Rate (%)
Cardiac output	↑ ↑ ↑ ↑	40
Stroke volume	↑ ↑ ↑	0–30
Heart rate	↑ ↑	15
Systolic blood pressure	↓	0–5 mm Hg
Diastolic blood pressure	↓ ↓	10–20 mm Hg
Total peripheral resistance	↓ ↓	15
Central venous pressure	+	0
Pulmonary wedge pressure	−	0
Ejection fraction	−	0

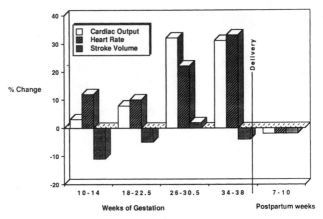

Figure 1–1 ■ Hemodynamic changes during pregnancy. (From Mashini IS, Albazzaz SJ, Fadel HE, et al: Serial noninvasive evaluation of cardiovascular hemodynamics during pregnancy. Am J Obstet Gynecol 156:1208–1213, 1987.)

Blood Volume

Blood volume increases by 35% during pregnancy compared with the nonpregnant state. The stimulus for this change is controversial. Increased mineralocorticoid levels seen during pregnancy will predispose to progressive sodium and water retention with consequent enlargement of the intravascular space (the "overfill" hypothesis).[1] Alternatively, primary enlargement of this space due to hormonal (prostaglandin, progesterone) vasodilation and placental arteriovenous shunting may be the stimulus for secondary renal sodium and water retention (the "underfill" hypothesis). Recent evidence seems to favor primary peripheral vasodilation early in the first trimester (underfill) as the etiology of subsequent blood volume expansion.[2]

Uterine Size and Vascularity

The gravid uterine blood flow is 20 to 40 times above the nonpregnant level, accounting for 20% of maternal cardiac output at term. Uterine vascular resistance is markedly reduced during gestation, producing a low-pressure "parallel" circuit in concert with an overall reduced maternal systemic vascular resistance.

The enlarged uterus will produce mechanical compression of surrounding vascular structures, known as aortocaval compression or the "maternal supine hypotensive syndrome." In the supine position, compression of the vena cava decreases venous return, resulting in decreased stroke volume and hypotension. A small percentage of women experience severe bradycardia in the supine position due to this decreased venous return. Compression of the aorta may decrease uterine perfusion, resulting in "fetal distress." Normal maternal compensatory response to aortocaval compression consists of tachycardia and both upper and lower extremity vasoconstriction.

Vascular Tone

Normal parturients demonstrate decreased responsiveness to vasopressor and chronotropic substances. Epinephrine, norepinephrine, isoproterenol, and angiotensin II all show dose-related blunting of effect during pregnancy.[3] Downregulation of α- and β-adrenergic receptors has been postulated as the etiology of this phenomena; however, the presence of vasodilatory prostaglandins may play a role as well because inhibitors of prostaglandin synthesis have been shown to reverse the vascular resistance to catecholamines and because patients with preeclampsia who manifest an abundance of vasoconstricting prostaglandins (e.g., thromboxane) demonstrate an increased sensitivity to exogenous catecholamines. Different vascular beds may react to vasopressors differently in the pregnant versus nonpregnant state. Uterine blood vessels show decreased responsiveness to ephedrine in pregnancy, whereas femoral vessels do not. Regional differences in nitric oxide synthetase in the different beds may explain these findings. This observation also explains, in part, the safety of ephedine when used to treat maternal hypotension.

Clinical Implications

Aortocaval compression should always be avoided. Parturients should not be allowed to rest in the supine position but rather encouraged to maintain uterine displacement by a right or left lateral tilt of the pelvis (Fig. 1–2). Sympathetic blockade due to spinal or epidural anesthesia will interfere with the mechanisms to compensate for aortocaval compression; thus, profound hypotension may ensue in the absence of adequate uterine displacement and intravascular volume expansion.

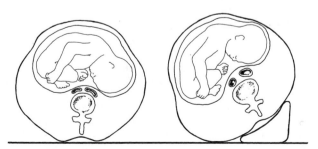

Figure 1–2 ■ Aortocaval decompression with left lateral tilt.

Conditions that predispose to a particularly large uterus (e.g., multiple gestation, polyhydramnios, diabetes mellitus) make those parturients especially susceptible to the risk and consequences of aortocaval compression.

■ **KEY POINT:** Compression of the aorta and inferior vena cava by the gravid uterus may precipitate profound hypotension. This hypotension may be worsened following initiation of spinal and epidural anesthesia. To minimize this risk, parturients undergoing cesarean section should have left uterine displacement initiated as soon as possible.

Engorgement of the epidural vasculature (Battson's plexus) makes puncture or cannulation of an epidural vein more likely than in the nonpregnant patient during initiation of epidural analgesia. Likewise, negative pressure in the epidural space may not be consistently found in the parturient. Hence, theoretically, the "hanging drop" technique for identification of the epidural space may be less successful in the pregnant patient than in the nonpregnant counterpart.

Patients with cardiac disease may tolerate pregnancy poorly. The increased blood volume and decreased systemic resistance may cause decompensation in patients with stenotic valvular lesions and may worsen right-to-left shunting in the presence of uncorrected congenital heart defects. In contrast, parturients with regurgitant valvular lesions usually do quite well during pregnancy. Although coronary artery disease is rare among women of childbearing age, a gradual trend to older parturients may increase the incidence of myocardial ischemia and/or infarction during gestation. The hypermetabolic demands of pregnancy suggest that invasive monitoring should be considered in parturients with known or suspected atherosclerotic, spastic, or thrombotic coronary artery disease.

RESPIRATORY SYSTEM

Upper Airway

Generalized peripheral edema is a common problem in pregnancy; however, edematous changes of the upper airway may be life threatening. Mucous membranes become extremely friable during the third trimester, and manipulation of the upper airway, such as may occur during insertion of nasal airways, nasogastric tubes, or nasotracheal intubation, should be done with great care because severe bleeding may result. Preeclamptic patients are particularly susceptible to airway and vocal cord edema. Difficult intubation and requirement for very small diameter endotracheal tubes (i.e., 6.0 mm or less) should always be considered when caring for such patients.

Respiratory Mechanics

The expanding uterus produces cephalad displacement of the diaphragm; thus, functional residual capacity (FRC) is decreased. Total lung capacity, vital capacity, and inspiratory capacity all remain unchanged as compensatory subcostal widening and increased anterioposterior diameter of the thoracic cage occurs (Table 1–2). The increased oxygen consumption of pregnancy is compensated by a 70% increase in alveolar ventilation at term. This is accomplished by increases in both tidal volume (40%) and respiratory rate (15%). Enhancement of tidal volume is largely due to rib cage volume displacement and less so to abdominal (diaphragmatic) movement. The rise in alveolar ventilation exceeds the oxygen demands of the parturient and is likely a result of elevated progesterone levels that increase the ventilatory response to carbon dioxide.

Gas Exchange

Ventilatory augmentation produces a respiratory alkalosis with compensatory renal excretion of bicarbonate and hence partial pH correction. Oxygenation is improved during normal pregnancy; arterial Po_2 values are typically slightly higher than in the nongravid state (Table 1–3). Physiologic dead space at term is decreased.[4] It is likely that increased cardiac output with favorable ventilation–perfusion matching in upper lung zones accounts for both the increased Po_2 values and decreased dead space (e.g., less unperfused alveoli).

■ Table 1–2
MATERNAL RESPIRATORY ALTERATIONS AT TERM

Variable	Change	Rate (%)
Minute ventilation	↑ ↑ ↑ ↑	50
Alveolar ventilation	↑ ↑ ↑ ↑ ↑	70
Tidal volume	↑ ↑ ↑	40
Respiratory rate	↑	15
Closing volume	± ↓	0
Airway resistance	↓ ↓	36
Vital capacity	±	0
Inspiratory lung capacity	±	0
Functional residual capacity	↓ ↓	20
Total lung capacity	±	0
Expiratory reserve volume	↓ ↓	20
Residual volume	↓ ↓	20
Oxygen consumption	↑ ↑	20

From Skaredoff MN, Ostheimer GW: Physiologic changes during pregnancy: effects of major regional anesthesia. Reg Anesth 6:28–40, 1981.

■ Table 1–3
ACID-BASE VALUES IN PREGNANCY VS. THE NONPREGNANT STATE

Variable	Nonpregnant State	Pregnancy
pH	7.38–7.42	7.38–7.42
P_{O_2}, mm Hg	90–100	100–110
P_{CO_2}, mm Hg	35–45	28–32

Clinical Implications

The decreased FRC is usually of little concern to the normal parturient. However, conditions that decrease closing volume (otherwise unchanged in normal pregnancy) such as smoking, obesity, or kyphoscoliosis may result in airway closure and increasing hypoxemia as pregnancy progresses. The relationship between FRC and closing volume may be further aggravated by the positions assumed during birth (Trendelenburg, lithotomy, and supine) and by induction of general anesthesia. The increased P_{O_2} values are seen consistently in pregnant women in the erect position; this finding is not always true in the supine position. Consequently, one should have a low threshold for administration of supplemental oxygen to the parturient in labor, particularly during episodes of fetal distress or before induction of general anesthetic. The decreased FRC should imply that oxygenation (denitrogenation) occurs more rapidly in the parturient than in the nonpregnant women, and indeed this is the case.[5] However, the marked increase in oxygen consumption contributes to the frighteningly rapid development of maternal hypoxemia during periods of apnea. The decrease in dead space serves to further enhance the reliability of noninvasive respiratory monitoring (capnography and/or mass spectrometery), as the gap between end-tidal and arterial gas measurements narrows.[6]

■ **KEY POINT:** Functional residual capacity begins to decrease in the second trimester and is decreased to 80% of the nonpregnant value at full term. This decrease in FRC causes maternal hypoxemia to develop very quickly following apnea associated with the induction of general anesthesia.

GASTROINTESTINAL SYSTEM

Elevated levels of circulating progesterone will decrease gastrointestinal motility, decrease food absorption, and lower esophageal sphincter pressure.[7] In addition, elevated gastrin levels (of placental origin) result in more acidic gastric contents. The enlarged uterus increases intragastric pressure and decreases the normal oblique angle of the gastroesophageal junction, facilitating reflux of gastric contents.

Clinical Implications

These gastrointestinal tract alterations mandate that the parturient always should be considered to have a full stomach, regardless of the actual number of hours elapsed since the last meal. Consequently, pregnant patients should always be considered to be at risk for aspiration of gastric contents (Mendelson's syndrome), and measures should be taken to minimize this risk. Moreover, pain, anxiety, and narcotic analgesics will serve to further retard gastric emptying during labor. Even opioids administered via the epidural or intrathecal route may retard gastric emptying. Maternal "bearing down" efforts and the lithotomy position during the second stage of labor and delivery coupled with incompetence of the lower esophageal sphincter mechanism may all increase the risk of silent regurgitation and aspiration.

■ **KEY POINT:** Gastric emptying is slowed during labor and the early postpartum period. If general anesthesia becomes necessary during those periods, the airway must be secured in order to minimize the risk of aspiration.

Our practice is to require oral administration of 30 mL of a nonparticulate antacid (0.3 M sodium citrate or its equivalent) before the initiation of any anesthetic. This agent will rapidly decrease the acidity of gastric contents and help ameliorate the consequences of aspiration. Histamine receptor (H_2) antagonists such as cimetidine (Tagamet) or ranitidine (Zantac) may be administered orally the evening before and orally or intravenously the morning of an elective procedure. Metoclopramide (Reglan) will stimulate gastric emptying, increase lower esophageal sphincter tone, and serve as a centrally acting antiemetic. Metoclopramide has been very useful for those parturients who have ingested a large meal shortly before arrival in the labor suite and in diabetic patients, whose disease results in inherently slow gastric emptying.

HEMATOLOGIC SYSTEM

Both plasma volume and red cell mass increase above prepregnant values, but the increase in the former far exceeds the increase in the latter. A "dilutional" anemia will therefore ensue (Table 1-4). Blood viscosity and oxygen content will

■ Table 1–4
MATERNAL HEMATOLOGIC ALTERATIONS AT TERM

Variable	Change	Rate (%)
Blood volume	↑ ↑ ↑	35
Plasma volume	↑ ↑ ↑ ↑	45
Erythrocyte volume	↑ ↑	20
Blood urea nitrogen	↓ ↓ ↓	33
Plasma cholinesterase	↓ ↓	20
Total protein	↑	18
Protein	↓	7
Albumin	↓	14
Globulin	±	0
AST, ALT, LDH	↑	
Cholesterol	↑	
Alkaline phosphatase (produced by placenta)	↑ ↑	

AST, ALT, aspartate and alanine aminotransferases; LDH, lactate dehydrogenase.

From Skaredoff MN, Ostheimer GW: Physiologic changes during pregnancy: effects of major regional anesthesia. Reg Anesth 6:28–40, 1981.

both decrease. Platelet count is usually elevated, as are coagulation factors VII, X, and XII and fibrinogen. Thrombocytopenia may, however, be seen in some normal pregnant patients in the absence of any other hematopathology. Systemic fibrinolysis is slightly increased, reflected by an increased concentration of fibrin degradation products and plasminogen. Levels of plasma proteins, especially albumin and acid-1-α glycoprotein decrease during pregnancy. A slight decrease in maternal colloid osmotic pressure is noted during pregnancy.

Clinical Implications

The physiologic "anemia of pregnancy" (normal hematocrit 35%) is usually of little concern to the normal parturient, because increases in cardiac output serve to actually increase oxygen delivery to tissues. The increase in coagulation factors (Table 1-5) renders pregnancy a "hypercoaguable" state, with a consequent increase in thrombotic events (e.g., deep venous and cortical vein thrombosis). Enhanced clotting coupled with the expanded blood volume affords teleologic protection to the parturient for blood loss incurred at the time of delivery. The free fraction of highly protein-bound drugs increases in pregnancy due to the decrease in plasma proteins, and an occassional dosing adjustment must be made. Plasma cholinesterase is slightly decreased (20%) at term. However, the intubating dose of succinylcholine should not be decreased, because this may result in inadequate intubating conditions. The small decrease in plasma cholinesterase levels will slightly

■ Table 1–5
COAGULATION FACTORS AND INHIBITORS
DURING NORMAL PREGNANCY

Factor	Nonpregnant	Late Pregnancy
Factor I (fibrinogen), mg/dL	200–450	400–650
Factor II (prothrombin), %	75–125	100–125
Factor V, %	75–125	100–150
Factor VII, %	75–125	150–250
Factor VIII, %	75–150	200–500
Factor IX, %	75–125	100–150
Factor X, %	75–125	150–250
Factor XI, %	75–125	50–100
Factor XII, %	75–125	100–200
Factor XIII, %	75–125	35–75
Antithrombin III, %	85–110	75–100
Antifactor Xa, %	85–110	75–100
Platelets		Slight ↑
Fibrinolysis		Slight ↓

From Shnider SM: Anesthesia for Obstetrics, 2nd ed. Baltimore, MD: Williams & Wilkins, 1987.

prolong the duration of action of succinylcholine, and this effect may be exacerbated if the patient is also receiving magnesium sulfate infusion.

RENAL SYSTEM

Renal hemodynamics undergo profound changes during gestation.[8] Marked increases in renal plasma flow (80% above normal) occur by the middle of the second trimester and then decline slightly by term. Glomerular filtration rate (GFR) increases to 50% above prepregnant values by the 16th gestational week and remains so until delivery (Fig. 1-3). Consequently, 24-hour creatine clearance values are elevated, a change discernible as early as the eighth week of gestation. Glycosuria is common in normal pregnancy due to both alterations in tubular reabsorptive capacity and the increased load of glucose presented by the increased GFR. Although these changes are noted in early pregnancy, implying a hormonal stimulus, the exact mechanism is as yet unknown. Increased levels of aldosterone, cortisol, and human placental lactogen all contribute to the multifactorial renal adaptations to pregnancy. Progesterone will cause dilatation of the renal pelvis and uterus; hence, the incidence of urinary tract infections is increased, particularly after instrumentation of the urinary bladder.

Clinical Implications

Laboratory determinations of renal function are so altered that great care must be exercised when "normal" nonpregnant

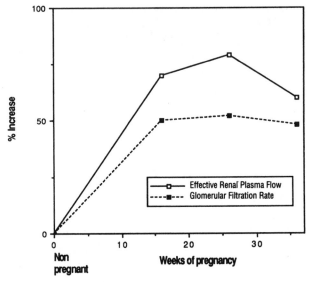

Figure 1–3 ■ Renal function during pregnancy. (Reproduced from Davison J: Overview: kidney function in pregnancy. Am J Kidney Dis 9:249, 1987.)

values are applied to the pregnant woman. For example, "normal" values of blood urea nitrogen and creatinine in a preeclamptic or diabetic patient may actually indicate a significant degree of renal compromise; in contrast, such values may indicate hypovolemia in a parturient with otherwise normal renal function.

> ■ **KEY POINT:** The increased GFR results in decreased blood concentrations of nitrogenous metabolites. At term in a healthy parturient, BUN concentration is 8–9 mg/dL and serum creatinine concentration is 0.5–0.6 mg/dL.

Although glucose excretion is enhanced during pregnancy, excessive administration of glucose to patients during labor may result in both maternal hyperglycemia and fetal hyperglycemia. Resultant fetal hyperinsulinemia persists after delivery and a reactive neonatal hypoglycemia may ensue.

Serum electrolyte values are unchanged during pregnancy. Expansion of plasma volume must therefore be accompanied by electrolyte retention. A primary resetting of thirst and vasopressin osmoreceptors allows the pregnant woman to maintain internal homeostasis during this volume expanded state, that is, the threshold for antidiuretic hormone secretion is reset at a lower level of plasma sodium, thus allowing volume expansion without an accompanying diuresis. The antecedent stimulus for this adaptation has yet to be elucidated. However, failure to appropriately expand plasma volume after conception has been correlated with early fetal wastage.

CENTRAL NERVOUS SYSTEM

The parturient should always be treated with compassion and respect. Pregnancy is a stressful experience, and wide mood swings during gestation, delivery, and the postpartum period can be expected. Emotional, social, and cultural overtones all contribute to the psychological milieu during labor and delivery. Hence, the interpersonal skills of the obstetric anesthesiologist are often acutely challenged. A hormonal basis for emotional lability has been proposed as progesterone and endogenous endorphins act as both neurotransmitters and analgesics.

The effect of progesterone and endorphins also serves to decrease minimal alveolar concentration of all inhaled anesthetic agents.[9] Reduced enzymatic degradation of opioids at term contributes to elevated pain thresholds. Reduced dosages of local anesthetic (LA) agents are required for spinal and epidural anesthesia compared with nonpregnant patients. Vascular congestion in the epidural space contributes to the decreased LA requirement by three mechanisms:

1. Reduced volume in the epidural space facilitates spread of a given dose of LA over a wider number of dermatomes;
2. Increased pressure within the epidural space facilitates dural diffusion and higher cerebrospinal fluid levels of LA;
3. Venous congestion of the lateral foramina decreases egress of LA via the dural root sleeves.

■ **KEY POINT:** Local anesthetic dose requirement for spinal and epidural anesthesia is reduced in the parturient.

The respiratory alkalosis of pregnancy may enhance LA action by increasing the relative concentration of uncharged molecules that facilitates penetration through neural membrane.[10] This decreased requirement for LA is seen as early as the first trimester; thus, hormonal changes may be operative as well, because progesterone has been shown to correlate with enhanced conduction blockade in isolated nerve preparations.

MISCELLANEOUS

Musculoskeletal

Production of the hormone relaxin (of placental origin) stimulates generalized ligamentous relaxation. Particularly notable is the widening of the pelvis in preparation for fetal passage. A resultant "head-down" tilt ensues when the parturient assumes the lateral position, and compensation should be made when performing regional anesthesia in this position (Fig. 1–4).

Generalized vertebral collagenous softening, coupled with the burden of a gravid uterus, increases lumbar lordosis. Technical difficulty with regional anesthesia may result. In addition, these changes account for the high incidence of back pain and sciatica during pregnancy, complaints that per se do not represent contraindications to regional anesthesia. Stress fractures of the weight-bearing bony pelvis have also been noted, especially during difficult deliveries.

Dermatologic

Hyperpigmentation of the face, neck (chloasma or "mask of pregnancy"), and abdominal midline (linea nigra) are due to the effects of melanocyte-stimulating hormone (MSH), a cogener of corticotropin. MSH levels increase markedly during the first trimester and remain elevated until after delivery.

Mammary

Breast enlargement is typical in normal pregnancy and is a result of placental lactogen secretion. The obese parturient

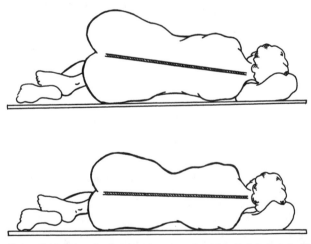

Figure 1–4 ■ Pelvic widening and resultant "head-down" tilt in lateral position during pregnancy. (*Top*, pregnant.)

with a short neck and enlarged breasts may predispose to difficult laryngoscopy and intubation. Use of a short-handled laryngoscope can be extremely helpful in these patients (Fig. 1-5).

Ocular

Conjunctival vasospasm and subconjunctional hemorrhage are occasionally seen, especially during maternal expulsive efforts and in preeclamptic patients. Intraocular pressure is lowered during pregnancy. The mechanism is believed to be a result of progesterone and relaxin effects, which facilitate aqueous outflow, and human chorionic gonadotropin, which depresses aqueous humor production.

The retina may manifest focal vascular spasm, detachment, and retinopathy associated with hypertensive disorders. Central serous choriodopathy or a breakdown of the blood–retinal barrier may occur in the absence of hypertension.

Corneal thickness, a manifestation of the generalized edema of pregnancy, may produce mild visual disturbances and contact lens intolerance during gestation.

INTRAPARTUM CHANGES

Active labor magnifies many physiologic variables already altered during gestation. The stresses of labor are usually well tolerated; however, the limited reserves of the term parturient may potentially be imposed upon in a way not always beneficial to mother or fetus.

Cardiovascular System

Cardiac output during active labor rises to approximately twice prelabor values, with the maximal increase seen in the

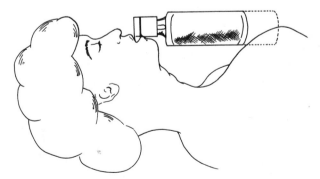

Figure 1–5 ■ Use of short-handled laryngoscope for large-breasted parturient. The dotted line indicates a traditional laryngoscope handle impinging on the breast.

immediate postdelivery period (Fig. 1–6). The rise in cardiac output is multifactorial. First, pain and anxiety during labor will increase maternal circulating catecholamines with a resultant tachycardia and increased stroke volume.[11] Second, uterine contractions result in cyclic autotransfusion and increased central blood volumes. This augmentation of preload in the setting of normal (or hyperdynamic) ventricular function contributes to increased cardiac output via Frank-Starling mechanisms.

Adequate regional anesthesia can ameliorate many of the pain-mediated hemodynamic consequences of labor. Uterine contractions, however, will still result in a transient autotransfusion of blood with elevation of central vascular pressures.

Respiratory System

Hyperventilation is common during labor. This may be a natural response to pain or the result of various prepared childbirth methods in which repetitive panting breathing techniques are used. Hyperventilation during labor in the setting of an already lowered maternal P_{CO_2} at term may result in dangerous degrees of alkalemia. Women who have received narcotic analgesics during labor may alternate periods of hyperventilation with marked hypoventilation between contractions, resulting in wide swings in P_{CO_2}. Uterine vascular response to hypocapnea is vasoconstriction and subsequent decreased placental perfusion. Thus, the potential for fetal compromise exists during episodes of maternal alkalemia, particularly if a fetus is already compromised for other reasons.[12]

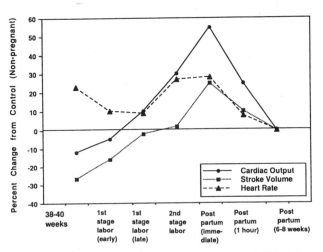

Figure 1–6 ■ Cardiovascular alterations during labor. (Reproduced from Shnider S, Levinson G: Anesthesia for Obstetrics, 2nd ed. Baltimore, MD: Williams & Wilkins, 1987.)

Regional anesthesia during labor will obviate the need for "breathing techniques" and eliminate pain-induced hyperventilation. Thus, patients whose disease process may produce marginal placental reserve (e.g., preeclampsia, diabetes, postdates pregnancy, small abruptio placentae) should be strongly considered as candidates for epidural analgesia during labor.

Metabolic Effects

The homeostatic millieu that slowly develops during gestation undergoes marked changes during labor. A metabolic acidosis may ensue for several reasons. First, prolonged labor, especially in the setting of inadequate intravenous hydration, may contribute to elevation of lactate and pyruvate levels. Second, muscular activity due to pain, shivering, or respiratory muscle demands will add to acidic metabolites in the maternal circulation. Third, maternal alkalemia may predispose to compensatory acid retention. Overall maintenance of normal acid-base status during labor is accomplished by the balance of what may be markedly altered (vs. nonpregnant) levels of acidemic and alkalemic mediators. Thus, situations that further aggravate pH balance (e.g., dehydration, vomiting, ketoacidosis, hypothermia, hemorrhage) may be poorly tolerated by the gravida in labor.

The common markers of physiologic stress (epinephrine, norepinephrine, and cortisol) have all been measured to increase during labor versus prelabor values. The magnitude of this increase can be blunted by regional anesthesia.

PUERPERAL RESOLUTION

Cardiac output acutely rises immediately after birth, because sustained contraction of the emptied uterus results in autotransfusion of 500 to 750 mL of blood, coincident with elimination of the placental arteriovenous shunt. The immediate postpartum period is a high-risk time for decompensation in patients with certain cardiac disease states. Cardiac output gradually returns to nonpregnant levels by 2 to 4 weeks after delivery.

Uterine evacuation and involution promotes rapid resolution of many pulmonary changes induced by mechanical compression of the diaphragm and lungs by the gravid uterus. Thus, FRC and residual volume rapidly return to normal. Rapid decline in blood progesterone levels is accompanied by a slow rise in arterial P_{CO_2}, and alveolar ventilation returns to normal by 2 to 3 weeks postpartum.

Postpartum diuresis is common; GFR, blood urea nitrogen, and creatinine levels return to normal in 1 to 3 weeks. This diuretic phase contributes to a gradual decline in plasma volume, although red cell mass remains constant. Thus, the "dilutional" anemia of pregnancy resolves, and the hematocrit rises to nonpregnant levels in 2 to 4 weeks. Situations where blood loss at delivery is excessive will markedly alter the course of hematologic resolution.

Mechanical effects on the gastrointestinal tract rapidly resolve by 2 to 3 weeks postpartum. Progesterone levels decrease rapidly after delivery. Precautions to minimize the risk and consequences of acid aspiration therefore should be used if surgery with anesthesia is planned during the immediate postpartum period.

REFERENCES

1. Schrier RW, Durr JA: Pregnancy: An overfill or underfill state. Am J Kidney Dis 9:284–289, 1987.
2. Schrier RW: Pathogenesis of sodium and water retention in high-output and low output cardiac failure, nephrotic syndrome, cirrhosis, and pregnancy. N Engl J Med 319:1127–1134, 1988.
3. Desimone CA, Leighton BL, Norris MC, et al: The chronotropic effect of isoproterenol is reduced in term pregnant women. Anesthesiology 69:626–628, 1988.
4. Shankar KB, Moseley H, Vemula V, et al: Physiological dead space during general anesthesia for caesarean section. Can J Anaesth 34:373–376, 1987.
5. Russell GN, Smith CL, Snowdon SL, et al: Preoxygenation and the parturient patient. Anaesthesia 42:346–351, 1987.
6. Shankar KB, Moseley H, Kumar Y, et al: Arterial to end-tidal carbon dioxide tension difference during anaesthesia for tubal ligation. Anaesthesia 42:482–486, 1987.
7. O'Sullivan GM, Sutton AJ, Thompson SA, et al: Noninvasive measurement of gastric emptying in obstetric patients. Anesth Analg 66:505–511, 1987.
8. Davison JM: Overview: kidney function in pregnant women. Am J Kidney Dis 9:248–252, 1987.
9. Palahniuic RJ, Shnider SM, Eger EI: Pregnancy decreases the requirement for inhaled anesthetic agents. Anesthesiology 41:82–87, 1974.
10. Datta S, Lambert DH, Gregus J, et al: Differential sensitivities of mammalian nerve fibers during pregnancy. Anesth Analg 62:1070–1072, 1983.
11. Jones CM, Greiss FC: The effect of labor on maternal and fetal circulating catecholamines. Am J Obstet Gynecol 144:149–153, 1982.
12. Moya F, Morishima HO, Shnider SM, et al: Influence of maternal hyperventilation on the newborn infant. Am J Obstet Gynecol 90:76–84, 1965.

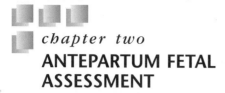

chapter two

ANTEPARTUM FETAL ASSESSMENT

Ramon Martin, MD

Anesthesia for the obstetric patient is an integral part of labor and delivery. For routine normal deliveries, this usually involves providing pain relief with an epidural or spinal technique. In pregnancies complicated by either maternal or fetal disease, the role of anesthesia is more central to patient care and can involve close monitoring with invasive lines during labor, fluid management, and discussion with the obstetricians about the timing and type of anesthesia. Equally important in the dialogue with obstetricians is an understanding of the techniques used to assess the fetus because this provides important information about how the fetus might tolerate labor and delivery. This chapter reviews the causes of perinatal mortality, the techniques available to assess the fetus, and the clinical application to labor and delivery.

PERINATAL MORTALITY

According to the National Center for Health Statistics,[1] the perinatal mortality rate (PMR) is defined as the number of late fetal deaths (>28 weeks gestation) plus early neonatal deaths (infants 0 to 6 days of age) divided by 1000 live births plus the fetal and neonatal deaths. In the United States, the PMR has declined by an average of 3% per year since 1965. Over the past 6 years, fetal death rate alone has decreased 16% and neonatal mortality has fallen 21%. Of all fetal deaths, 22% occur between the 36th and 40th weeks of gestation and another 10% occur beyond the 41st week of gestation.

Congenital anomalies account for 25% of perinatal mortality and are the leading cause. Premature labor and delivery was the most common event leading to death in this group. Overall, prematurity with associated respiratory distress syndrome (RDS) was the next most common cause of perinatal death. Intrauterine hypoxia and birth asphyxia account for 3% of the PMR and placenta or cord complications account for 2% of the PMR. Several associated factors, identified by Lammer et al.,[2] were race (African-American), marital status (single), age (>34 and <20 years), parity (more than five), and lack of prenatal care. Multiple gestations were associated with 10% of all fetal deaths. This gives a PMR of 50 in 1000, which is seven times that of singleton pregnancies. Over half of all fetal deaths were associated with asphyxia or maternal causes such as pregnancy-induced hypertension (PIH) or placental abruption.

If the first step to reduce the PMR further is recognizing the causes, then the next step is prevention. A study of perinatal mortality in the Mersey region of England showed that of 309 perinatal deaths, 182 or 58.9% were due to avoidable causes, primarily a delayed response to abnormalities of the progress of labor or fetal heart rate tracing during labor and delivery, maternal weight loss with a resulting growth-retarded fetus, and reductions in fetal movement.[3] Antepartum fetal monitoring is the means to decrease these fetal deaths. This is most useful when targeting specific groups of parturients who are at increased risk of perinatal mortality (Table 2–1).

TECHNIQUES OF ANTEPARTUM FETAL ASSESSMENT

■ **K E Y P O I N T :** Antepartum fetal monitoring is most useful when targeting high-risk parturients.

Maternal Assessment of Fetal Activity

Having a parturient count the fetal activity over a period of time is a simple and sensitive test of fetal well-being. It is based on the fact that from 28 weeks of gestation on, the fetus makes approximately 30 body movements each hour (about 10% of the total time) and the parturient is able to appreciate most of these. Although fetal movement is reassuring, lack of movement can indicate either a quiet period, which can usually last 20 minutes (but can last as long as 75 minutes), or fetal compromise secondary to asphyxia. Factors that can decrease maternal appreciation of fetal activity are an anterior placenta, polyhydramnios, and obesity.

■ Table 2–1
PARTURIENTS AT INCREASED RISK OF PERINATAL MORTALITY

Postdate gestation
Diabetes
Previous stillbirth
Pregnancy-induced hypertension
Maternal age > 35 yr
Maternal weight loss
Premature labor

Amniocentesis

Performed before 15 weeks gestation, early amniocentesis is an alternative to chorionic villus sampling to obtain fetal cells for diagnosis of genetic or morphologic abnormalities. Although the success of obtaining cells is the same as for chorionic villus sampling, the disadvantages are primarily due to the withdrawal of amniotic fluid. The volume of fluid removed is a much greater proportion of the total fluid volume, and this could increase fetal loss.

After 16 weeks gestation, midtrimester amniocentesis with ultrasound guidance is safe, with a rate of fetal loss of 0.5 to 1.0%. The amniotic fluid is used to grow fetal cells, which in turn are used to scan for chromosomal aberrations. During the third trimester, amniocentesis is used to obtain fluid to assess fetal lung maturity.

Chorionic Villus Sampling

Performed between 9 and 12 weeks of gestation, chorionic villus sampling allows early determination of chromosomal abnormalities. Under ultrasound guidance, this technique is simply the aspiration of villi either through the cervix or the abdomen. Because actual tissue is obtained, results from cells are available as early as 24 to 48 hours and can also be analyzed for abnormalities in DNA or specific enzymatic reactions. Fetal loss was 2.3 to 2.5% in one randomized trial.[4] Limb reduction defects and oromandibular hypogenesis have been reported in a small number of infants after chorionic villus sampling,[5] but other studies[6, 7] have not demonstrated any difference between the expected rates of appearance of these developmental aberrations.

Percutaneous Umbilical Blood Sampling

Starting at 18 weeks gestation, fetal blood can be obtained transabdominally under ultrasound guidance by needle puncture of the umbilical cord. This is useful in diagnosing a range of problems:

1. Hematologic abnormalities, such as hemoglobinopathies, isoimmunization, thrombocytopenia, and coagulation factor deficiencies;
2. Inborn errors of metabolism;
3. Infections by viruses, bacteria, or parasites;
4. Chromosomal abnormalities, especially mosaicism.

The risk to the fetus is greater than other tests, with an increase in fetal loss of 2%. As a result, this test is usually reserved for situations where information cannot be obtained by other means.

Ultrasonography

Over the past two decades, ultrasound has become an important method of antepartum fetal assessment. Useful throughout gestation, it gives an accurate measurement of gestational age and provides an assessment of fetal growth and developmental abnormalities. It is also an important guide in the performance of amniocentesis, chorionic villus sampling, and cordocentesis. Real-time ultrasound permits a dynamic assessment of fetal well-being by following, over time, fetal breathing activity, movements, and tone.

Despite its importance as a method of fetal assessment, there is still controversy about the routine use of ultrasound in pregnancy. In Helsinki, Finland, which like many other European countries advocates routine ultrasound screening, a randomized trial showed a significant decrease in perinatal mortality in the screened group compared with the control group.[8] This was primarily due to early detection of fetal malformations. A number of other studies have not found a benefit from routine ultrasound screening.[9, 10] A recent large-scale study of 15,151 pregnant women demonstrated no difference in adverse perinatal outcome. Subgroups of women with postdate gestation, multiple pregnancies, or infants who are small for gestational age did not differ in perinatal outcome between the control and study populations.[11] This controversy is also fueled by the desire to contain medical costs by decreasing unnecessary testing.

During the first trimester, ultrasonography, particularly transvaginal sonography, can help determine whether a fetus is viable, when there is vaginal bleeding, or determine the presence of other processes: ectopic pregnancy, uterine anomaly, or an adnexal mass. In addition, it can provide the first measurement of fetal crown–rump length as a measure of fetal age. During the second trimester, ultrasound assessment of biparietal diameter becomes an accurate measure of gestational age. From 12 to 28 weeks of gestation, the relation between biparietal diameter and gestation is linear. Ultrasonic assessment of fetal growth, when continued into the third trimester, is important in diagnosing deviations from normal growth such as growth retardation, macrosomia, or developmental anomalies. Diagnoses of oligohydramnios or polyhydramnios are made by ultrasound. As mentioned previously, real-time ultrasound measures variables that are the components of the biophysical profile (amniotic fluid volume, fetal breathing, limb movement, and tone). These measurements can have an effect on the course of labor and delivery.

Analysis of Maternal Serum

Maternal serum is routinely sampled during the first trimester to assess the possibility of neural tube defects and Rh sensitization. Neural tube defects are one of the most frequent congenital abnormalities, with an incidence of 1 to 2 per 1000 live births in the United States. α-Fetoprotein (AFP) is elevated in the fetal serum during the first trimester when the neural tube fails to close, resulting in anencephaly, meningomyelocele, or encephalocele. AFP passes through the placenta into the maternal serum and can be measured with a radioimmunoassay. AFP is also elevated in malformations of the gastrointestinal and genitourinary tracts and in fetal death, decreasing the specificity of the test. Despite this, it is still used as a general screening test. With any abnormal values, ultrasonography and amniocentesis are performed for confirmation.

Rh sensitization occurs in Rh (D)-negative women who are carrying an Rh-positive fetus. Sensitization of the mother occurs from a prior delivery when fetal cells enter the maternal circulation and stimulate formation of maternal antibodies to fetal erythrocyte Rh antigens. With a subsequent pregnancy, the antibodies traverse the placenta and destroy fetal erythrocytes. This results in the syndrome of erythroblastosis fetalis, which is characterized by severe hemolytic anemia that leads to edema, jaundice, and congestive heart failure. Rh titers are measured early and serially throughout the pregnancy in Rh-negative mothers. Rising or elevated titers are followed up with amniocentesis.

Assessment of Fetal Lung Maturity

Because fetal chronologic age does not necessarily correlate with functional maturity, particularly of the pulmonary system, methods of assessing fetal maturity are important adjuncts in clinical decision making. Most perinatal morbidity and mortality results from complications of premature delivery. The most frequently seen complication is RDS. This disorder is due to a particular deficiency of a surface-active agent (surfactant) that prevents alveolar collapse during expiration. Phospholipids, produced by fetal alveolar cells, are the major component of lung surfactant and are produced in sufficient amounts by 36 weeks gestation. The most commonly used technique measures the lecithin-sphingomyelin (L/S) ratio. The concentration of lecithin, a component of surfactant, begins to rise in the amniotic fluid at 32 to 33 weeks gestation and continues to rise until term. The concentration of sphingomyelin remains relatively constant, so that the ratio of the two provides an estimate of surfactant production that is not affected by variations in the volume of amniotic fluid. The risk of neonatal RDS when the L/S ratio is greater than 2 is less than 1%. If the ratio is less than 1.5, approximately 80% of neonates will develop RDS.

> ■ **K E Y P O I N T :** In an effort to decrease the risk of RDS, assessment of fetal lung maturity may be performed. The most commonly used technique measures the L/S ratio. The risk of RDS when the L/S ratio is greater than 2 is less than 1%.

Disaturated phosphatydylcholine (SPC) is the major component of fetal pulmonary surfactant. The technique that separates SPC from lecithin in the amniotic fluid is complicated, and the results can be altered by abnormalities in amniotic fluid production and excretion (i.e., oligohydramnios or polyhydramnios). A value greater than 500 μg/dL amniotic fluid for SPC concentration is consistent with mature fetal lungs and a small risk of RDS.

The disadvantages in measuring the L/S ratio include the long turnaround time, the use of toxic chemicals, a lack of technical expertise, and the inability to standardize the test. As a result, few hospitals are able to perform the test. Another method, the TDx fetal lung maturity test, is automated and avoids the technical involvement in sample preparation and measurement. The test relies on the fluorescence polarization of a dye added to a solution of amniotic fluid that is then compared with values on a standard curve to determine the relative concentration of surfactant and albumin. The determined values are expressed in milligrams of surfactant per gram of albumin. With a cutoff of 50 mg/g for maturity, the TDx test was equal in sensitivity (0.96) and more specific (0.88 vs. 0.83) when compared with the L/S ratio in one multicenter study.[12]

Biophysical Profile

The biophysical profile involves evaluation of immediate biophysical activities (fetal movement, tone, breathing movements, and heart rate activity) and semiquantitative assessment of amniotic fluid. The biophysical parameters reflect acute central nervous system (CNS) activity and when present correlate positively with the lack of depression (secondary to asphyxia) of the CNS. Amniotic fluid volume represents longterm or chronic fetal compromise. Major indications for referral for biophysical profile include suspected intrauterine growth retardation, hypertension, postdate gestation, and diabetes.

The biophysical evaluation of the fetus is done by ultrasound with the sole purpose of detecting changes in fetal activity due to asphyxia. As has been mentioned previously, changes in fetal breathing movements, heart rate, and body movements are indicators of the state of fetal oxygenation. Superimposed on these factors are the nonrandom pattern of CNS output and the sleep state, with effects that might be mistaken for hypoxia. However, extending the period of observation to find a period of normal recovery for the latter conditions helps to differentiate asphyxia from normal variants.

The scoring of the fetal biophysical profile is an assessment of five variables (Table 2-2), four of which are monitored simultaneously by ultrasound. The variables are said to be normal (score of 2) or abnormal (score of 0). The nonstress test (NST) is monitored after the biophysical evaluation. When the test score is normal, conservative therapy is indicated, with some exceptions:

1. Postdate gestation with a favorable cervix;
2. Growth-retarded fetus with mature pulmonary indices and a favorable cervix;
3. Insulin-dependent diabetic woman at 37 weeks gestation or more with mature pulmonary indices;
4. Class A diabetic woman at term with a favorable cervix;
5. Women with medical disorders (e.g., asthma, preeclampsia, pregnancy-induced hypertension) that might pose a threat to maternal and fetal health.

Table 2-3 lists recommendations for management of biophysical profile scores.

Several prospective studies,[13-16] summarized in Table 2-4, have shown that most women studied (>97%) have normal test results and delivery outcome. Perinatal mortality varies inversely with the last score before delivery. In 1981 and 1985, in large groups of patients, Manning et al.[17, 18] found that the gross perinatal mortality rate decreased from 11.7 to 7.4 per 1000 and the corrected value decreased from 5 to 1.9 per 1000. In Manitoba, since the use of this testing, the stillbirth rate has decreased by 30%. A stillbirth occurring

■ Table 2–2
BIOPHYSICAL PROFILE SCORING

Variable	Score = 2	Score = 0
Fetal breathing movements	1 episode, 30-s duration in 30 min	Absent
Gross body movement	3 discrete body/limb movements in 30 min	<2 episodes in 30 min
Fetal tone	1 episode of extension/flexion of hand, limb, or trunk	Absent or slow movement
Fetal heart rate	2 episodes of acceleration with fetal movement in 30 min	<2 episodes
Amniotic fluid volume	1 pocket, 1 × 1 cm	No amniotic fluid or a pocket <1 × 1 cm

■ Table 2–3
INTERPRETATION AND MANAGEMENT OF BIOPHYSICAL PROFILE SCORE

Score	Interpretation	Recommended Management
8–10	Normal infant	Repeat test in 1 wk*
6	Suspect asphyxia	Repeat test in 4-6 hr†
4	Suspect asphyxia	If >36 weeks, deliver
		If <36 weeks, repeat in 24 hr
0–2	Probable asphyxia	Deliver

*Repeat test twice a week if diabetic or >42 weeks gestation.
†Deliver if oligohydramnios is present.

within a week of a normal test result is defined as a false negative. This ranges from 0.41 to 1.01 per 1000 with a mean of 0.64 per 1000.

The false-negative rate, although small, directly reflects the negative predictive accuracy of the test. Manning et al.[13] calculated from a study of 19,221 pregnancies a negative predictive accuracy of 99.224%, or the probability of fetal death after a normal test result as 0.726 per 1000 patients.

Because the ideal testing method would result in no false-negative deaths, the biophysical profile is not perfect. The cause of the imperfection is the probability of change in the fetal status from either a chronic condition or an acute variable. Although more frequent testing of all patients would decrease the false-negative rate, this has not been attempted due to the increased workload. The proper selection of patients requiring more vigilant monitoring (those judged to be at risk, e.g., an immature fetus with growth retardation, preeclampsia, diabetes, etc.) would render this more feasible.

Nonstress Testing

Nonstress testing is the external detection of fetal heart rate and fetal movement in relation to uterine contractions, noting

■ Table 2–4
BIOPHYSICAL PROFILE AND PERINATAL MORTALITY

Study	No. Patients	No. Deaths	Perinatal Mortality
Manning et al.[13]	19,221	141	1.92
Baskett et al.[14]	5,034	32	3.10
Platt et al.[15]	286	4	7.0
Schifrin et al.[16]	158	7	12.6

accelerations of fetal heart rate with fetal movement. These parameters are predictors of fetal outcome.

With the parturient recumbent in the semi-Fowler's position and left lateral tilt (to displace the uterus from the inferior vena cava and aorta), 20 minutes of consistent fetal heart rate tracing is followed, and a tocodynamometer is used to measure uterine contractions. Fetal movement is noted either by the mother by external palpation of the maternal abdomen or by spikes in the tocodynamometer tracing.

The test is usually interpreted as either

1. Reactive—at least two fetal movements in 20 minutes with acceleration of the fetal heart rate to at least 15 beats/min, with long-term variability of at least 10 beats/min and a baseline rate within the normal range (Fig. 2-1);
2. Nonreactive—no fetal movement or acceleration of the fetal heart rate with movement, poor to no long-term variability, and baseline fetal heart rate may be within or outside the normal range (Fig. 2-2);
3. Uncertain reactivity—fewer than two fetal movements in 20 minutes or acceleration to less than 15 beats/min, long-term variability amplitude less than 10 beats/min, and baseline heart rate outside of normal limits.

Fetuses have sleep or inactive cycles that can last up to 80 minutes. The test administrator can either wait for a while or manually stimulate the infant.

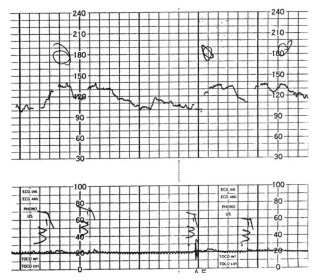

Figure 2-1 ■ Reactive nonstress test, characterized by acceleration in the fetal heart rate with fetal movement (FM).

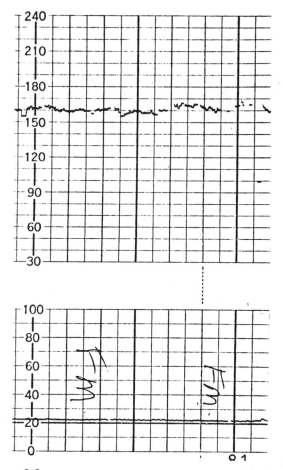

Figure 2–2 ■ Nonreactive nonstress test, with no accelerations in fetal heart rate with fetal movement (FM).

A reactive test is associated with survival of the fetus for 1 or more weeks in more than 99% of cases. A nonreactive test is associated with poor fetal outcome in 20% of cases. Although the false-positive rate of this technique is high (80%), further evaluation needs to be done when a nonreactive result is obtained. The next step is usually a contraction stress test (CST). Similarly, an uncertain reactive pattern needs to be followed up with either another NST or a CST.

Contraction Stress Test

As its name implies, the CST assesses the fetal response (heart rate pattern) to regular uterine contractions. Using the same technique as the NST, the CST requires three adequate contractions within a 10-minute period, each with a duration of 1 minute. If there are not enough spontaneous contractions, augmentation with intravenous oxytocin is indicated. Beginning at a rate of 1.0 mU/min, the infusion is increased every 15 minutes until the requisite number of contractions are obtained. It is rarely necessary to exceed 10 mU/min.

Certain clinical situations present contraindications to CSTs: prior classic cesarean section, placenta previa, and women at risk of premature labor (premature rupture of membranes, multiple gestations, incompetent cervix, and women undergoing treatment for preterm labor).

CSTs are interpreted as

1. Negative—no late deceleration and normal baseline fetal heart rate;
2. Positive—persistent late decelerations (even when the contractions are less frequent than three contractions within 10 minutes), possible absence of fetal heart rate variability;
3. Suspicious—intermittent late deceleration or variable decelerations, abnormal baseline fetal heart rate;
4. Unsatisfactory—poor-quality recording or inability to achieve three contractions within 10 minutes;
5. Hyperstimulation—excessive uterine activity (contractions closer than every 2 minutes or lasting longer than 90 seconds) resulting in late decelerations or bradycardia.

A negative CST is associated with fetal survival for a week or more in 99% of cases, whereas a positive CST is associated with poor fetal outcome in 50% of cases. Like the NST, the CST also has a high false-positive rate (50%), but the treatment, if delivery is indicated, can be a trial of induction of labor.

■ **KEY POINT:** In low-risk pregnancies, fetal well-being can be assessed by having the parturient count the fetal activity. In high-risk pregnancies more sophisticated techniques (nonstress test, biophysical profile, contraction stress test) can be used.

TECHNIQUES OF INTRAPARTUM FETAL MONITORING

Fetal Heart Rate Monitoring

In conjunction with fetal scalp sampling to measure acid-base balance, fetal heart rate monitoring provides the main method of evaluating the fetus during labor and delivery and is also part of nonstress testing, contraction stress testing, and biophysical profile during the antepartum period. A review by

Fenton and Steer[19] documents the historical use of fetal heart rate auscultation. First described by Marsac in 1650, a number of clinical studies have shown that perinatal morbidity and mortality are increased when the fetal heart rate is greater than 160 to 180 beats/min or less than 100 to 120 beats/min. Begining in the 1940s, fetal heart rate was followed over a period of time as a more sensitive indicator of fetal well-being. This developed into continuous fetal heart rate monitoring, which charted beat to beat changes in the fetal heart rate.

Intermittent auscultation of the fetal heart rate is still a widely used means to monitor the fetus. In low-risk patients, this is done every 30 minutes, listening for 30 seconds during and after a contraction, when the parturient is in the first stage of labor and every 15 minutes during the second stage of labor. In high-risk patients, the frequency of listening is shortened to every 15 minutes during the first stage of labor and every 5 minutes during the second stage. Auscultation with a fetoscope or Doppler is able to detect changes in basal heart rate, variability, and decelerations in relation to uterine contractions. When abnormalities are noted, either fetal scalp sampling or continuous fetal heart rate monitoring are indicated.

Continuous fetal heart rate monitoring entails measuring each fetal heart beat and the interval between two beats, calculating the fetal heart rate, and then plotting each successive rate. This can be done externally on the mother's abdo-

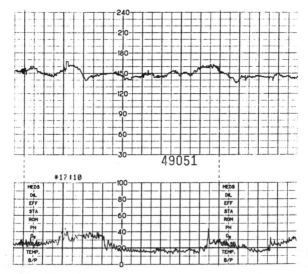

Figure 2–3 ■ Normal heart rate pattern. The heart rate (140 beats/min) and short-term and long-term variability are normal. There are no periodic changes.

men with a Doppler ultrasound, a phonocardiographic monitor, or an electrocardiogram. An electrode attached to the fetal scalp after rupture of the amniotic membranes provides an internal or direct recording of fetal heart rate. Similarly, uterine contractions are measured either externally with a tocodynamometer or internally with a saline-filled catheter placed into the uterine cavity.

Fetal Heart Rate Patterns

The fetal heart rate pattern is characterized by its baseline between contractions and periodic changes in association with uterine contractions. The baseline and periodic changes are further broken down into fetal heart rate and variability. This section will consider the baseline fetal heart rate and its variants and variability.

Fetal heart rate is normal from 120 to 160 beats/min between contractions (Fig. 2-3). Rates greater than 160 beats/min are described as tachycardia (Fig. 2-4) and those less than 120 beats/min as bradycardia (Fig. 2-5). If the alteration in rate is less than 2 minutes in duration, it is called either an acceleration or deceleration.

The usual initial response of the normal fetus to acute hypoxia or asphyxia is bradycardia. A heart rate between 100 and 120 beats/min might signify either a compensated mild hypoxic stress or may be idiopathic and benign. When the heart rate falls below 60 beats/min, the fetus is in distress and

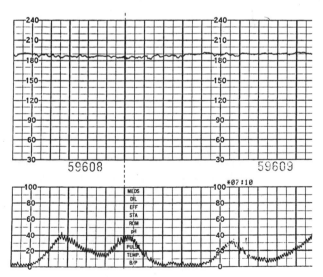

Figure 2–4 ■ Tachycardia. In this case there was a maternal fever secondary to chorioamnionitis.

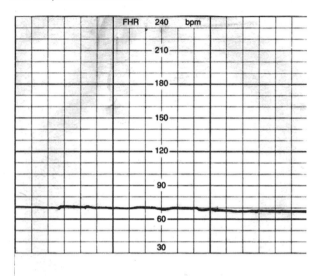

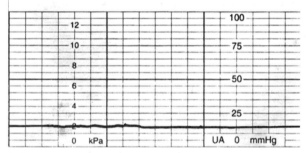

Figure 2–5 ■ Bradycardia, accompanied by absence of fetal heart rate variability.

requires either reversal of the cause of the bradycardia or emergency delivery. Other causes of bradycardia that are non-asphyxic in origin are bradyarrhythmias, maternal drug ingestion (especially beta-blockers), and hypothermia. Tachycardia is occasionally seen with fetal asphyxia or with recovery from asphyxia but is more likely seen secondary to

1. Maternal or fetal infection, especially choriamnionitis;
2. Maternal ingestion of β-mimetic or parasympathetic blockers;
3. Tachyarrhythmias;
4. Prematurity;
5. Thyrotoxicosis.

Variability in the fetal heart rate tracing describes the irregularity or the difference in interval from beat to beat. If the interval between heart beats were identical, then the tracing would be smooth (Fig. 2–6). In most healthy fetuses, one notes an irregular line. This is thought to be secondary to an intact nervous pathway through the cerebral cortex, midbrain, vagus nerve, and the cardiac conduction system. It is thought that when asphyxia affects the cerebrum, there is decreased neural control of the variability. This is made worse by the failure of fetal hemodynamic compensatory mechanisms to maintain cerebral oxygenation. So with normal variability, irrespective of the fetal heart rate pattern, the fetus is not suffering cerebral anoxia.

Variability is described as being either short term or long term. Short-term variability is the beat to beat difference, and it requires accurate detection of the heart rate. Because this can only be obtained with the fetal electrocardiogram, external monitors cannot be used to describe short-term variability, which is characterized as either present or absent. Long-term variability looks at a wider window of the fetal heart rate, between 3 and 6 minutes. It can be detected using either internal or external methods of fetal heart rate monitoring and is described by the approximate amplitude range in beats/min as

1. Normal—the amplitude range is 6 beats/min or greater;
2. Decreased—the amplitude range is between 2 and 6 beats/min;
3. Absent—the amplitude range is less than 2 beats/min;
4. Saltatory—the amplitude is greater than 25 beats/min.

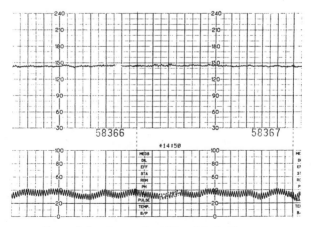

Figure 2–6 ■ Decreased variability of the fetal heart rate.

In addition to asphyxia, there are other causes of altered variability, such as anencephaly, fetal drug effect (secondary to morphine, meperidine, diazepam, and magnesium sulphate), vagal blockade (due to atropine or scopolamine), and interventricular conduction delays (complete heart block).

Periodic changes in fetal heart rate occur in association with uterine contractions. Early accelerations occur concomitantly with a uterine contraction. They have a smooth contour and are a mirror image of the contraction (Fig. 2-7). The descent of the fetal heart rate is usually never more than 20 beats/min below the baseline. The cause is presumed to be due to a vagal reflex caused by a mild hypoxia but is not associated with fetal compromise. Late decelerations are also smooth in contour and mirror the contraction, but they begin 10 to 30 seconds after the onset of the contraction (Fig. 2-8). The depth of the decline is inversely related to the intensity of the contraction. Late decelerations have been classified as either reflex or nonreflex. Reflex late decelerations are due to maternal hypotension, which acutely decreases uterine perfusion to an otherwise healthy fetus. A uterine contraction on top of this insult further reduces oxygen flow, causing cerebral hypoxia, which then leads to the deceleration. In between contractions, the fetal heart rate returns to baseline with good variability. The nonreflex late deceleration is due to prolonged hypoxia that leads to myocardial depression. Cerebral function is also depressed. This is seen with preeclampsia, intrauterine growth retardation, and prolonged repetitive late decelerations. Fetal heart rate variability is either decreased or absent.

Variable decelerations differ in duration and shape, and they decrease in fetal heart rate from contraction to contraction. The abrupt onset and cessation of the deceleration is thought to be due to increased vagal firing in response to

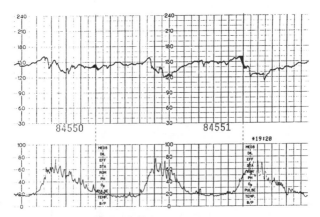

Figure 2–7 ■ Early decelerations.

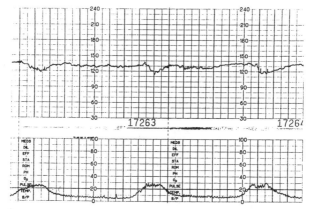

Figure 2–8 ■ Late decelerations, with decreased variability of the fetal heart rate between contractions.

compression of either the umbilical cord (during early labor) or dural stimulation with head compression (during the second stage of labor). The vagal activity causes bradycardia, which decreases cardiac output and umbilical blood flow. Variable decelerations are described as severe when they fall to 60 beats/min below the baseline fetal heart rate or last longer than 60 seconds (Fig. 2–9). Otherwise, they are classified as mild to moderate (Fig. 2–10). The normal fetus is generally able to tolerate mild to moderate variable decelerations for prolonged periods of time; however, severe variable

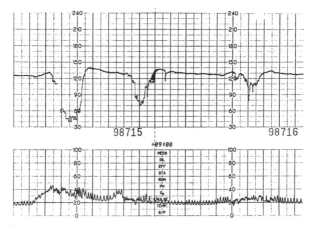

Figure 2–9 ■ Severe deep variable decelerations, with decreased variability of the fetal heart rate between contractions.

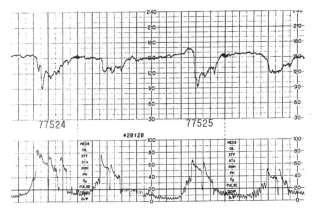

Figure 2–10 ■ Mild to moderate variable decelerations with pushing during the second stage of labor.

decelerations eventually result in fetal compromise unless reversed.

Accelerations with uterine contractions represent the greater effect of sympathetic activity over the parasympathetic nervous system (Fig. 2-11). They indicate a reactive healthy fetus and have a good prognostic significance.

The components of fetal heart rate described earlier comprise a normal pattern of a baseline rate of 120 to 160 beats/min, which has a variability of greater than 6 beats/min. One can see either no decelerations, early decelerations, or accelerations with contractions. This is associated with a good fetal outcome (i.e., Apgar score > 7 at 5 minutes). Depending on the severity and duration of the stress, there are other fetal heart rate patterns seen.

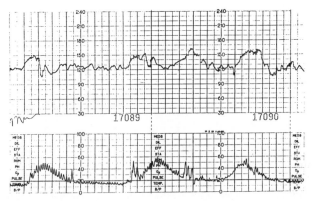

Figure 2–11 ■ Accelerations with uterine contractions.

The acute stress pattern is a compensatory reaction in an otherwise healthy fetus to a short-lived period of asphyxia or hypoxia. The fetal heart rate usually demonstrates bradycardia, although tachycardia is also seen, but the most important fact noted is that variability remains normal. There can be either late or variable decelerations. The fetal outcome is generally good, because the impact of the asphyxia is brief, with possible depression from carbon dioxide narcosis, which is rapidly reversible.

When the stress persists, bradycardia is more profound and is associated with decreased variability and late and/or deep variable decelerations. This is a prolonged stress pattern that indicates mounting hypoxic damage to the heart and brain, resulting in the loss of compensatory mechanisms. Unless corrected, fetal death in utero can occur.

■ **KEY POINT:** The presence of FHR variability is predictive of fetal well-being and early neonatal health. FHR accelerations signal fetal well-being, whereas late decelerations are suggestive of fetal hypoxia.

For a growth-retarded fetus, already compromised by a placenta with marginal function, persistent asphyxia results in a sinister pattern characterized by absent variability. The fetal heart rate displays severe variable or late decelerations, with a smooth rather than abrupt decrease and recovery in heart rate. Persistent bradycardia without variability is also called sinister.

TREATMENT OF FETAL HEART RATE PATTERNS

The first step in treatment is to recognize and describe an abnormal fetal heart rate pattern. Then the cause must be identified and corrected as quickly as possible. Causes and treatment of fetal heart rate patterns are presented in Table 2-5. If the pattern does not improve with these measures, then one needs to get more direct evidence of the fetal status (i.e., fetal scalp sampling) or deliver the fetus immediately.

Electronic fetal heart rate monitoring is now an important part of fetal assessment during the antepartum period. Its use to diagnose fetal distress, whether acute or chronic, has directly affected labor and delivery practice in an attempt to decrease fetal morbidity and mortality. A review of the literature over the past 10 years, however, suggests that electronic monitoring has poor sensitivity in identifying morbidity and limited sensitivity in predicting its absence.[20] To determine if

■ Table 2–5
TREATMENT OF FETAL HEART RATE PATTERNS

Pattern	Cause	Treatment
Bradycardia, late decelerations	Hypotension	Intravenous fluids, ephedrine, change position
	Uterine hyperstimulation	Decrease oxytocin, administer tocolytic
Variable decelerations	Umbilical cord compression	Change position
	Head compression	Continue pushing if variability good
Late decelerations	Decreased uterine blood flow	Change position, O_2 for mother
Decrease in variability	Prolonged asphyxia	Change position, O_2 for mother

neonatal neurologic damage could be correlated with fetal heart rate tracing, this review looked at 10 studies and found that

1. There were several definitions of fetal heart rate patterns, making a comparison of data from various centers difficult;
2. Fetal heart rate patterns had a poor predictive value on outcome;
3. A significant number of neonates with poor outcome had no monitoring abnormalities;
4. Monitoring fetal heart rate did not lead to effective treatment that had a significant impact on neonatal morbidity.

Although electronic fetal heart rate monitoring has been used for over 30 years, there is no standard associating brain damage with a specific fetal heart rate tracing. There has not been a study yet to demonstrate whether fetal heart rate monitoring predicts or prevents neurologic morbidity. This does not deny the fact that electronic fetal heart rate monitoring is without merit. Rather, it needs to be further refined, standardized, and applied to particular clinical situations where physiologic correlations are possible.

■ **KEY POINT:** Despite current controversy, many obstetricians routinely use continuous electronic fetal heart rate monitoring. The term "fetal distress" should not be used to describe an FHR pattern because it is an imprecise term with little positive predictive value.

Fetal Scalp Sampling

Since it was first introduced by Saling and Schneider in 1967,[21] fetal blood sampling has become the final determinant in making a diagnosis of fetal hypoxia or asphyxia. The fetal blood sample is obtained from the presenting part (scalp or buttock) during labor. The instrumentation and technique of fetal blood collecting are described in many standard textbooks. In this brief discussion, mention is made of the indications for sampling and the prognostic significance of values obtained.

Although a full set of blood gas determinations (pH, P_{CO_2} and P_{O_2}) can be done on as little as 0.25 mL of blood, most institutions obtain a minimal amount of blood for pH determination. Having the pH value alone does not allow differentiation between respiratory and metabolic acidosis. Treatment of the causes of acidosis are theoretically different. Metabolic acidosis requires immediate delivery, whereas respiratory acidosis should respond to standard resuscitation. In reality, the initial resuscitation measures (oxygen for the mother, uterine displacement, intravenous fluid bolus) are generally begun immediately with any severe deceleration. If a deceleration does not respond quickly to resuscitation, the clinical situation (stage of labor, presence of meconium, estimated fetal weight, gestation age, parity, etc.) will determine whether fetal scalp sampling is needed and/or if delivery is necessary immediately.

In human newborns, there is good correlation between the pH of scalp blood taken shortly before delivery and that of umbilical cord samples. Beard et al.,[22] correlating scalp blood pH and 2-minute Apgar scores, showed that a scalp pH above 7.25 was associated with an Apgar score greater than 7 in 92% of infants. When the scalp pH was less than 7.15, the Apgar score was less than 6 in 80% of cases. Fetal heart rate decelerations have also been found to correlate with pH values (Table 2–6).[23] This correlation is not always close, so fetal scalp sampling is used when there is any question about the fetal heart rate tracing.

■ Table 2–6
CORRELATION OF FETAL SCALP pH AND FETAL HEART RATE PATTERN

Deceleration Pattern	Scalp pH
Early mild variable	7.30 ± 0.04
Moderate variable	7.26 ± 0.04
Mild moderate late variable	7.22 ± 0.06
Severe late variable	7.14 ± 0.07

From Kubli FW, Hon EW, Khazin AF, et al: Observations on heart rate and pH in the human fetus during labor. Am J Obstet Gynecol 104:1190, 1969.

There are other fetal heart rate patterns that signal the need for fetal scalp sampling in addition to persistent late decelerations:

1. Absent or decreased short-term variability, which might be due to CNS depressants given to the mother;
2. Variable deceleration when combined with reduced or absent short-term variability;
3. Severe persistent variable decelerations.

The clinical situation provides indications for fetal scalp sampling, especially if there is decreased variability or severe decelerations.

Pulse Oximetry

Reflectance pulse oximetry is a refinement of conventional pulse oximetry, which requires transmitted light and provides a noninvasive method to assess fetal oxygenation. A study by Dildy et al.[24] demonstrated in healthy parturients in labor, when the sensor was placed between the cervix and the fetal presenting part, a significant correlation between fetal oxygen saturation and umbilical vein saturation and pH and umbilical artery pH. The relationship of umbilical artery pH and saturation to fetal O_2 saturation was not significant. The range of the values was large: For a fetal oximetry value of 60% the umbilical vein saturation ranged from 30 to 70% and the pH from 7.25 to 7.38. Values for fetal pulse oximetry varied from 40 to 90% when, with delivery, the umbilical vein pH was generally greater than 7.24. Although there were statistical correlations, the wide range of values suggests a low specificity of the oximeter. In this same study, fetal O_2 saturation was measured after giving a parturient supplemental oxygen and found a rise in fetal O_2 saturation; however, one third of the patients were excluded because of poor signal quality. Even more patients were excluded because of caput formation, fetal anemia, and meconium staining. Dildy et al.[24] studied 73 healthy parturients in labor and were unable to obtain a reliable signal 50% of the time. These preliminary studies suggest technical problems to be overcome; thus, the oximeter is not yet a useful clinical tool.

SUMMARY

The reduction of perinatal morbidity and mortality is the sole purpose of fetal assessment, which spans the three trimesters of gestation. Chromosomal and developmental abnormalities are the focus of first and early second trimester studies. During the late second and third trimesters, the emphasis shifts to causes of asphyxia and hypoxia. These problems tend to occur more frequently in parturients who have underlying diseases such as diabetes, PIH, drug addiction, malnutrition, and obesity.

REFERENCES

1. Friede A, Rochat R: Maternal mortality and perinatal mortality: definitions, data and epidemiology. In: Sachs B; ed. Clinical Obstetrics. Littleton, MA: PSG Pub. Inc., 1985:35.
2. Lammer EJ, Brown LB, Anderka MT, et al: Classification and analysis of fetal deaths in Massachusetts. JAMA 261:1757–1762, 1989.
3. Mersey Region Working Party on Perinatal Mortality: Perinatal health. Lancet 1:491–494, 1982.
4. Jackson LG, Zachary JM, Fowler SE; et al: A randomized comparison of transcervical and transabdominal chorionic villus sampling. N Engl J Med 327:594–598, 1992.
5. Burton BK, Schulz CJ, Burd LI: Limb anomalies associated with chorionic villus sampling. Obstet Gynaecol 79:726–730, 1992.
6. Monni G, Ibba RM, Lai R, et al: Limb-reduction defects and chorionic villus sampling. Lancet 337:1091, 1991.
7. Mahoney MJ: Limb abnormalities and chorionic villus sampling. Lancet 337:1422–1423, 1991.
8. Saari-Kemppainen A, Karjalainen O, Ylostalo P, et al: Ultrasound screening and perinatal mortality: controlled trial of systemic one-stage screening in pregnancy. The Helsinki Ultrasound Trial. Lancet 336:387–391, 1990.
9. Ewigman B, LeFevre N, Hesser J: A randomised trial of routine prenatal ultrasound. Obstet Gynaecol 76:189–194, 1990.
10. Bakketeig LS, Eik-Nes SH, Jacobsen G, et al: Randomised controlled trial of ultrasonographic screening in pregnancy. Lancet 2:207–211, 1984.
11. Ewigman B, Crane JP, Frigoletto FD, et al: Effect of prenatal ultrasound screening on perinatal outcome. N Engl J Med 329:821–827, 1993.
12. Russell JC, Cooper CM, Ketchum CH, et al: Multicenter evaluation of TDx test for assessing fetal lung maturity. Clin Chem 35:1005–1010, 1989.
13. Manning FA, Morrison I Harmon CR, et al: Fetal assessment by fetal BPS: experience in 19,221 referred high-risk pregnancies. II. The false negative rate by frequency and etiology. Am J Obstet Gynaecol 157:880–884, 1987.
14. Baskett TF, Allen AC, Gray JH, et al: The biophysical profile score. Obstet Gynaecol 70:357–360, 1987.
15. Platt LD, Eglington GS, Scorpios L, et al: Further experience with the fetal biophysical profile score. Obstet Gynaecol 61:480–485, 1983.
16. Schifrin BS, Guntes V, Gergely RC, et al: The role of real-time scanning in antenatal fetal surveillance. Am J Obstet Gynaecol 140:525–530, 1981.
17. Manning FA, Baskett TF, Morrison I, et al: Fetal biophysical profile scoring: a prospective study in 1184 high-risk patients. Am J Obstet Gynaecol 140:289–294, 1981.
18. Manning FA, Morrison I, Lange IR, et al: Fetal assessment based on fetal biophysical profile scoring: experience in 12,620 referred high-risk pregnancies. I. Perinatal mortality by frequency and etiology. Am J Obstet Gynaecol 151:343–350, 1985.
19. Fenton AN, Steer CM: Fetal distress. Am J Obstet Gynaecol 83:354, 1962.
20. Rosen MG, Diskensen JC: The paradox of electronic fetal monitoring: more data may not enable us to predict or prevent infant neurologic morbidity. Am J Obstet Gynaecol 168:745–751, 1993.
21. Saling E, Schneider D: Biochemical supervision of the foetus during labor. J Obstet Gynaecol Br Commonw 74:799–811, 1967.
22. Beard RW, Morris ED, Clayton SE: pH of fetal capillary blood as an indicator of the condition of the foetus. J Obstet Gynaecol Br Commonw 74:812–822, 1967.
23. Kubli FW, Hon EW, Khazin AF, et al: Observations on heart rate and pH in the human fetus during labor. Am J Obstet Gynaecol 104:1190–1206, 1969.
24. Dildy GA, Clark SL, Loucks CA: Preliminary experience with intrapartum fetal pulse oximetry in humans. Obstet Gynaecol 81:630–635, 1993.

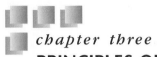

chapter three

PRINCIPLES OF PERINATAL PHARMACOLOGY

Gerald A. Burger, MD

OVERVIEW

Perinatal pharmacology is the study of the physiologic and biochemical effects of endogenous and exogenous compounds during the development of the human being from conception through the first 28 days of neonatal life. As anesthesiologists, we understand that most if not all drugs we administer to a pregnant woman may potentially have far-reaching effects on the developing fetus. Drugs may have not only a direct pharmacologic impact from placental transfer but may also have an impact on the environment in utero. Like it or not, by virtue of our role in obstetrics, we must have a basic understanding of how our medications and interventions affect the fetus. We must ensure that our actions are as safe as possible for both the mother and child in utero. Safety can result only if we understand how our actions affect the mother and fetus or, in other words, have a thorough understanding of perinatal pharmacology.

ANATOMY OF THE MATERNAL-PLACENTAL-FETAL UNIT

The circulations of the mother and the fetus come together in the placenta. Because the two circulatory systems are so vastly different, their juncture at the placenta is quite complex. For this reason, the pharmacologic and physiologic interactions between the mother and fetus are most easily discussed using a model, the maternal-placental-fetal unit, and dividing the process into its three main elements (Fig. 3–1).

■ **KEY POINT:** The placenta is a dynamic organ that brings the maternal and fetal circulations into close interface. In addition to the exchange of materials that occurs, the placenta produces numerous enzymes, proteins, and hormones.

The Maternal Component

Every maternal biologic system is dramatically altered during pregnancy. Alterations in the maternal cardiovascular system

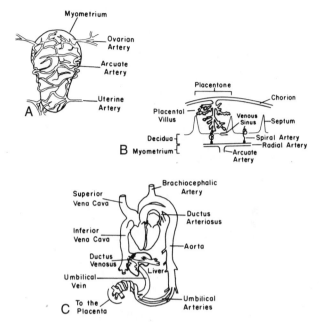

Figure 3–1 ■ The maternal-placental-fetal unit. *A,* The maternal component; *B,* the placental component; *C,* the fetal component.

and uterine anatomy are reviewed because they are particularly important to our understanding of the unit.

Maternal Cardiovascular and Hemodynamic Changes

1. Increased total blood volume (25 to 40%) resulting from increased plasma volume (40 to 50%) and increased red cell mass (20%).
2. Increased cardiac output (30 to 50%) resulting from increased heart rate (12 to 15 beats/min), increased stroke volume (30%), and decreased systemic vascular resistance (15%).
3. Increased uterine blood flow and a redistribution of uterine perfusion to the placenta.

These changes in the cardiovascular system have broad-reaching influence on the pharmacologic characteristics of maternally administered drugs by affecting the volume of distribution, kinetics, and absorption from tissue depots.

Uterine Blood Flow and Distribution

In the nonpregnant uterus, blood flow averages 50 mL/min, increasing with pregnancy to 700 mL/min. This change represents a 10-fold increase in blood flow, accounting for 10% of maternal cardiac output. In addition to flow changes, the pattern of uterine perfusion also changes in pregnancy, with the placenta receiving more than 80% of the uterine blood flow, whereas the myometrium receives only 20%.

Changes in Uterine Anatomy

The gravid uterus is an enlarging abdominal mass requiring an enlarging vascular supply. During gestation, the uterus grows from about 50 g to over 1100 g, excluding placental tissue. Arterial supply to the gravid uterus is provided by the uterine arteries, which arise from the hypogastric (internal iliac) arteries (85%) and ovarian arteries (15%). These vessels in turn arise from the abdominal aorta.

Anastomoses occur between uterine and ovarian arteries along the lateral border of the gravid uterus in the broad ligament. Uterine vessels then penetrate the myometrium, forming a circular ring of vessels (the arcuate arteries) in the middle third of the myometrium. These vessels further divide to form the radial arteries that penetrate the remaining myometrium, forming spiral arteries (named for their appearance) as they enter the intervillous space between the maternal and fetal placental plates. As the uterine vascular supply subdivides, its characteristics change. The arcuate and radial arteries are muscular, whereas the spiral arteries are not. For this reason, the spiral artery is more prone to occlusion. This fact becomes important in the discussion of the regulation of uteroplacental perfusion.

Venous drainage of the gravid uterus begins in decidual veins, which empty into larger conduits leading to the uterine and ovarian veins, which accompany the uterine and ovarian arteries. Ultimately, these veins join the inferior vena cava.

The Placental Component

The placenta is an organ present only in gestation. It is composed of both maternal and fetal tissues. The placenta may be viewed as a semipermeable membrane that provides an interface for maternal and fetal circulation.

Gross Anatomy

The placenta is a disc consisting of two plates: a basal plate of maternal tissue and a chorionic plate of fetal tissue. These two plates join at the periphery in a ring of connective tissue, the ring of Waldeyer. Placental tissue is grossly divided into lobulations known as cotyledons. In a normal gestation, the placenta weighs about one sixth as much as the fetus (500 g), but its size may be affected by acute or chronic disease (i.e., preeclampsia, diabetes).

Microscopic Anatomy

The basal plate of the placenta is composed of decidual tissue and blood vessels. The chorionic plate is made up of three tissue layers that form the fetal chorionic villi, the interface for the fetus. The space separating the basal and chorionic plates is the intervillous space. The intervillous space is subdivided by a series of decidual tissue septa. The chorionic villi and the spiral arteries protrude into the intervillous space, forming placentones.

The chorionic villi mature as gestation proceeds, altering their microscopic anatomy. Initially, the villi are smooth, consisting of an external layer of cuboidal cells (the syncytiotrophoblasts) and an internal layer of cells (the cytotrophoblasts). These two layers separate the intervillous space from the fetal umbilical capillaries. As maturation occurs, the villi become branched and the two cell layers flatten, reducing the distance between the intervillous space and the fetal umbilical capillaries.

Placental Blood Flow

There are several hundred spiral arteries that divide the placenta into its primary functional units, placentones. A placentone consists of the spiral artery, surrounding intervillous space, and at least one fetal chorionic villus. Maternal blood flows into the intervillous space from the spiral artery in a fountain pattern, bathing the fetal chorionic villi in the vicinity. At the same time, fetal blood traverses the umbilical capillaries within the chorionic villus. Placental transfer from mother to fetus occurs across the chorionic membrane. The pattern of blood flow in the human placenta (villous stream pattern) differs from other mammalian placentas where countercurrent exchange is most common. Although the mechanics of villous stream exchange are poorly understood, there are similarities with the pulmonary alveolus. Each placentone, like its structural counterpart in the lung, may receive an unequal portion of the uteroplacental blood flow. At any one time, approximately 100 spiral arteries (out of several hundred) are patent. The remaining spiral arteries act as a shunt just as in the lung. Current theory about the regulation of shunt in the placenta focuses on altered sensitivity of placental vessels to endogenous vasodilators and nonuniform release of these vasodilators: prostaglandin, nitric oxide, and steroids (estrogen).

The Fetal Component

Fetal Blood Flow Through the Placenta

The umbilical-placental circulation receives 50% of the combined ventricular output of the fetus. The fetal blood flow is 75 mL/kg/min (approximately 250 mL/min at term), much less than maternal uteroplacental flow. Approximately 20% of the total umbilical-placental flow is functionally shunted. Although the two dissimilar circulatory patterns are mismatched in flow and pressure, placenta transfer is rapid for most substances. Although maternal uteroplacental perfusion varies in response to many factors, the fetal umbilical–placental circulation remains quite constant, with changes being less predictable, less measurable, and less preventable. Additionally, the response of the fetal circulation to asphyxia and pharmacologic manipulation varies substantially with the gestational age.

> ■ **KEY POINT:** Exchange in the placenta occurs in the intervillous space, where maternal blood contacts fetal tissue. About 80% of the uterine blood flow passes through the intervillous space.

Fetal blood enters the placenta via the two umbilical arteries, which arise from the internal iliac arteries. The umbilical arteries continue through the umbilical cord and enter the placenta, where they subdivide to form smaller vessels and finally the umbilical capillaries. The umbilical capillaries traverse the chorionic villi separated from maternal blood in the intervillous space by the two cellular layers, the cytotrophoblast and the epithelioid syncytiotrophoblast. Poorly oxygenated fetal blood containing the byproducts of metabolism enters the umbilical arteries, traverses the umbilical capillaries, and returns cleansed and oxygenated via the single umbilical vein.

Approximately 50% of the returning blood enters the portal circulation and perfuses the fetal liver, with the remainder going to the inferior vena cava. The proportion of fetal umbilical blood flow entering the fetal portal circulation is variable due to the reactivity of the ductus venosus. For example, in fetal acidosis the ductus venosus closes, shunting a greater fraction of umbilical blood flow into the inferior vena cava than into the portal circulation. From the inferior vena cava, blood enters the right atrium and mixes with poorly oxygenated blood from the head and upper extremities that is returning via the superior vena cava. In the right atrium, most of the blood is shunted across the foramen ovale into the left atrium. A small fraction of right atrial flow proceeds through the right ventricle and out the pulmonary outflow tract to the fetal lungs. Because the fetal lungs have no respiratory function, their perfusion is not a priority. From the left atrium, flow continues to the left ventricle and out into the aorta where blood from the fetal lungs joins via the ductus arteriosus. The body is perfused and the cycle is completed with the blood returning to the placenta via the umbilical arteries.

Regulation of the Umbilical-Placental Circulation

Regulation of the umbilical-placental circulation may occur via two mechanisms: fetal physiologic reflex changes and alterations in the fetal neuroendocrine axis. Because the umbilical-placental circulation provides a wide margin of safety for the fetus, a significant challenge to fetal survival (i.e., asphyxia) must be present for these changes to occur. The most common expression of alterations in the umbilical-placental circulation is in fetal heart rate anomalies.

Reflex Changes in the Fetal Circulation. The fetal circulation is a low-resistance system that relies on fetal cardiac output to maintain umbilical-placental circulation. In the developing fetus, cardiac output is determined primarily by the fetal heart rate (FHR) because alterations in stroke volume and peripheral resistance are not possible. As the fetus matures, FHR declines and fetal blood pressure rises, indicating a transition of the circulatory pattern and a maturation of peripheral resistance control. The transition corresponds closely to development of the aortic chemoreceptors. In early gestation, the fetus responds to asphyxia by increasing heart rate without changing blood pressure. As the fetus matures, the response to asphyxia is bradycardia with a concomitant increase in blood pressure, suggesting a reflex mechanism. In the immature fetus, central nervous system control and/or catecholamine release are presumed to be responsible for the regulation of these circulatory responses, whereas the aortic chemoreceptors appear responsible in the more mature fetus.

Alterations in the Neuroendocrine Axis. Although reflex changes contribute significantly to the regulation of umbilical-placental perfusion in the mature fetus, they are not entirely responsible. In the immature and the mature fetus, certain substances found in the neuroendocrine system, such as vasopressin, prostaglandins, endorphins, and catecholamines, have been implicated in the regulation of umbilical-placental perfusion.

Peripartum Events That Influence the Umbilical-Placental Circulation

Direct Effects on Umbilical Vessels. The umbilical vessels are lengthy, redundant, and muscular with sparse innervation (before entry into the fetal abdomen). Umbilical-placental perfusion may be altered through

1. Mechanical compression from cord prolapse or compression by fetal parts;
2. Vasospasm from local anesthetics, vasopressors, or maternal hypocarbia;
3. An increase in intervillous pressure from a tetanic uterine contraction limiting blood flow through the chorionic villi in the intervillous space (Starling resistor effect).

Drug Effects on the Fetal Neuroendocrine Axis. The administration of certain drugs may produce changes in the fetal neuroendocrine system. Although these changes are well documented, their etiology and specific mechanism of action are unclear. For example, administration of morphine or benzodiazepines to the mother results in a decrease in the variability of the FHR. Similarly, adrenergic agents used to halt labor may lead to fetal tachycardia, presumably through an autonomic nervous system mechanism.

PHYSIOLOGY OF THE MATERNAL-PLACENTA-FETAL UNIT

The coordinated function of these two very dissimilar circulatory patterns is vital to the survival and well-being of the developing fetus. Anesthetic drugs and techniques have the potential to adversely affect the fetus by altering the in utero milieu on either the maternal or the fetal side of the placenta. These alterations, known as *indirect effects,* can often be influenced by the anesthesiologist. Adverse changes in uteroplacental perfusion must be rapidly addressed to avoid fetal compromise. A discussion of the general principles follows.

Uteroplacental Circulation

Uterine Perfusion Equation

Under normal conditions, the uterine vascular bed is maximally dilated. There is no autoregulation, and flow depends on perfusion pressure. Oxygen transfer and carbon dioxide elimination in the fetus are directly related to uteroplacental blood flow, making preservation of optimal flow vital to the fetus.

Seventy to 90% of uterine blood flow passes through the intervillous space. Investigations in animals suggest that the normal placenta has a 50% "safety factor," that is, uterine blood flow can decrease to 50% of normal before fetal hypoxia and acidosis develop. This safety factor is generally adequate to protect the fetus from the stresses of normal pregnancy, labor, and delivery. However, this safety factor is present only in normal gestations. In pathologic situations, the margin may be greatly reduced or absent, as with pregnancy-induced hypertension or diabetes.

Uteroplacental blood flow is described by the following relationship:

$$UBF = \frac{MMAP - UP}{UVR} = \frac{PPP}{UVR}$$

where UBF is uteroplacental blood flow, MMAP is maternal mean arterial blood pressure, UP is uterine venous pressure or intervillous pressure (whichever is greater), PPP is placental perfusion pressure, and UVR is uterine vascular resistance.

Maternal Factors That Influence Uterine Blood Flow

Position. Compression of both the abdominal aorta and the inferior vena cava occurs in the supine pregnant patient as a result of mechanical compression by the gravid uterus, a phenomenon referred to as aortocaval compression. Compression of the aorta occurs above the origin of the hypogastric (internal iliac) arteries that supply the uterine arteries, reducing uteroplacental perfusion. Compression of the inferior vena cava leads to an increase in uterine venous pressure with a concomitant decrease in the perfusion pressure in the intervillous space and a decrease in maternal cardiac output from diminished venous return to the heart. Aortocaval compression can markedly reduce uterine blood flow and is best avoided in the lateral decubitus or sitting positions. When a supine posture or lithotomy is required, left uterine displacement should always be used.

Hypotension. Pressure in the uterine arteries equals MMAP (without aortocaval compression). A fall in MMAP of 20 to 25% or an MMAP below 100 mm Hg systolic may be associated with a significant reduction in uteroplacental blood flow. Most commonly, hypotension in the peripartum setting is seen after sympathetic blockade from major regional anesthesia or in a severe form of aortocaval compression known as the supine hypotensive syndrome. Blood pressure changes in the mother demand prompt therapy to prevent fetal compromise. Therapy may include positioning, intravenous fluids, and vasopressors (ephedrine or phenylephrine), depending on the clinical circumstances.

Alterations in Uterine Tone. Increases in uterine tone severely alter uteroplacental perfusion by raising uterine vascular pressure (UVP), reducing the intervillous perfusion pressure and increasing UVR through compression of the arcuate and radial arteries. Although uterine tone is normally altered during the physiologic process of parturition, certain drugs used in obstetrics and obstetric anesthesia (ketamine, intrathecal sufentanil, and Pitocin) may also increase uterine tone and must be administered carefully. Some pathologic obstetric conditions may also alter uterine tone or lead to frank tetanic uterine contractions (abruptio placentae).

■ **KEY POINT:** Uterine contractions decrease uterine blood flow as a result of increased uterine venous pressure.

Maternal Respiratory Alterations. Severe hypoxia, hypercarbia, or hypocarbia are all associated with a decrease in uteroplacental perfusion. Moderate alterations do not appear, however, to affect uteroplacental blood flow.

Catecholamines. Exogenous and endogenous catecholamines decrease uteroplacental perfusion by augmenting UVR. Of the vasopressors used in anesthetic practice, ephedrine appears to best maintain uteroplacental perfusion without significantly altering UVR. The increase in MMAP with administration of ephedrine is presumed to be due to central nervous system stimulation rather than catecholamine release or direct effect.

Fetal Circulation and Respiratory Gas Exchange

Oxygen. Fetal oxygen delivery is determined by factors that affect umbilical blood flow and umbilical vein oxygen content. Studies in animals suggest that reductions in oxygen delivery of as much as 40 to 50% are tolerated by the fetus without adverse effects on fetal oxygen consumption. This suggests the existence of a fetal reserve and other compensatory mechanisms. In animals, fetal oxygen delivery averages 24 mL/min/kg and oxygen consumption averages 8 mL/min/kg. A reduction in oxygen delivery is compensated for by an increase in oxygen extraction. When oxygen delivery drops below 12 to 14 mL/min/kg, fetal oxygen consumption decreases and the fetus incurs an oxygen debt, resulting in an increased base deficit. Redistribution of blood flow to vital organs occurs.

■ **KEY POINT:** The transfer of oxygen from mother to fetus depends on rates of blood flow as well as oxygen tension in maternal and fetal blood.

Carbon Dioxide. Carbon dioxide elimination depends on blood flow. In the fetus, a condition analogous to respiratory acidosis develops when there is a decrease in either uterine or umbilical blood flow. In such circumstances, carbon dioxide acutely rises and the pH decreases without changes in fixed acid.

It is postulated that maternal hypocapnia may cause uterine arterial vasoconstriction, which leads to a decrease in uterine blood flow. Additionally, maternal-fetal alkalosis results in a shift to the left of the oxygen-hemoglobin dissociation curve, which leads to decreased oxygen delivery to fetal tissues.

Obstetric Factors in Uteroplacental Blood Flow

1. Uterine contraction produces a decrease in blood flow. This occurs in response to the increase in uterine venous pressure caused by the increase in transuterine pressure. There also may be decreases in uterine arterial pressure with contractions. Uterine hypertonus results in a decrease in uteroplacental blood flow by the same mechanism.

2. Uterine blood flow depends on perfusion pressure. Thus, any condition that results in hypotension, such as sympathetic block, hypovolemic shock, or supine hypotensive syndrome (aortocaval compression), causes decreased uteroplacental blood flow.
3. Hypertension, either essential or pregnancy induced, results in a decrease in uteroplacental blood flow due to high vascular resistance in the uterine vessels and narrowing placental vascular beds.
4. Vasoconstrictors, either endogenous or exogenously administered, increase uterine vascular resistance, leading to a decrease in uteroplacental blood flow.
5. Uteroplacental blood flow is decreased in postmature pregnancy and is potentially compromised in diabetic mothers.

Measurement of Uteroplacental Blood Flow

There is no practical direct method of monitoring uteroplacental blood flow in humans. In clinical practice we infer changes in uteroplacental blood flow by monitoring FHR and acid-base status (fetal scalp pH). In the late 1970s, Rekonen et al.[3] developed a quantitative method to measure intervillous blood flow using the clearance of xenon 133 (^{133}Xe) administered intravenously. Although extremely useful, this technique has not become popular because of the perceived risks of radiation exposure to both the mother and the fetus.

More recently, Doppler ultrasound examinations of maternal uterine and fetal umbilical arterial velocity waveforms have been used to measure the effects of interventions on uteroplacental and umbilical blood flow. A 4-MHz Doppler probe is positioned over the abdomen and the vessel of interest is identified. An amplitude versus frequency characteristic of the Doppler return is calculated and displayed as amplitude and frequency versus time.[4] The ratio of the systolic to the diastolic peaks of this waveform is thought to be reflective of the vascular resistance, providing an indirect assessment of perfusion. A high ratio is thought to correlate with poor perfusion.

Despite these advances, most information regarding uteroplacental blood flow is extrapolated from animal studies. Animals are chronically instrumented, which allows precise measurement of changes in uterine and placental blood flow and their effect on fetal acid-base status (Fig. 3-2). Uterine blood flow is measured by one of many techniques, including electromagnetic flow probes, steady-state diffusion techniques (Fick principle), and injection of radioactive tracers. Animal studies are criticized for the following issues:

1. Most animal model studies involve chronic instrumentation of the maternal-placental-fetal unit. Instrumentation certainly introduces error into studies by altering both anatomy and physiology.

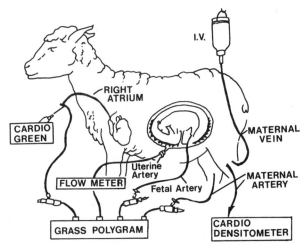

Figure 3–2 ■ Animal model with chronically implanted maternal and fetal intravascular catheters and an electromagnetic flow probe around a branch of the uterine artery. (From Ralston DH, Shnider SM, deLorimer AA: Effect of equipotent ephedrine, metaraminal, mephentermine and methoxamine on uterine blood flow in the pregnant ewe. Anesthesiology 40:354, 1974.)

2. Variables known to alter the physiology of the maternal-placental-fetal unit have not been standardized. As a result, data obtained may vary greatly from one study to another.
3. Most studies in the animal models have required general anesthesia or heavy sedation to complete, potentially altering the physiology of the maternal-placental-fetal unit.
4. Although animal models are selected for their similarity to the human, none is a perfect replica of the human.

Anesthetic Agents and Uteroplacental Blood Flow

General Anesthesia

Barbiturates. Animal studies with thiopental and thiamylal in clinical doses (4 mg/kg) demonstrated reduced maternal systolic and diastolic blood pressure and decreased uterine blood flow. The onset, as one might expect, was within 20 to 30 seconds of injection and the effect lasted from 3 to 8 minutes. These changes were associated with transient fetal hypoxia and acidosis. Methohexital showed similar findings, although these effects were smaller in magnitude, shorter in duration, and were not associated with changes in fetal Pao_2 or acid-base status.

Ketamine. In the near-term ewe, ketamine administered intravenously at doses of 5 mg/kg produced a 15% increase in mean blood pressure with a concomitant 10% increase in uterine blood flow.[1] Intrauterine pressures in postpartum humans demonstrate a dose-related increase in uterine tone with increasing doses of ketamine.[2] For general anesthesia, induction doses of up to 1 mg/kg appear to have little effect on uterine blood flow.

Volatile Anesthetics. The volatile agents are potent uterine relaxants. Uteroplacental flow with halothane at 1 to 1.5 minimal alveolar concentration (MAC) is essentially unchanged. However, at 2 MAC, there is a resultant decrease in cardiac output and blood pressure, leading to a decrease in uteroplacental blood flow. Isoflurane and enflurane are essentially identical to halothane in their effects on uterine blood flow. Light planes of anesthesia do not decrease uterine blood flow, but deeper planes do.

Enflurane, when studied in acidotic fetuses at concentrations of 1% or higher, produced a dose-related maternal and fetal bradycardia, a decrease in uterine blood flow, and fetal acidosis.[5]

Nitrous Oxide. Nitrous oxide can increase sympathetic activity, which theoretically can lead to a decrease in placental perfusion. However, when combined with volatile anesthetics, as in our clinical practice, the increases in sympathetic activity are blunted.

Local Anesthesia

Greiss et al.[6] studied local anesthetics and their effects on uteroplacental blood flow. Local anesthetic was infused directly into the uterine artery of nonpregnant ewes. The threshold level at which uterine blood flow was first noted to decrease was 1 μg/mL for bupivacaine and 3 to 4 μg/mL for lidocaine, mepivacaine, and procaine. The point at which there are severe reductions in uterine blood flow is much higher than would be expected clinically with epidural or subarachnoid anesthesia, unless associated with an intravascular injection.

Concentrations of this magnitude, however, can be seen locally with a paracervical block. Some investigators have suggested that the fetal bradycardia associated with paracervical block is due to decreases in oxygenation secondary to vasoconstriction of uterine arteries and possibly uterine hypertonus, resulting in diminished uteroplacental blood flow.

Regional Anesthesia

Epidural anesthesia in pregnant sheep has been shown to have no effect on uteroplacental perfusion unless associated with decreases in systemic blood pressure. In a classic study in humans during normal labor, increases in intervillous blood flow were demonstrated after epidural anesthesia.[7] Preeclamptic patients appear to benefit greatly from epidural anesthesia, with some studies showing an increase in intervillous blood flow of as much as 77% after epidural anesthesia.[8]

In the absence of intravascular injection, local anesthetics

■ Table 3–1
VASOPRESSOR EFFECTS ON
UTEROPLACENTAL PERFUSION

	α	β
Ephedrine	+ +	+ + +
Mephentermine	+	+ +
Metaraminol	+ + +	+
Methoxamine	+ + + + +	0
Phenylephrine	+ + + + +	0

containing epinephrine seem to have little or no effect on uteroplacental perfusion. However, when studied in animals, as little as 15 μg of epinephrine injected intravascularly can result in a 50% decrease in uterine blood flow.[9] Because it is not uncommon to unintentionally enter an epidural vessel in gravid patients during the placement of an epidural catheter, these data suggest epinephrine-containing local anesthetics should be administered carefully when initiating an epidural block in gravid patients.

Vasopressors

Vasopressors may have a primary α, β, or mixed effect (Table 3–1). In their classic study with normotensive pregnant ewes, Ralston et al.[10] demonstrated that ephedrine affected uterine blood flow the least compared with other vasopressor agents. Phenylephrine was not evaluated in this study. More recently, investigators studied the use of ephedrine versus phenylephrine in treating hypotension secondary to epidural and spinal anesthesia[11] in healthy women undergoing elective cesarean delivery and detected no abnormalities in fetal acid-base status.

In patients with normal placental reserve who are not in labor, decreases in blood pressure are generally well tolerated by the fetus despite limited changes in uteroplacental blood flow. Most measures used to increase maternal blood pressure will, for the most part, restore uteroplacental blood flow to an adequate level. The fetus should experience little effect because there is significant fetal reserve.

If there is preexisting placental insufficiency or superimposed labor, particularly if contractions are prolonged, the decreases in maternal blood pressure may have very adverse effects on uterine blood flow and α-agents used to restore blood pressure may have questionable effects. In these situations, it may be more efficacious to use a β-specific agent to increase maternal blood pressure.

■ **K E Y   P O I N T :**   Animal studies have suggested that vasopressors with predominantly α-adrenergic activity cause a reduction in uterine blood flow that can adversely affect the fetus. Studies in humans undergoing elective cesarean sections have not confirmed the animal data and have suggested that small doses of phenylephrine may improve the mother's hemodynamics without having an adverse impact on the fetus.

PLACENTAL TRANSFER OF ANESTHETICS

In addition to their effects on placental perfusion, all drugs administered to the mother cross to the fetus to some extent, potentially affecting either fetal development or neonatal behavior (see Fig. 3–2). The administration of diethylstilbestrol to mothers in the 1960s to prevent abortion with the subsequent development of vaginal carcinoma in many of their female progeny remains a painful reminder of the far-reaching effects of drugs administered during gestation. Similarly, neurobehavioral testing of the neonate has detected evanescent behavioral changes secondary to the maternal administration of drugs commonly used in anesthesia. Behavioral and developmental changes noted in the fetus or neonate that can be ascribed to a particular compound are known as *direct effects.* The extent of the direct effect is assumed to be directly related to the quantity of the drug or metabolite transferred across the placenta. Using the concept of placental transfer, we can predict the extent of drug transfer from mother to fetus and predict how likely it is that a drug will affect the fetus.

CLINICAL IMPLICATIONS OF THE PLACENTAL TRANSFER OF DRUGS

Placental transfer of drugs can occur by several mechanisms including simple diffusion, facilitated diffusion, active transport, bulk flow, and direct diffusion through breaks in the placental or, more accurately, the chorionic membrane. Factors related to drug transfer across this membrane include the diffusion constant for the particular drug, the surface area and the thickness of the chorionic membrane across which the drug will diffuse, and the diffusion gradient from maternal to fetal tissues. These factors can be related by the Fick equation for simple diffusion:

$$Q/t = \frac{K \times A \times (C_m - C_t)}{D}$$

where Q/t is the amount of drug transferred per unit of time, K is the diffusion coefficient or constant of the drug studied,

A is the total surface area of the chorionic membrane available for transfer, $(C_m - C_f)$ is the diffusion gradient (maternal drug concentration minus fetal drug concentration), and *D* is thickness of the chorionic membrane.

The diffusion coefficient (K) depends on several variables, including the molecular weight, lipid solubility, and protein binding of the drug. A molecular weight of 1000 appears to be the maximal size for drugs to cross the placenta by simple diffusion. Most analgesic and anesthetic drugs have molecular weights below 500 (Table 3-2), allowing them to cross the placenta by simple diffusion. Many of these drugs exist in both ionized and non-ionized forms. The non-ionized form is more lipid soluble and passes through the membrane more readily. Because the neonate's blood is more acidotic than the mother's blood, basic drugs may achieve a higher blood

▪ Table 3–2
MOLECULAR WEIGHT OF DRUGS USED IN OBSTETRICS

Drug Classification	Molecular Weight
Induction agents	
Etomidate	244
Ketamine	238
Propofol	178
Sodium thiopental	264
Neuromuscular drugs	
Succinylcholine chloride	361
Gases	
Enflurane	184
Halothane	197
Isoflurane	184
Nitrous oxide	44
Oxygen	32
Anticoagulants	
Sodium warfarin	330
Heparin	6000+
Local anesthetics	
Bupivacaine	288
Chloroprocaine	271
Etidocaine	276
Lidocaine	234
Mepivacaine	246
Prilocaine	220
Procaine	236
Tetracaine	264
Narcotics	
Fentanyl	336
Meperidine	247
Methadone	309
Morphine	285
Tranquilizers	
Midazolam	325

concentration in the neonate. This can occur as a result of ion trapping and occurs more frequently if the fetus develops distress with a very low blood pH. Increased protein binding may decrease drug transfer, as only the bound drug can pass the placenta. However, this may not be significant, because binding is a reversible process and any unbound drug that crosses the placenta will promote drug release from the bound form.

■ **K E Y   P O I N T :**   Placental transfer of drugs depends on the dose and route of administration, the rate of absorption, the maternal and fetal pH, the pKa of the drug, protein binding, and uteroplacental blood flow.

The important factor of time must be kept in mind when evaluating drug transfer. The more time allowed, the more drug transferred. Finally, one must bear in mind that placental transfer is a dynamic process that continues in both directions across the chorionic membrane until birth.

The Fetal/Maternal Ratio

The placental transfer of drugs in both human and animal model studies is difficult to determine. The maternal-placental-fetal unit is pharmacologically dynamic and multicompartmented. A simple approach to determining the ease with which a drug crosses the placenta and its uptake by the fetus has been to administer the drug maternally and obtain serum concentrations of the drug in the mother (either arterial or venous samples) and in the fetus (usually umbilical venous and arterial samples at delivery) at an arbitrary time. Given the dynamic nature of placental transfer and the many variables involved, the validity of this technique must be questioned. Past studies using this technique have demonstrated the following limitations:

1. Any one-time determination of fetal and maternal serum drug levels does not reflect the dynamic nature of placental transfer.
2. Maternal venous and arterial concentrations and umbilical venous and arterial concentrations are not equivalent if an equilibrium state has not been achieved. Studies are not usually done at equilibrium.
3. Because of differences in fetal and maternal protein binding and tissue/blood partition characteristics, fetal sequestration of a drug may not be reflected by the fetal/maternal ratio.

These inadequacies raise the question of the utility of the fetal/maternal ratio as a tool in perinatal pharmacologic research.

Neurobehavioral Studies

Since its introduction in 1953, the Apgar score[12] has become the most frequently used method for evaluating neonatal well-being and the effects of maternally administered medications on the neonate. Although subjective, the scoring system is rapidly administered and reproducible (Table 3–3). The five evaluations are essentially a set of vital signs that can be used to describe the healthy neonate's condition and can serve as a guide to success during neonatal resuscitation or as a description of the neonate's condition at specified times after delivery. The 1-minute score is thought to be a reflection of the acid-base status of the neonate. However, this correlation is not strong. The 5-minute score is thought to be a predictor of both survival and neurologic abnormalities, although the latter correlation has not held up to scrutiny.

So, although the Apgar score has encouraged us to look more objectively at the neonate, the value of the Apgar score to predict neonatal acidosis and neurologic abnormalities is poor. By itself, a low score indicates neonatal depression. However, the reason for a low score may include inaccurate scoring, prematurity, drug effects, congenital abnormalities, endotracheal intubation, nasopharyngeal suctioning, and/or asphyxia. Another problem with the Apgar score is that only the most severe neonatal depression from excessive or poorly timed maternal medications can be detected at birth using the score.

To better evaluate the more subtle effects of maternally administered drugs, other neurobehavioral tests were developed. Neurobehavioral assessment is not a standard part of the neonatal examination but has been used to assess the neonate's response to its environment and again the effects of maternally administered drugs. The three most popular

■ Table 3–3
APGAR SCORE

Score	0	1	2
Heart rate	Absent	<100	>100
Respiratory effort	Absent	Irregular, shallow	Good, crying
Reflex irritability	No response	Grimace	Cough, sneeze
Muscle tone	Flaccid	Good tone	Spontaneous flexed arms/legs
Color	Blue, pale	Body pink, extremities blue	Entirely pink

neurobehavioral tests for this purpose are Brazelton's Neonatal Behavior Assessment Scale,[13] Scanlon et al.'s Early Neonatal Neurobehavioral Scale[14] (ENNS), and the Neonatal Neurologic and Adaptive Capacity Score of Amiel-Tison et al.[15]

■ **KEY POINT:** The Neurologic and Adaptive Capacity Score (NACS) has become a very popular test of central nervous system depression in the neonate. Although NACS scores are of scientific and academic interest, they are of questionable clinical value.

The neonate's state of consciousness (deep sleep, light sleep, drowsy, alert, active, crying) is probably the most important element of these behavioral examinations, because the neonate's responses to external stimuli depend on his or her state of consciousness. Tests are usually repeated for several days during the neonatal period to make the results more predictive.

A period of 3 to 4 weeks of training is needed to become adequately trained in performing the Brazelton examination. About 45 minutes is required to perform each test. As a result of the amount of training needed and the time required to perform this test, the Brazelton examination is not as widely used today as the other tests discussed below. It is, however, considered a gold standard for neurobehavioral evaluations, particularly in the research setting.

In 1974, Scanlon et al.[14] developed a neurobehavioral examination, ENNS, in an attempt to simplify neurobehavioral testing and to assess the neonatal effects of epidural anesthesia. The main advantages of this examination are that it is simple and rapid to perform (it takes only 5 to 10 minutes) and personnel can be trained to 85% reliability in only 2 to 3 days.

In 1982, Amiel-Tison et al.[15] introduced another neurobehavioral test called the Neonatal Neurologic and Adaptive Capacity Score. This examination takes less time than the ENNS, places greater emphasis on motor tone, and avoids the use of noxious stimuli.

These neurobehavioral assessments were designed to evaluate the neonate in the first few hours to days after delivery. Carefully controlled studies using these neurobehavioral tools identify causes of abnormal behavior in the early neonatal period that can influence the interaction between the caregiver and the infant, thus improving the safety of anesthetic medications and techniques.

REFERENCES

1. Levinson G, Shnider SM, Gildea JE, et al: Maternal and foetal cardiovascular and acid base changes during ketamine anesthesia in pregnant ewes. Br J Anaesth 45:1111, 1973.

2. Marx GF, Hwang HS, Chandra P: Postpartum uterine pressures with different doses of ketamine. Anesthesiology 50:163, 1979.
3. Rekonen A, Luotola H, Pitanen M, et al: Measurement of intervillous and myometrial blood flow by intravenous ^{133}Xe method. Br J Obstet Gynaecol 83:732, 1976.
4. O'Rourke MF: Vascular impedance in studies of arterial and cardiac function. Physiol Rev 62:570, 1982.
5. Cosmi EV: Drugs, anesthetics and the fetus. In: Scarpelli EM, Cosmi EV, eds. Reviews in Perinatal Medicine. Vol. I. Baltimore: University Park Press, 1976:191.
6. Greiss F, Still JG, Anderson SG: Effects of local anesthetic agents on the uterine vasculatures and myometrium. Am J Obstet Gynecol 124:889, 1976.
7. Hollmén AI, Jouppila R, et al: Effect of extradural analgesia using bupivacaine and 2-chloroprocaine on intervillous blood flow during normal labor. Br J Anaesth 54:837, 1982.
8. Jouppila P, Jouppila R, Hollmén AI, et al: Lumbar epidural analgesia to improve intervillous blood flow during labor in severe pre-eclampsia. Obstet Gynecol 59:158, 1982.
9. Hood DD, Dewan DM, James FM III: Maternal and fetal effects of epinephrine in gravid ewes. Anesthesiology 64:610, 1986.
10. Ralston DH, Shnider SM, deLorimer AA: Effect of equipotent ephedrine, metaraminol, mephentermine and methoxamine on uterine blood flow in the pregnant ewe. Anesthesiology 40:354, 1974.
11. Ramanathan S, Grant GJ: Vasopressor therapy for hypotension due to epidural anesthesia for cesarean section. Acta Anesth Scand 32:559, 1988.
12. Apgar V: A proposal for a new method of evaluation of the newborn infant. Anesth Analg 32:260, 1953.
13. Brazelton TB: Neonatal behavioral assessment scale. In: Clinics in Developmental Medicine, No. 50. London: Spastics Int Med Publ., William Heinemann Medical Books, 1973.
14. Scanlon JW, Brown WU Jr, Weiss JB, et al: Neurobehavioral responses of newborn infants after maternal epidural anesthesia. Anesthesiology 40:121, 1974.
15. Amiel-Tison C, Barrier G, Shnider SM, et al: A new neurologic and adaptive capacity scoring system for evaluation of obstetric medications in full term newborns. Anesthesiology 56:340, 1982.

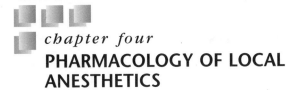

chapter four

PHARMACOLOGY OF LOCAL ANESTHETICS

Esther M. Yun, MD

STRUCTURE

A local anesthetic usually has an aromatic moiety (benzene ring) on one end of the molecule and an amino group on the other separated by an intermediate alkyl chain (Fig. 4–1). The benzene ring is the lipophilic portion that allows the local anesthetic to penetrate lipid membranes, such as those found surrounding nerves. The hydrophilic "tail" is the amino group, usually a tertiary amine, which becomes charged (ionized) in the presence of hydrogen ions. The intermediate alkyl chain connects the two ends with either an ester or an amide linkage. The type of link is important because it determines metabolism and nomenclature.

■ **KEY POINT:** With the exception of cocaine, all local anesthetics contain a desaturated carbon ring and a tertiary amine connected by an intermediate alkyl chain.

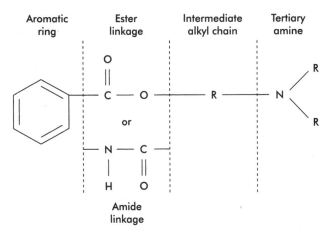

| Aromatic ring | Ester linkage | Intermediate alkyl chain | Tertiary amine |

Figure 4–1 ■ Structure of a local anesthetic molecule. (From Santos A, Pedersen H, Finster M: Local anesthetics. In Chestnut DH (ed): Obstetric Anesthesia Principles and Practice. St. Louis, MO: Mosby, 1994:203.)

COMMON FEATURES

Local anesthetics act as weak bases because their pK_a is greater than 7.4. In their tertiary un-ionized form, local anesthetics are poorly soluble in water but when combined with acids to form hydrochloride salts, they become quite hydrophilic. For that reason, local anesthetics are formulated for clinical use in an acidic solution (pH 4 to 7). However, at a lower pH, the molecule is more highly ionized. Both the ionized and non-ionized moieties are necessary for action. The non-ionized tertiary amine is the lipid-soluble moiety that penetrates the axonal membrane, whereas the ionized cation is the hydrophilic form necessary for binding to the sodium channel receptors.

MECHANISM OF ACTION

Resting Neuron

At rest, the neuronal membrane is relatively impermeable to sodium (Na^+) but highly permeable to potassium (K^+). The net result is that the extracellular concentration of sodium is large, whereas the intracellular concentration of potassium is large. At rest, this ionic gradient across the membrane is maintained by the sodium–potassium ATPase-dependent pump. The resting membrane potential is approximately -90 mV.

Excitation/Depolarization

During neuronal excitation, membrane sodium channels open, allowing sodium ions to enter into the cell and thus resulting in depolarization. The threshold level for depolarization is approximately -60 mV, at which point there is a sharp influx of sodium ions into the cell and propagation of the action potential at adjacent sites.

After depolarization, sodium channels close, making the membrane no longer permeable to sodium, and potassium channels open, resulting in an efflux of K^+ from the cell. At this point, sodium is actively transported extracellularly by the ATPase-dependent pump, whereas potassium ions move back into the cell along their concentration gradient. In this way, the initial concentrations of sodium and potassium are restored and the resting membrane potential is reestablished.

Mechanism of Local Anesthetics

Local anesthetics produce reversible inhibition of nerve conduction by interfering with sodium channel function and preventing the intracellular flow of sodium during excitation. Specific membrane receptors may be affected by different local anesthetics. The most commonly used clinical agents bind the sodium channel receptor on the inner surface of the nerve membrane. In contrast, biotoxins with local anesthetic activity, such as tetrodotoxin, act on the external surface of the nerve membrane. Other highly lipid-soluble local anesthetics, such as benzocaine, block sodium channels by penetration and physical expansion of the cell membrane, which mechanically interferes with the ability of the sodium channel to open.

Regardless of the site of action, local anesthetic inhibition of sodium ion influx into the neuronal cell slows the rate of depolarization, and the threshold for the action potential is not achieved. It is important to note that local anesthetics do not affect either the resting membrane or the threshold potentials.

■ **KEY POINT:** Interference with sodium ion conductance is considered to be the mechanism by which local anesthetics inhibit action potential propagation.

PHYSICOCHEMICAL PROPERTIES

Potency

Generally speaking, the degree of lipid solubility directly correlates with anesthetic potency[1] (Figs. 4-2 and 4-3). Agents with high lipid solubility, such as bupivacaine and etidocaine, are highly potent anesthetics and produce conduction blockade at lower concentrations than less lipid-soluble agents, such as lidocaine and mepivacaine.

Speed of Onset

The pK_a of a local anesthetic may determine the speed with which conduction block develops[1] (Figs. 4-2 and 4-4). The pK_a of a drug is that pH at which the concentration of the ionized and un-ionized forms are equal. The onset of action is directly related to the amount of drug in the non-ionized lipid-soluble form and inversely related to the local anesthetic's pK_a. Stated in a different way, drugs with a pK_a close to physiologic pH have a faster onset of action than drugs with a higher pK_a. For example, lidocaine (pK_a 7.74) has a faster onset of action than bupivacaine (pK_a 8.1) because the non-ionized form of lidocaine is 35% compared with 15% for bupivacaine at physiologic pH.

■ **KEY POINT:** The Henderson-Hasselbalch equation predicts the relative proportions of local anesthetic that exist in the ionized versus un-ionized form. The higher the pK_a relative to physiologic pH, the smaller the proportion in an un-ionized form.

Agent	Chemical configuration			Physicochemical properties			Pharmacologic properties		
	Aromatic lipophilic	Intermediate chain	Amine hydrophilic	Molecular weight (base)	pKₐ (36°C)	Octonal/buffer partition coefficient (25°C)	Onset	Relative potency	Duration
Esters									
Procaine		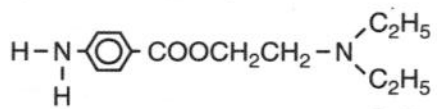		236	8.9	81	Slow	1	Short
Chloroprocaine		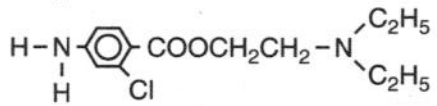		271	9.1	720	Fast	1	Short
Tetracaine		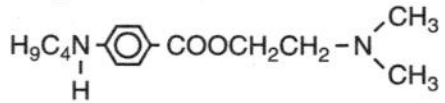		264	8.4	3615	Slow	8	Long
Amides									
Mepivacaine		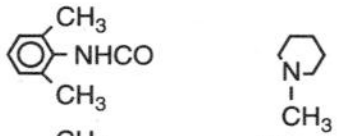		246	7.7	90	Fast	2	Moderate
Prilocaine		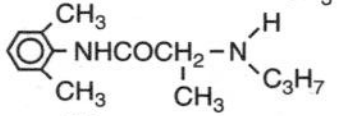		220	7.8	129	Fast	2	Moderate
Lidocaine		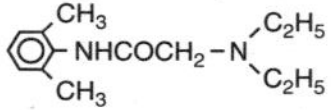		234	7.8	30	Fast	2	Moderate
Ropivacaine		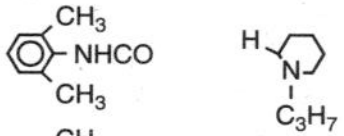		274	8.1	775	Moderate	8	Long
Bupivacaine		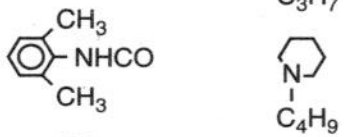		288	8.1	2565	Moderate	8	Long
Etidocaine		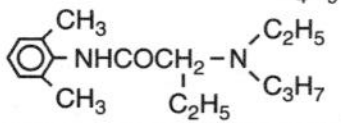		276	7.9	4900	Fast	6	Long

Figure 4–2 ■ Physicochemical and pharmacologic properties of local anesthetic agents. (From Covino B: Clinical pharmacology of local anesthetic agents. In Cousins MJ, Bridenbaugh PO (eds): Neural Blockade. Philadelphia: J.B. Lippincott, 1988:1236.)

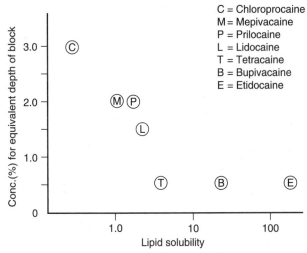

Figure 4–3 ■ Relationship between lipid solubility and potency of local anesthetic agents. (From Covino B: Clinical pharmacology of local anesthetic agents. In Cousins MJ, Bridenbaugh PO (eds): Neural Blockade. Philadelphia: J.B. Lippincott, 1988:114.)

Duration of Action

The degree of protein binding may affect the duration of action[1] (see Figs. 4-2 and 4-4). Agents with greater affinity for proteins remain at the receptor site for longer periods, thus producing a greater duration of block. Procaine, which

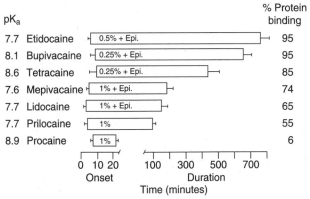

Figure 4–4 ■ Relationship between pK_a and onset of anesthesia *(left)* and between protein binding and duration of anesthesia *(right)*. (From Covino B: Clinical pharmacology of local anesthetic agents. In Cousins MJ, Bridenbaugh PO (eds): Neural Blockade. Philadelphia: J.B. Lippincott, 1988:115.)

exhibits low protein binding, has a short duration of action, whereas bupivacaine, a highly protein-bound drug, has a long duration of action. Indeed, a brachial plexus block using procaine results in 30 to 60 minutes of anesthesia, compared with bupivacaine, which can last for approximately 10 hours.[2]

FACTORS AFFECTING BLOCKADE

Vasoconstrictor Properties of Local Anesthetics

The degree of intrinsic vasodilation can also affect the duration of action. Drugs that are potent vasodilators are absorbed from the injection site to a greater degree than less-potent dilators. With the exception of cocaine and the new single levorotary formulations of amides, all local anesthetics are vasodilators at the concentrations used in clinical practice.[3] This results in local anesthetic diffusion away from the receptor site, thus decreasing the duration of block.

The addition of a vasoconstrictor, such as epinephrine or phenylephrine, to a local anesthetic may increase the depth and duration of block by decreasing the rate of vascular absorption from the injection site. It may also reduce the risk of systemic toxicity by decreasing vascular absorption and the resultant peak plasma level of drug. Epinephrine 1:200,000 (5 μg/mL) is most frequently used as an adjuvant for this purpose.

The effects of the addition of epinephrine vary with the individual local anesthetic used and its site of injection. For example, epinephrine prolongs the duration of action of lidocaine, mepivacaine, and procaine in all types of blocks,[4-6] whereas it only prolongs the duration of action of bupivacaine when used for infiltration and peripheral nerve blocks but not for epidural blockade.[6] The apparent differences in the effects of epinephrine may be related to the high lipophilic property of bupivacaine that results in high absorption into epidural fat.

Sodium Bicarbonate

The addition of sodium bicarbonate to most local anesthetics immediately before their use hastens the onset of block. Alkalization of local anesthetic solutions increases the pH of the solution that in turn increases the concentration of the nonionized drug and facilitates penetration of cell membranes. For every 10 mL of 2-chloroprocaine, lidocaine, and bupivacaine, bicarbonate at doses of 1, 0.7, and 0.1 mEq, respectively, may be added.

The effect of bicarbonate on latency may be even more pronounced with commercially prepared local anesthetic solutions containing epinephrine because these are formulated to be more acidic than plain solutions for the stability of epinephrine.

■ **KEY POINT:** Alkalinization of a local anesthetic solution shortens the latency of neural blockade.

Dosage

The concentration of local anesthetic used can also affect the depth of the block. An increase in the total dose of drug can result from increasing the volume and/or concentration. In general, increasing the concentration but keeping the volume constant speeds the onset, increases the depth, and prolongs the duration of block.[1] On the other hand, the volume of anesthetic solution injected affects the spread of block and level of anesthesia.

Site of Injection

The onset and duration of block also depend on the site of injection. For example, the onset of a spinal block is much faster than that of an epidural block because the spinal nerves lack a dural layer. The vascularity of the anatomic site may also affect the duration of action. For instance, a brachial plexus block lasts longer than a paracervical block, in part because of a lower rate of vascular absorption.

Local Anesthetic Mixtures

The use of a local anesthetic with a fast onset of action in conjunction with one that has a long duration of action may be of benefit. However, the effects of such mixtures are inconsistent. A combination of chloroprocaine and bupivacaine for brachial plexus block has been reported to produce a faster onset of action than bupivacaine alone and longer duration of action than chloroprocaine.[7] Unfortunately, when given by epidural injection, the duration of action of such a mixture was shorter than when only bupivacaine was administered.[8] Because of the availability of various local anesthetics for clinical use and the availability of adjuvants such as bicarbonate and epinephrine, which may shorten latency and prolong the block, anesthetic mixtures are not often used.

METABOLISM

Ester-linked local anesthetics are inactivated by plasma cholinesterase. Chloroprocaine is hydrolyzed approximately four times faster than tetracaine by pseudocholinesterase. The in vitro half-life of chloroprocaine has been reported to be only

21 seconds in plasma for adults and 43 seconds in plasma for newborns.[9] It is therefore one of the safest local anesthetics for clinical use. However, the half-life of an ester-linked local anesthetic may be prolonged in patients having atypical pseudocholinesterase, thus risking toxicity. Paraminobenzoic acid, a byproduct of ester metabolism, has been implicated in hypersensitivity reactions.[8]

The metabolism of amide-linked local anesthetics is more complex. The local anesthetic must first be absorbed into the circulation from the injection site and then transported to the liver where it is degraded enzymatically. Both hepatic blood flow and drug extraction may affect the metabolism of amide-linked local anesthetics. Therefore, factors that decrease hepatic blood flow (e.g., general anesthesia, propranolol, cimetidine) and hepatic drug extraction (e.g., congestive heart failure, cirrhosis) may reduce the metabolism of amide-linked local anesthetics.

SYSTEMIC TOXICITY

Direct adverse effects of local anesthetics are most often related to high plasma levels of drug. Some factors affecting the plasma level of drug have already been discussed.

> ■ **KEY POINT:** True allergy to a local anesthetic is very rare. If it occurs, it is most often a response to ester agents in patients who are allergic to PABA.

Site of Injection

Plasma level may depend, in part, on the site of injection. Generally speaking, the greater the vascularity of the injection site, the greater the absorption of drug. The highest plasma levels of local anesthetics are observed with intercostal and intrapleural blocks, both very vascular areas, followed by paracervical, caudal, epidural, brachial plexus, and finally subarachnoid block.

Central Nervous System Toxicity

The initial signs and symptoms of central nervous system (CNS) toxicity are due to CNS excitation and are manifested by perioral numbness, lightheadedness, diplopia, tinnitus, muscular twitching, tremors, and, with increasing plasma levels, generalized convulsions (Fig. 4–5). Convulsions are due to a selective inhibition of cortical pathways resulting in unopposed activity of brainstem facilitatory neurons.

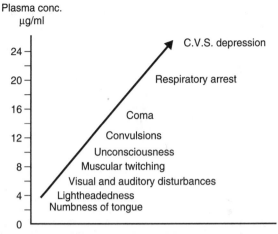

Plasma conc.
µg/ml

Figure 4–5 ■ Relationship of signs and symptoms of local anesthetic toxicity to plasma concentrations of lidocaine. CVS, cardiovascular system. (From Covino B: Clinical pharmacology of local anesthetic agents. In Cousins MJ, Bridenbaugh PO (eds): Neural Blockade. Philadelphia: J.B. Lippincott, 1988:122.)

■ **KEY POINT:** Pregnancy does not reduce the seizure threshold for amide local anesthetics.

With further increases in plasma level, CNS depression may occur due to inhibition of both inhibitory and facilitatory pathways. Clinical manifestations at this point may include the cessation of seizure activity, progressing to coma and, finally, cardiorespiratory arrest.

Treatment of seizures includes protection of the airway and ensuring adequate oxygenation and ventilation. Avoiding marked hypercarbia is important because it can further lower the convulsant threshold. Seizures may be terminated with the administration of small doses of thiopental (50–100 mg) or diazepam (5–10 mg) by intravenous injection.

Cardiovascular Toxicity

Increasing plasma levels of local anesthetics may increase the PR and QRS intervals. At even higher concentrations, spontaneous electrical activity is decreased, resulting in sinus bradycardia, atrioventricular conduction block, and even sinus arrest. Myocardial depression may also occur.

Long-acting potent local anesthetics, such as bupivacaine and etidocaine, are considered to be more cardiotoxic than less-potent agents, such as lidocaine and mepivacaine. Several cases of cardiac arrest, with patients often refractory to resuscitation, have been reported after unintended intravenous injection of bupivacaine and etidocaine.[10] Bupivacaine is different from other local anesthetics in this regard because bupivacaine rapidly blocks Na^+ channels during systole but dissociates from Na^+ channels at a much slower rate during diastole than, for instance, lidocaine. Studies examining whether pregnancy itself enhances the cardiotoxicity of bupivacaine have been conflicting.[11, 12] Nonetheless, the use of bupivacaine 0.75% for epidural anesthesia in pregnant women has been proscribed by the U.S. Food and Drug Administration.

■ **K E Y   P O I N T :**   Laboratory studies evaluating the effects of pregnancy on bupivacaine toxicity have been contradictory. The most recent study on sheep, however, which involved more rigorous methods and a larger number of sheep, reported that pregnancy did not enhance the cardiotoxicity of bupivacaine.

OBSTETRIC USE OF LOCAL ANESTHETICS

Lower Drug Requirement

Pregnant women as early as in the first trimester require less local anesthetic to achieve an effect as compared with nonpregnant women.[13] This is most likely due to progesterone-related increases in the sensitivity of nerve fibers to local anesthetics.[14] In the latter part of pregnancy, further decreases in drug requirement may be related to decreased cerebrospinal fluid volume and engorgement of the epidural veins.

Placental Transfer

Local anesthetics cross the placenta readily. The amount of placental transfer is determined by the degree of ionization, lipid solubility, protein binding, molecular size of the local anesthetic, and the blood concentration gradient of drug between the mother and fetus.

Ion Trapping

Fetal acidosis may cause accumulation of local anesthetic in the fetus. A lower fetal pH relative to the mothers may result in greater ionized levels of drug to become trapped in the fetus. Ion trapping is of least concern with chloroprocaine because it is rapidly metabolized by the fetus.

Local Anesthetics for Obstetric Use

Lidocaine

Lidocaine has had a long history of safe and flexible use in obstetrics. It has a relatively fast onset of action with intermediate duration of action. Because of its profound motor-blocking capability, it is generally no longer used for labor epidural analgesia but provides excellent surgical block for cesarean delivery. Bicarbonate, epinephrine, and opioids are often used as adjuvants with lidocaine.

Recently, there has been concern over the use of 5% hyperbaric lidocaine for spinal injection because of reports of transient neurologic symptoms involving the lower back and extremities.[15] Although lidocaine's concentration, osmolarity, and its additives, such as dextrose and epinephrine, have been implicated as a possible cause of neurologic dysfunction, the exact mechanism remains unknown. Diluting hyperbaric lidocaine with equal volumes of cerebrospinal fluid and fast injection of lidocaine intrathecally have been suggested to decrease pooling in the caudad areas.

Chloroprocaine

Chloroprocaine is an ester-linked agent with low potency, rapid onset, and short duration of action. It is one of the safest agents for obstetric use because of its rapid metabolism (half-life < 45 seconds). Because of its rapid onset of action, it is also an excellent choice for use in emergency cesarean delivery when there is a preexisting epidural catheter in place.

In the past, there have been reports of arachnoiditis associated with inadvertent intrathecal administration of large volumes of chloroprocaine. This was due to a combination of sodium bisulfite (antioxidant) and a low pH in the formulation of 2-chloroprocaine used at the time. In a new formulation, disodium ethylenediamine-tetraacetic acid (EDTA) replaced sodium bisulfite as a preservative; however, this has been associated with back pain and muscle spasm probably due to EDTA binding of calcium and hypocalcemic tetany of the paraspinous muscles. The latest formulation of chloroprocaine contains no preservatives, and spontaneous hydrolysis of the drug is prevented by packaging in colored bottles.

Bupivacaine

Despite its narrow margin of safety, bupivacaine has become popular for use in obstetric anesthesia. It has a longer duration of action than other amide local anesthetics and thus requires less frequent administration. At the low concentrations used for epidural analgesia during labor, bupivacaine produces a motor-sparing block.

New Amide Local Anesthetics

Concern over the cardiotoxicity of bupivacaine has led to a search for new amide local anesthetics with blocking properties similar to bupivacaine but with a wider margin of safety.

Most amide local anesthetics are known as chiral compounds because they can exist as mirror images of each other.

The isomers are named according to the direction in which the compound rotates polarized light: dextrorotatory rotates light to the right (+ or rectus) and levorotary rotates to the left (− or sinister). Different isomers of the same compound can have different biologic activity. In general, the levo isomers have greater vasoconstrictor activity but are less toxic and have a longer duration of action than the dextro forms of the drug.[16] Although the clinical formulations of local anesthetics in clinical use contain a racemic mixture of both the S and R forms of the drug, recent technologic advances have led to the formulation of single S isomer preparations of drug.

Ropivacaine

Ropivacaine is a homologue of mepivacaine and bupivacaine. It was the first single S isomer formulation of local anesthetic (99.5% levo isomer) to be developed for clinical use. Ropivacaine's physicochemical characteristics are intermediate between those of mepivacaine and bupivacaine. However, it is considerably less lipid soluble than bupivacaine and thus less potent. Nevertheless, the available clinical evidence suggests that ropivacaine is similar to bupivacaine with respect to its blocking properties. Pregnancy does not enhance the systemic toxicity of ropivacaine.[12] The use of ropivacaine for labor epidural analgesia results in a block that is virtually indistinguishable from that of bupivacaine.[17] However, the intensity and duration of motor blockade is shorter with ropivacaine than with bupivacaine for epidural anesthesia for cesarean delivery.[18] Neonatal condition and mode of delivery are also similar with both drugs.

Levobupivacaine

Levobupivacaine, the other drug currently being investigated for clinical use, is the single levo isomer of bupivacaine. Levobupivacaine appears to be closer in potency to bupivacaine than is ropivacaine.

Systemic toxicity is less with levobupivacaine than with the racemate. The convulsant dose range for levobupivacaine was greater than for racemic bupivacaine in human volunteers.[19] Levobupivacaine has been shown to be less arrhythmogenic than the dextro or racemic forms of the drug.[20] Although limited data are available, levobupivacaine appears to be a promising drug for use in obstetrics.

■ **KEY POINT:** Single levorotary isomer formulations of amide local anesthetics have a lower potential for cardiotoxicity than does racemic bupivacaine.

REFERENCES

1. Covino BG: Pharmacology of local anaesthetic agents. Br J Anaesth 58:701–716, 1986.
2. Scott DB, Cousins MT: Clinical pharmacology of local anesthetic agents. In: Cousins MJ, Bridenbaugh PO, eds. Neural Blockade. Philadelphia: J.B. Lippincott, 1980:80.
3. Blair MR: Cardiovascular pharmacology of local anesthetics. Br J Anaesth 47:247–252, 1975.
4. Albert J, Lofstrom B: Bilateral ulnar nerve block for the evaluation of local anaesthetic agents. Tests with a new agent, prilocaine and lidocaine in solutions with and without epinephrine. Acta Anaesthesiol Scand 9:203–211, 1965.
5. Swerdlow M, Jones R: The duration of action of bupivacaine, prilocaine, and lignocaine. Br J Anaesth 42:335–339, 1970.
6. Keir L: Continuous epidural analgesia in prostatectomy: comparison of bupivacaine with and without adrenaline. Acta Anaesthesiol Scand 18:1–4, 1974.
7. Cunningham NL, Kaplan JA: A rapid onset long acting regional anesthetic technique. Anesthesiology 41:509–511, 1974.
8. Cohen SE, Thurlow A: Comparison of a chloroprocaine–bupivacaine mixture with chloroprocaine and bupivacaine used individually for obstetric epidural analgesia. Anesthesiology 51:288–292, 1979.
9. O'Brien JE, Abbey V, Hinsvark O, et al: Metabolism and measurement of 2-chloroprocaine, an ester-type anesthetic. J Pharmacol Sci 68:75–78, 1979.
10. Albright GA: Cardiac arrest following regional anesthesia with etidocaine or bupivacaine. Anesthesiology 51:285–287, 1979.
11. Morishima HO, Pederson H, Finster M: Bupivacaine toxicity in pregnant and nonpregnant ewes. Anesthesiology 63:134–139, 1985.
12. Santos AC, Arthur GR, Wlody D: Comparative systemic toxicity of ropivacaine and bupivacaine in nonpregnant and pregnant ewes. Anesthesiology 82:734–740, 1995.
13. Fagraeus L, Urban BJ, Bromage PR: Spread of epidural analgesia in early pregnancy. Anesthesiology 58:184–187, 1983.
14. Datta S, Lambert DH, Gregus J: Differential sensitivities of mammalian nerve fibers during pregnancy. Anesth Analg 62:1070–1072, 1983.
15. Schneider M, Ettlin T, Kauffmann M, et al: Transient neurologic toxicity after hyperbaric subarachnoid anesthesia with 5% lidocaine. Anesth Analg 76:1154–1157, 1993.
16. Aps C, Reynolds F: An intradermal study of the local anaesthetic and vascular effects of the isomers of bupivacaine. Br J Clin Pharmacol 6:63–68, 1978.
17. Stienstra R, Tonker TV, Bourdez P: Ropivacaine 0.25% versus bupivacaine 0.25% for continuous epidural analgesia in labor: a double-blind comparison. Anesth Analg 80:285–289, 1995.
18. Datta S, Camann W, Bader A, et al: Clinical effects on maternal and fetal plasma concentrations of epidural ropivacaine versus bupivacaine for cesarean section. Anesthesiology 82:1346–1352, 1995.
19. Mather LM, Huang YF, Veering BT, et al: Cardiovascular and central nervous system toxicity of bupivacaine and levobupivacaine in sheep. Presented at Symposium on Levobupivacaine, World Congress of Anaesthesiologists, Sydney, 1996.
20. Graf BM, Martin E, Bosnjak ZJ, et al: Stereospecific effect of bupivacaine isomers on atrioventricular conduction in the isolated perfused guinea pig heart. Anesthesiology 86:410–419, 1997.

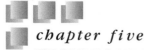

chapter five

TECHNIQUES OF NEURAXIAL ANALGESIA FOR LABOR

Kathleen Leavitt, MD, and David J. Birnbach, MD

PAIN PATHWAYS DURING PARTURITION

During the first stage of labor, the pain of uterine contractions together with cervical dilation and effacement is transmitted by afferent fibers that enter the spinal cord through the posterior roots of the T-11 and T-12 nerves and some fibers from the T-10 and L-1 nerves. During the second stage of labor, pain resulting from distention of the birth canal, vulva, and perineum is conveyed by afferent fibers of the posterior roots of the S2–4 nerves. These pathways must be blocked to achieve satisfactory analgesia during labor and vaginal delivery (Fig. 5–1).[1]

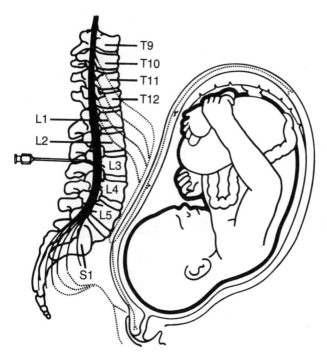

Figure 5–1 ■ Pain pathways during parturition.

LUMBAR EPIDURAL ANALGESIA

Indications

Lumbar epidural analgesia extending from the level of T-10 through S-5 provides effective pain relief during labor and vaginal delivery. Usually, an epidural catheter is placed and medication is injected intermittently or by continuous infusion so that analgesia can be extended throughout labor and into the postdelivery period or for a cesarean section, should that eventuality arise.

Segmental epidural analgesia makes it possible to individualize the epidural block according to the stage of labor by adjusting the volume and concentration of local anesthetic administered. For the first stage of labor, a dilute concentration of local anesthetic (often combined with an opioid) is used to extend the block to the lower three thoracic and the upper lumbar segments (Fig. 5-2). This helps preserve motor function in the lower extremities and muscle tone to the pelvic floor, the latter of which is thought to be important for proper rotation and descent of the fetal presenting part. Most importantly, segmental epidural blockade spares the sacral fibers, leaving the urge to bear down (Ferguson's reflex) intact as the parturient progresses to the second stage of labor.

During the second stage of labor, the block can be extended into the lower sacral nerve roots by using a larger volume of a more concentrated local anesthetic solution (Fig. 5-3). This may, however, produce motor blockade to the lower extremities and perineal relaxation. Although this perineal anesthesia may be disadvantageous, it becomes necessary

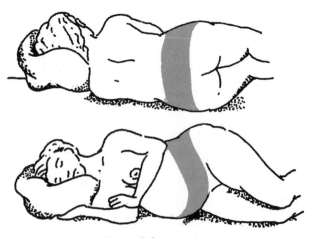

Figure 5–2 ■ First stage.

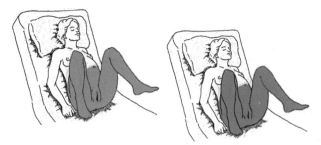

Figure 5–3 ■ Early second stage and late second stage.

if vacuum or forceps delivery is attempted. Because it may be difficult to provide dense anesthesia to the perineum with an epidural catheter inserted in the lumbar region, it is sometimes necessary for the obstetrician to supplement the epidural blockade at the time of delivery by injecting local anesthetic directly into the perineum or, rarely, by performing a pudendal block.

> ■ **KEY POINT:** Neuraxial analgesia is the most effective and least depressant form of intrapartum analgesia available today.

Because of the versatility of lumbar epidural analgesia in terms of extent of blockade and duration of effect, it is particularly beneficial for parturients with a high risk of cesarean section or with any of the following:

- Prolonged labor;
- Cervical dystocia;
- Oxytocin augmentation of labor;
- Vaginal birth after cesarean (VBAC)
- Pregnancy complicated by maternal disease (preeclampsia, diabetes, or cardiovascular or pulmonary disease).

Please refer to Chapter 14 for a complete description of these situations.

Contraindications

Although there are numerous "relative contraindications" to regional anesthesia in the parturient, each case must be determined individually, assessing the risks and benefits of regional anesthesia and comparing these with the risks and benefits of alternative techniques of analgesia or anesthesia. There are very few "absolute" contraindications to regional anesthesia in the hands of an experienced anesthesiologist, except

- Infection over the site of needle puncture;
- Blood coagulopathies;
- Hypovolemic shock;
- Patient refusal.

Patient Preparation

If possible, a brief history and physical examination should be performed by the anesthesiologist on *all* patients admitted to the labor and delivery ward, with emphasis on airway examination, medication allergies, body habitus, prior history of anesthetic complications (difficult intubation, malignant hyperthermia susceptibility), presence of scoliosis or prior back surgery with instrumentation, and last oral intake.

An early attempt should be made to identify in each patient the risk factors that may predispose her to emergency cesarean delivery (i.e., severe preeclampsia, intrauterine growth retardation, VBAC, etc.). In an effort to decrease the need for general anesthesia and the increased morbidity associated with it,[2] any patient considered at high risk for operative delivery should be counseled about the benefits of epidural placement.

■ **KEY POINT:** Any parturient may require an emergency cesarean section. The early examination of all parturients allows better planning for the parturient with problems that might have an impact on the anesthetic.

All patients receiving a neuraxial block must first have an intravenous catheter inserted. They should all receive prehydration using a nonglucose-containing balanced salt solution.[3] The volume of prehydration becomes more important if more dense local anesthetics that produce sympathetic blockade are used. All parturients should receive a nonparticulate antacid such as 30 mL of 0.3 mol/L sodium citrate[4] before initiation of any neuraxial block.

The parturient receiving neuraxial analgesia should be monitored with an automatic blood pressure cuff (NIBP) applied to the upper extremity. Baseline maternal blood pressure and heart rate should be monitored and recorded frequently (every 2 to 5 minutes) for a minimum of 20 minutes after administration of local anesthetic/narcotic medications. It has also been suggested that maternal heart rate is monitored using a pulse oxymeter when epinephrine-containing test doses are used.

Before placement of a regional anesthetic, the fetal heart

rate tracing should be reviewed and discussed with the obstetricians if abnormalities are present. According to American College of Obstetricians and Gynecologists guidelines, continuous fetal heart rate monitoring during placement of a regional anesthetic is not mandatory in the absence of an underlying abnormality. Although internal monitoring will allow continued observation regardless of patient position during placement of the block, external monitoring is not always possible when the parturient is in the sitting position. However, even with external fetal heart rate monitoring, it is often possible to continue fetal heart rate monitoring if the monitor is held in place by hand. If continuous fetal heart rate monitoring is abandoned during the initiation of a neuraxial blockade, it is important to recheck the fetal heart rate periodically if epidural placement is prolonged.

Figure 5–4 illustrates proper patient positioning. The sitting position is advantageous when performing a combined spinal-epidural technique, in obese patients with poorly defined landmarks, and in patients with scoliosis. Position the patient on a flat surface and consider supporting her feet on a stool to minimize lumbar lordosis. The patient should be leaning slightly forward with her shoulders slouched and her chin resting on her chest. A nurse or assistant should steady the patient from the front to prevent the patient from falling should neurogenic syncope occur. Although placement of the epidural is often easier with the patient in the sitting position, the lateral decubitus position offers several advantages: a reduction in the risk of syncope, the ability to continue external fetal monitoring, and patient comfort. Occasionally, the lateral position will be required if the patient suffers severe discomfort or exhibits fetal heart rate abnormalities in the sitting position. The patient's back should be placed as close to the edge of the bed as possible with her knees drawn close to her chest. Flex the neck so that the chin almost touches the chest. Ask the patient to tilt her pelvis forward or "push out" her back in the lumbar area to open the vertebral interspaces.

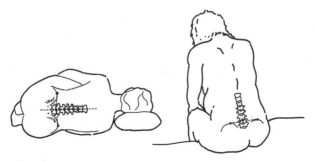

Figure 5–4 ■ The right lateral and sitting positions for epidural block.

Materials

Full cardiopulmonary resuscitative equipment must be immediately available, as is customary for any regional block. A disposable epidural anesthetic tray should contain the items listed in Table 5-1. In addition, proper attire, including a hat, face mask, and sterile gloves, must be worn by the anesthesiologist performing the block. Antiseptic solution (such as povidone iodine) should be available to disinfect the skin. Sterile adhesive dressings and tape should be accessible to secure the epidural catheter.

Anatomy and Landmarks

The spinal cord in the adult usually ends at L-1 and rarely extends below the vertebral body of L-2; however, it may end at L-3 or lower (Fig. 5-5).[5] The dural sac, however, usually ends at the level of S1-2. Surrounding the dural sac, delineated by the dura mater on one side and the periosteum of the vertebral bodies and the ligamentum flavum on the other, is the epidural space. It extends from the foramen magnum superiorly to the sacral hiatus caudally. Therefore, in theory, epidural anesthesia may be administered at any level between C-1 and S-5. The L2-5 interspaces are usually chosen for obstetric epidural blockade.

The anatomic landmarks for epidural anesthesia are the same as for subarachnoid anesthesia: An imaginary line drawn between the right and left iliac crests crosses either the spinous process of the L-4 vertebra or the L4-5 vertebral interspace (Fig. 5-6). The selected vertebral interspace for the epidural block can be pinpointed by locating this interspace and then palpating the desired interspace in the cephalad

■ Table 5–1
MATERIALS INCLUDED IN A DISPOSABLE EPIDURAL ANESTHETIC TRAY

- Perforated sterile drape (clear plastic is preferable)
- Sterile gauze pads
- One 25-gauge ⅝-inch needle for skin infiltration
- One 22-gauge 1½-inch needle for deep infiltration
- One 18-gauge needle (to draw up medications or create an opening in the skin)
- One 17- to 19-gauge epidural needle with stylet
- One 3-mL syringe
- One 5-mL syringe (glass is preferable to other materials)
- One 20-mL syringe
- One polyamide epidural catheter with connector

Optional materials

- Local anesthetic for skin infiltration (lidocaine HCl 1%)
- Preservative-free sodium chloride (0.9%)
- Epinephrine-containing solution

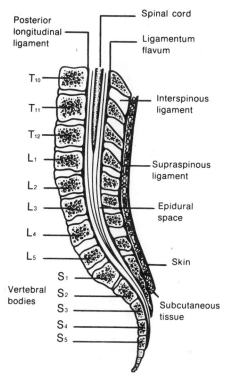

Figure 5–5 ■ The vertebral column.

direction. For lumbar epidural analgesia, the L2-3, L3-4, or L4-5 interspaces are most commonly used. Many anesthesiologists find the L2-4 interspaces to be the most suitable because of diminished lordosis at this level.

Technique

Table 5-2 summarizes the technique of continuous lumbar epidural placement.

Identify the Midline of the Back

Open the epidural tray and check the expiration date of any medications to be used. Prepare the skin of the back with a disinfectant such as povidone iodine, used as per manufacturer's suggestions. The epidural should be performed in a sterile manner, using a face mask and gloves. After waiting for the disinfectant to dry, excess solution should be removed with sterile gauze or towel. Locate the desired interspace by palpating the *spinous process* with the second and third fingers of the nondominant hand. These fingers are used to

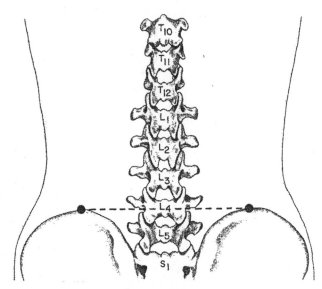

Figure 5–6 ■ The lumbar area. A line drawn between the right and left iliac crests crosses either the spinous process of the L-4 vertebra or the L4-5 vertebral interspace.

produce two-point tactile discrimination, giving a better indication of the midline. Many anesthesiologists choose to leave these fingers on the spinous process to identify the midline until the epidural needle has been inserted into the interspinous ligament.

■ Table 5–2
TECHNIQUE FOR EPIDURAL CATHETER PLACEMENT

1. Identify the midline of the back.
2. Anesthetize the skin.
3. Insert the epidural needle into the interspinous ligament.
4. Locate the epidural space by
   Intermittent loss-of-resistance technique;
   Continuous loss-of-resistance technique;
   Confirmatory tests.
5. Aspirate through the epidural needle.
6. Thread an epidural catheter and remove the needle.
7. Aspirate through the epidural catheter.
8. Administer intrathecal and intravascular test dose through the catheter.
9. Secure the catheter.
10. Initiate the block with fractionated doses of local anesthetic/opioid.
11. Maintain the block with a continuous infusion of local anesthetic/ opioid.

Anesthetize the Skin

Perform an intradermal injection of local anesthetic in the midline toward the inferior border of the interspace. Xylocaine 1% is often used for this purpose. Some anesthesiologists inject an additional 1 to 2 mL of local anesthetic into the subcutaneous tissue and interspinous ligament with a longer needle, but unless the patient is obese or a difficult needle placement is anticipated, this practice may be unnecessary because the skin is usually the only structure contacted by the epidural needle that carries pain fibers. Although some anesthesiologists inject local anesthetic into the paramedian area, this practice causes needless discomfort to the patient and should only be performed when it is unclear where the midline of the back is located or if a paramedian approach is expected. The insertion of an 18-gauge needle through the local anesthetic skin wheal to prevent tissue plugging of the epidural needle is also unnecessary, because a well-fitted stylet will prevent coring of the skin.

Insert the Epidural Needle Into the Interspinous Ligament

Figure 5–7 illustrates the hand position used at the Brigham and Women's Hospital and favored by the late Gerard W. Ostheimer, MD, for the initial insertion of the epidural needle.

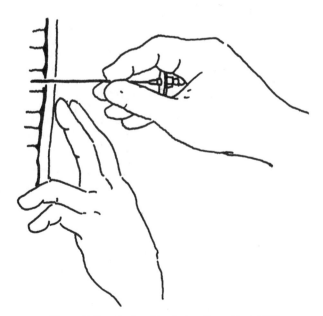

Figure 5–7 ■ Hand position for inserting epidural needle.

Cradle the hub of the needle in the palm of the hand and wrap the thumb, index, and middle finger around the needle bore. While the nondominant hand palpates the spinous process, firmly insert the epidural needle through the skin wheal at the inferior border of the interspace and angle the needle slightly cephalad. Although most anesthesiologists insert the epidural needle perpendicular to the spinal axis, a few authors still suggest inserting the epidural needle with the bevel directed parallel to the spinal axis so that if unintentional dural puncture occurs, the severity of postdural puncture headache will be decreased. Recent studies, however, document higher rates of accidental dural puncture with this method, due to dural puncture at the time that the epidural needle is rotated within the epidural space to allow appropriate threading of the catheter. Most anesthesiologists insert the epidural needle with the bevel directed cephalad to avoid the need for rotation once the epidural space is located.

The depth of the epidural space from the skin varies considerably from patient to patient.[6] Figure 5–5 illustrates the tissue layers and ligaments encountered as the needle is advanced 1.2 to 3.7 cm (sometimes deeper), to a point where the tissue resistance of the interspinous ligament is felt. The needle should feel firmly engaged, located perfectly midline, and directed slightly cephalad.

Locate the Epidural Space

Once the epidural needle is firmly engaged in the interspinous ligament, remove the stylet and attach a syringe filled with either air or saline. There are two loss of resistance methods currently used to identify the epidural space: the intermittent loss-of-resistance technique and the continuous loss-of-resistance technique.

Intermittent Loss-of-Resistance Technique. This technique is usually performed using the winged (Weiss modification) Touhy needle. Proper hand position is shown in Figure 5–8. Grasp the wings with the thumb and index finger of both hands. Place both middle fingers on the shaft of the

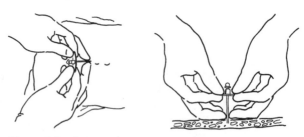

Figure 5–8 ■ Hand position for intermittent loss-of-resistance technique.

needle close to the insertion site at the skin. Rest the volar surfaces of the ring and little fingers of both hands against the patient's back. Attach a glass syringe with 2 to 3 mL of air or saline and advance the needle slowly, intermittently checking resistance on the plunger. Increased resistance on the plunger will be encountered when the needle is located within the ligamentum flavum, and a sudden loss of resistance indicates the needle tip has entered the epidural space. Minimal force exerted on the plunger will allow the air contained within the syringe to be expelled into the epidural space. No more than 0.5 to 1.0 mL of air should spontaneously move back into the syringe after it is injected into the epidural space.

Continuous Loss-of-Resistance Technique. Attach a saline-filled syringe to the epidural needle. A right-handed anesthesiologist holds the epidural needle firmly between the index finger and the thumb of the left hand, as illustrated in Figure 5–9. Rest the volar surface of the left hand firmly against the patient's back. This steadies the left hand so that it has fine control over the advancement of the needle. The right hand controls the syringe. Place the body of the syringe between the right index and middle finger and apply hard *steady* pressure to the plunger with the thumb while advancing the epidural needle with the left hand. None of the syringe contents will be expelled when the needle tip is located within the interspinous ligament or ligamentum flavum. However, as soon as the needle enters the epidural space, the tissue resistance suddenly disappears and the entire contents of the syringe are discharged. Apply countertraction with the left hand to control further advancement of the needle.

Confirmatory Tests. Consider performing the following confirmatory tests, especially when the subjective sensation of loss-of-resistance is equivocal:

- Inject 2- to 3-mL normal saline with a small (0.2-mL) air bubble incorporated into the solution. Compression of the air bubble indicates resistance on the end of the epidural needle and not within the epidural space.
- Compress the soft tissue of the back at the site of insertion

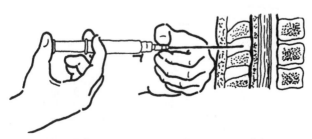

Figure 5–9 ■ Hand position for loss-of-resistance technique.

of the epidural needle while injecting normal saline or air. Increased resistance to injection indicates the needle tip is located in a compressible tissue space, not the epidural space.

■ After injection of 2 to 3 mL of saline through the epidural needle, recheck the loss of resistance with another 1 to 2 mL of air. If the resistance to air has increased, the solution was probably injected into a loose areolar tissue plane or ligament, not the epidural space. This is a helpful maneuver to perform any time a false loss of resistance is suspected. The solution "firms up" the ligament or tissue, and the epidural needle can be advanced without much danger of imminent dural puncture.

Aspirate Through the Epidural Needle

It is important to perform gentle aspiration to rule out intravascular or intrathecal placement of the epidural needle. If blood is aspirated or freely flows without aspiration, it is likely that the needle has entered one of the veins of the epidural venous plexus. If this occurs, remove the epidural needle and repeat the procedure at a different interspace.

If cerebrospinal fluid (CSF) is aspirated, there are two courses of action. First, consider threading a catheter and provide continuous *spinal* analgesia for labor. Alternatively, remove the epidural needle and repeat the procedure at a different interspace. If the latter option is chosen, be aware of the following:

■ Dural puncture with a 17- or 18-gauge epidural needle may result in rapid CSF accumulation within the epidural space. When epidural placement is performed at a different interspace, a *small* amount of CSF may be aspirated.

■ The dural tear may facilitate transdural passage of medications subsequently administered through an epidural catheter and produce exaggerated clinical effects. Consider modifying the dosages of epidural medications when inadvertent dural puncture has occurred.

■ The loss of resistance to air technique during an epidural replacement immediately after an accidental dural puncture may cause pneumocephalus and severe postdural puncture headache. Therefore, if the epidural is to be resited after a "wet tap," a loss of resistance to saline technique should be used.

■ **KEY POINT:** Following unintentional dural puncture with an epidural needle, the method of threading the epidural catheter into the spinal space offers many advantages as compared to re-siting the epidural at another interspace.

Insert an Epidural Catheter and Remove the Needle

Before beginning, make sure the epidural catheter is compatible with the epidural needle being used. Epidural catheters vary in terms of size (18 to 20 gauge), configuration of the tip (open versus closed), and number of lumens (single versus multiorifice).

Examine the epidural catheter for imperfections and note the depth markings. Hold the catheter 5 cm from the tip with the thumb and index finger of the dominant hand. Place the volar surface of the left hand against the patient's back and stabilize the epidural needle by grasping it with the thumb and index finger. Insert the tip of the catheter through the hub of the epidural needle, using a threading-assist guide if applicable. If possible, both the bevel of the epidural needle and the curve of the catheter should be directed cephalad. When the catheter is advanced to the first marking, sudden resistance may be felt as it contacts the directional bevel of the epidural needle. Gently but aggressively overcome this resistance to advance the catheter beyond the needle tip until it projects 3 to 5 cm within the epidural space.

Remove the needle over the catheter by firmly holding the catheter 2 to 3 cm from the hub of the needle with the dominant hand. Place the volar surface of the other hand against the patient's back and grasp the bore of the epidural needle close to the hub with the thumb, index, and middle fingers. Hold the catheter in place by applying forward pressure while carefully withdrawing the needle until the thumbs of the two hands meet (about 2 cm). Repeat this maneuver by grasping the catheter another 2 to 3 cm distal to the hub of the needle and apply forward pressure as the needle is withdrawn another 2 cm. When the needle finally emerges from the skin, firmly grasp the catheter at the site of skin insertion and finish withdrawing the needle over the catheter. Move the left hand distally along the catheter as the needle is withdrawn. If the catheter has been advanced during removal of the needle, withdraw the catheter so that 3 to 5 cm lies within the epidural space. Attach a syringe adapter to the end of the catheter (Fig. 5-10).

Patients may experience transient paresthesias, especially when the catheter first enters the epidural space. If a paresthesia occurs, determine its character and location and reassure the patient there is little cause for concern. If a paresthesia persists or is severe, the catheter may be impinging upon a nerve root and should be removed. Repeated attempts to thread the epidural catheter may result in peripheral nerve injury. If a catheter cannot be threaded, remove the epidural needle and catheter *as a unit* and attempt epidural placement at a different interspace. *Never* withdraw the catheter alone once it has been advanced even slightly beyond the tip of the epidural needle. Likewise, *never* reposition the epidural

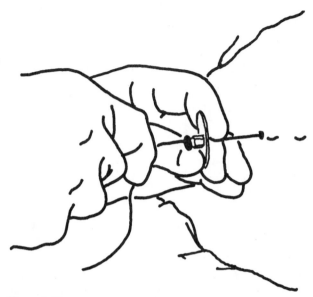

Figure 5–10 ■ Insertion of the epidural catheter and removal of the epidural needle over the epidural catheter.

needle once the catheter has been advanced beyond the tip. Both of these maneuvers may cause shearing of the epidural catheter.

Aspirate Through the Epidural Catheter

Before securing the epidural catheter, it is important to rule out intravascular or subarachnoid catheter placement by gentle aspiration. However, epidural veins are thin walled and easily collapse when subjected to negative pressure. A more sensitive test is to hold the open end of the catheter below the level of insertion and watch for passive return of blood or CSF. Continue to hold the catheter below the level of insertion, attach a small syringe, and perform gentle aspiration.

Administer a Test Dose Through the Epidural Catheter

Many anesthesiologists inject a test dose using lidocaine with epinephrine, bupivacaine, or ropivacaine to rule out *intrathecal* catheter placement. Ask the patient to report any sensory changes in the lower extremity. These may take up to 5 minutes to develop. Sympathetic blockade may be more readily apparent (within 1 minute) so cycle the automatic blood pressure cuff while injecting the local anesthetic and compare this reading to baseline.

To detect *intravascular* needle or catheter placement, a

much larger volume of local anesthetic would have to be administered to produce signs and symptoms of systemic local anesthetic toxicity. Because the volume and concentration of local anesthetic used to initiate labor analgesia is relatively small, intravascular injection of local anesthetic is difficult to detect. The optimal test to rule out the presence of an *intravascular* catheter in a patient during labor is very controversial. Although epinephrine-containing test doses are used by many anesthesiologists, epinephrine has limitations. Although epinephrine (15 μg) is considered a sensitive and specific marker of intravascular injection in the nonpregnant surgical population, in the obstetric population it has the potential to cause uterine artery vasoconstriction and reduction in uterine blood flow. In addition, epinephrine has been found to have an inhibitory effect on uterine contractility and may also be an unreliable marker of intravascular injection due to cyclic changes in maternal heart rate. Alternatives to the epinephrine test dose, such as the injection of air (Doppler test), have been proposed.[7] Although it has been recently suggested that test doses are unnecessary when injecting dilute local anesthetics through multiorificed catheters,[8] it should be remembered that in the event of an emergent cesarean section, the catheter that is receiving a dilute solution will be injected with a dense local anesthetic and failure to recognize intravenous placement of the catheter being used for cesarean section can lead to seizures, cardiovascular, collapse, and death.[9]

Therefore, consider *every* injection through the epidural catheter to be an intravascular test dose and adhere to the following recommendations:

- Carefully aspirate through the catheter before each injection.
- A negative aspiration does not rule out an intravascular or subarachnoid catheter, and the patient must be observed closely.
- Fractionate doses of local anesthetics into 3- to 5-mL aliquots.
- Frequently assess the patient for signs and symptoms of local anesthetic toxicity.
- Monitor the patient for the onset of appropriate analgesia. Suspect intravascular injection if the appropriate sensory level of analgesia does not develop or wears off in a parturient receiving a continuous epidural infusion.
- If in doubt, replace the epidural catheter rather than risk the development of systemic toxicity through repeated injections of local anesthetic.

Secure the Catheter

Cover the insertion site of the catheter with a clear sterile adhesive dressing. Tape the dressing and the catheter along the patient's back to the shoulder. In the obese patient, consider placing the patient in the lateral position before finally taping the catheter.[10]

Initiate the Block with Fractionated Doses of Local Anesthetic/Narcotic

Place the patient in a semisitting position or partially lateral position, with a wedge under the right hip to displace the uterus to the left. If vital signs remain stable and no significant analgesia develops after the test dose, initiate labor analgesia with a total of 10 mL of local anesthetic, given in divided doses. Table 5–3 outlines suggested medications and dosages. Although there are numerous "recipes" for initiation of epidural analgesia for labor, we usually inject 3- to 5-mL aliquots of 0.125% bupivacaine (or 0.1% ropivacaine) with 50 μg of fentanyl at 2-minute intervals to a total dose of 10 mL. Others prefer to omit narcotic in the initial dose of epidural medication so that systemic analgesia does not mask an inadequate epidural block.

Wait 15 to 20 minutes and then assess the patient's sensory level with a pinprick or alcohol swab. Expect a band of decreased sensation from approximately T-10 to L-2. Inform the patient (and her obstetric care provider) that her sensation may be fairly intact during vaginal examinations during the early stages of labor due to sparing of the sacral fibers. Assure the patient that the block can be extended into the perineum during the second stage of labor by injecting additional local anesthetic.

Measure maternal blood pressure every 3 to 5 minutes during initiation of epidural blockade. If maternal hypotension occurs,

■ Change maternal position to more pronounced right or left lateral decubitus to eliminate aortocaval compression;

■ Table 5–3
SUGGESTED DOSAGES FOR CONTINUOUS LUMBAR EPIDURAL ANALGESIA

Drug	Initial Injection	Continuous Infusion
Bupivacaine	10–15 mL of a 0.25–0.125% solution	0.0625–0.125% solution @ 8–15 mL/hr
Ropivacaine	10–15 mL of a 0.1–0.2% solution	0.5–0.2% solution @ 8–15 mL/hr
Fentanyl	50–100 μg given in a 10-mL volume	1–4 μg/mL
Sufentanil	10–25 μg given in a 10-mL volume	0.03–0.05 μg/mL
Epinephrine		1:200,000–1:800,000 concentration

- Rapidly infuse intravenous fluid;
- Administer intravenous ephedrine (5- to 10-mg boluses);
- Consider maternal oxygen administration to augment fetal oxygen delivery during transient uterine hypoperfusion.

Maintain Analgesia with a Continuous Infusion of Local Anesthetic/Narcotic

Maintain labor analgesia with a dilute mixture of local anesthetic combined with a narcotic administered by intermittent bolus injection, continuous infusion, or patient-controlled epidural analgesia (PCEA; demand dosing with or without a continuous background infusion).

Use of intermittent bolus injections should be reserved for situations when delivery is imminent. In most cases, a continuous infusion of dilute local anesthetic/narcotic solution is initiated once a bilateral T-10 sensory level of analgesia is established. A continuous infusion offers the advantages of a stable level of analgesia, increased maternal hemodynamic stability, and less risk of intravascular toxicity from repeated bolus doses of local anesthetic. Table 5–3 outlines suggested medications and infusion rates for continuous lumbar epidural analgesia.

PCEA consists of a background continuous infusion combined with intermittent demand dosing controlled by the patient. Patient-controlled demand dosing alone is sometimes used.[11] Table 5–4 outlines suggested dosages for PCEA, and potential advantages include greater patient satisfaction from an increased sense of autonomy and diminished local anesthetic requirement in some patients.

Whichever modality is used to maintain epidural analgesia during labor, the following parameters should be assessed on an hourly basis:

- Maternal hemodynamics (blood pressure and heart rate);
- Fetal heart rate;
- Sensory level of analgesia;
- Degree of motor blockade.

▪ Table 5–4
SUGGESTED REGIMENS FOR PCEA

Mode	Epidural Solution	Basal Infusion Rate (mL/hr)	Bolus Dose (mL)	Lockout Interval (min)	Hourly Maximum (mL)
Demand only	Bupivacaine (0.125–0.25%)	0	4	10–20	15–20
Continuous infusion plus demand	Bupivacaine (0.0625–0.125%)	4–8	2–4	10–20	15–20

Complications

Diminishing Analgesia

Progressive diminution of sensory block and loss of analgesia can be caused by several factors:

- Pump malfunction or tubing disconnection;
- Inadequate rate of infusion;
- Migration of the catheter out of the epidural space;
- Migration of the catheter into an epidural vein.

First, recheck the infusion setup. Next, disconnect the infusion, attach a small syringe to the epidural catheter, and gently aspirate. Remember, negative aspiration does *not* rule out intravascular catheter migration. At typical infusion rates, bupivacaine (and ropivacaine) will not produce characteristic central nervous system symptoms of intravascular injection. If aspiration of the catheter is negative, consider the use of an air or epinephrine-containing test dose before reinforcing the block with an additional bolus of local anesthetic and increasing the infusion rate. If the block cannot be reestablished, assume the catheter has migrated out of the epidural space and replace the catheter at another interspace.

High Sensory Block or Significant Motor Block

Progressive increase in the sensory level of analgesia or significant motor blockade may indicate subarachnoid migration of the epidural catheter. Disconnect the infusion, attach a small syringe to the end of the epidural catheter, and gently aspirate. A negative aspiration, however, does *not* always rule out intrathecal catheter migration. If clear fluid is aspirated from the catheter, CSF can usually be differentiated from local anesthetic by performing the following tests:

- Local anesthetic usually forms a precipitate when mixed with thiopental; CSF will not.
- Use a urine dipstick to measure the glucose and protein content of the solution. Typically, CSF tests positive for glucose and protein; local anesthetic does not.

Inadequate Analgesia

When the parturient complains of discomfort while receiving a continuous epidural infusion, it is important to assess the following *before* injecting additional medication:

- Sensory level of analgesia to pinprick or alcohol;
- Cervical dilatation and stage of labor;
- Uterine contraction and fetal heart rate tracing;
- Bladder size.

Possible etiologies of inadequate analgesia include the following.

1. *The patient has progressed to the second stage of labor.* Ask the patient to characterize the nature of her discomfort. The second stage of labor is heralded by the sensation of rectal pressure. If cervical examination reveals complete dilatation, the patient is ready to begin pushing. Often, it is not necessary to administer an additional dose of epidural medication early in the second stage of labor because the act of pushing itself relieves much of the discomfort. As the fetal head descends, the sensation of rectal pressure becomes more intense. The sacral fibers (S2) involved in pain transmission during the second stage of labor are large-diameter heavily myelinated nerves that require a large volume of more concentrated local anesthetic solution to achieve successful blockade. The injection of 10 to 12 mL of 0.25% bupivacaine or 0.2% ropivacaine will usually produce analgesia for the second stage. When delivery is imminent, the injection of a total of 10 to 15 mL of pH-adjusted 2% lidocaine or 3% 2-chloroprocaine (in divided doses) provides a faster onset and shorter duration of analgesia. Table 5–5 lists recommended dosages to supplement analgesia during the second stage of labor.

2. *The patient has developed an asymmetric or patchy block.* Determine the sensory level of analgesia to pinprick or alcohol. Adequate analgesia for the first stage of labor requires a bilateral T-10 to L-1 sensory level. Encourage the parturient who is receiving a continuous epidural infusion to turn from side to side each hour to prevent the development of a unilateral block. Sometimes, despite appropriate patient positioning, the sensory level is higher on one side of the body than the other. If aspiration of the catheter is negative, reinforce the block with an additional bolus of local anesthetic. Although there is no scientific data to prove a gravitational effect on epidural blockade, many anesthesiologists believe that asking the patient to lie on the inadequately blocked side during and after injection will help even the block. Table 5–5 lists recommended dosages used to reinforce labor analgesia. Consider increasing the epidural infusion rate if the reinforcement is successful. If the block remains inadequate after administration of additional local anesthetic, consider partially withdrawing and reassessing the catheter or replacing the epidural catheter at another interspace.

3. *The patient has a high analgesic requirement.* There is tremendous variability in anesthetic requirements among laboring patients. Anesthetic requirements are influenced by numerous factors, including social and psychological factors, parity, oxytocin augmentation and duration of labor, and fetal size and presentation. Tachyphylaxis to epidural analgesia may develop when labor is exceedingly long. Painful labor seems to correlate with a higher inci-

■ Table 5–5
**SUGGESTED DOSAGES FOR
SUPPLEMENTATION OF INADEQUATE LABOR
ANALGESIA ACCORDING TO
THE STAGE OF LABOR**

Drug	First Stage of Labor	Second Stage of Labor
Bupivacaine	5–10 mL of a 0.125–0.25% solution	8–15 mL of a 0.25% solution
Ropivacaine	5–10 mL of a 0.1–0.2% solution	8–15 mL of a 0.2% solution
Lidocaine	5–10 mL of a 1.0–1.5% solution	8–15 mL of a 2% solution with or without epinephrine 1:200,000 (pH adjusted)
2-Chloroprocaine		8–15 mL of a 3% solution (pH adjusted)

dence of cesarean section for dystocia. A persistent occiput posterior presentation of the fetal head correlates with low back pain during labor. When any of these conditions are present, consider using either PCEA, an increased concentration and rate of local anesthetic infusion, or additional boluses of fentanyl 50 μg diluted in 10 mL of preservative normal saline every 2 to 4 hours.

4. *Severe and unrelenting pain may indicate uterine rupture or placental abruption.* Parturients who complain of severe unrelenting pain despite an adequate sensory level of analgesia to pinprick should be evaluated for the presence of uterine rupture or placental abruption. Severe pain occurring between contractions is particularly ominous. Because these conditions are generally associated with fetal bradycardia, examine the uterine contraction and fetal heart rate tracing before any epidural injection and alert the obstetrician to any suspicious finding. This is a clinical situation where good communication is essential.

5. The catheter may have migrated out of the epidural space. Because catheters may migrate into the intravascular space, they must be aspirated prior to injection of supplemental medication.

CAUDAL ANALGESIA

Despite reports of high success rates with few complications, caudal techniques have been largely replaced by lumbar epidural analgesia. The pitfalls associated with caudal techniques include an unacceptably high failure rate (especially for the first stage of labor), the need for larger volumes of local anesthetic, and, because of the rich vasculature of the caudal space, a greater risk of local anesthetic toxicity. In addition, the blockade of the sacral nerve roots may result in malrotation of the fetal head and an increased need for instrumental or operative delivery. Although caudal anesthesia can often be successfully used either alone or as part of a two-catheter technique, spinal or lumbar epidural techniques offer many advantages compared with caudal techniques.

COMBINED SPINAL EPIDURAL ANALGESIA

The first report of combined spinal epidural (CSE) described placing an epidural catheter at one interspace and subsequently initiating a spinal anesthetic at a second interspace. This and subsequent reports suggested that CSE provided the fast onset and optimal operative conditions associated with a one-shot spinal but also offered the flexibility of an epidural catheter for extending the duration of the block and providing postoperative analgesia. The disadvantages of this technique, as it was originally described, was that it necessitated two separate anesthetics at two different interspaces and used a "traumatic" spinal needle. The evolution of CSE has been in the direction of a sequential technique, accomplished via a needle-through-needle technique. A recent review article describes the evolution of this technique from its introduction to its present use.[12]

■ **KEY POINT:** CSE is now widely recognized as a technique of neuraxial blockade that provides greater flexibility and reliability than can be achieved with either spinal or epidural analgesia alone.

CSE can be safely used to provide labor analgesia in any patient who is to receive an epidural for labor. There are, however, many patients who will greatly benefit from this technique. These include patients in early or late labor. Patients in early labor can be made comfortable with spinal opioids (such as sufentanil or fentanyl) that will last for approximately 2 to 3 hours, during which time the patient will not have a motor block and will be able to ambulate. If the CSE is performed on a patient in early labor, it is likely that she will be in the active phase of labor by the time the spinal narcotic wears off and additional medication is necessary. The major advantage of CSE for patients in late labor is the almost immediate pain relief. Because CSE allows ambulation of the parturient, it has been called the "walking epidural."

CSE analgesia for labor is usually achieved using a short-acting lipid-soluble narcotic such as fentanyl or sufentanil. Although morphine has been described as an intrathecal opiate for labor, it has several disadvantages, including slow onset, incomplete analgesia, prolonged nausea and pruritus, and delayed respiratory depression. Although pruritus is often associated with the lipid-soluble opioids, it is usually mild and short lived and does not generally need to be treated. A recent review of the complications associated with CSE has concluded that CSE is as safe a technique as conventional epidural technique and is associated with greater patient satisfaction.[13]

Sufentanil 2.5 to 10 μg and Fentanyl 10 to 25 μg are most often used to produce analgesia in the laboring patient. It has been reported that subarachnoid sufentanil provides much more profound analgesia than the same drug administered epidurally. Unfortunately, lipid-soluble opioids, even administered via the subarachnoid route, may not always provide adequate analgesia if given to the parturient who is in advanced labor. In cases where second stage of labor is imminent, the subarachnoid administration of a combination of local anesthetic plus opioid should be considered. The combination of sufentanil 5–10 μg plus bupivacaine 2.5 mg provides rapid analgesia without motor block, alleviates the pain of the second stage of labor, and lasts longer than sufentanil alone.[14]

■ **KEY POINT:** The intrathecal administration of lipid-soluble opioids provides excellent analgesia for the first stage of labor. For advanced labor, it is advisable to add a low dose of local anesthetic to the opioid.

Possible Complications and Side Effects of Intrathecal Opioids for Labor

Side effects and complications can occur after CSE and include

- Pruritus;
- Nausea/vomiting;
- Hypotension;
- Urinary retention;
- Uterine hyperstimulation and fetal bradycardia;
- Maternal respiratory depression.

Uterine Hyperstimulation/Fetal Bradycardia

It has been suggested that spinal opioids, perhaps due to their associated decrease in maternal catecholamines, may precipitate uterine hypertonicity and fetal bradycardia. Several recent reports have evaluated the incidence of fetal bradycardia and emergency cesarean section after CSE and have not found an increase in these complications.

Postdural Puncture Headache

Because the CSE technique includes a dural puncture, there has been concern regarding the potential for postdural puncture headache. The use of a small-bore atraumatic spinal needle such as the Sprotte, Whitacre, or Gertie Marx needles will greatly reduce the incidence of postdural puncture headache in patients receiving CSE. In addition, it has been suggested that the incidence of unintentional dural puncture is less in CSE patients than in patients receiving conventional epidurals. One possible explanation for this finding is that as part of the CSE technique, the spinal needle may be used for verification of correct placement of the epidural needle when there is inconclusive loss of resistance.

Subarachnoid Migration of the Epidural Catheter

This risk has been extensively studied and does not seem to be a major complication of the CSE technique, as compared with conventional epidural techniques. Holmstrom et al.[15] found in a cadaver study that it is almost impossible to pass an epidural catheter through a single dural hole made by a 25-g spinal needle. Special epidural needles with a separate port for the spinal needle are now available and should totally prevent the unintentional subarachnoid threading of the epidural catheter. Regardless of needle used, all epidural doses should be incremental.

Subarachnoid Spread of Epidurally Administered Drugs

Leighton et al.[16] demonstrated that after a CSE, a dose of epidural local anesthetic will produce a higher dermatomal level, presumably due to subarachnoid effect of the drug. In addition, animal evidence has also demonstrated the subarachnoid flux of epidurally administered drugs after dural puncture.

Respiratory Depression

Sufentanil and fentanyl-induced central respiratory depression has been reported. Although some reported cases of respiratory depression might have resulted from potentiation of the respiratory depressant effect of a parenterally administered opioid, respiratory depression after spinal opioids may also occur in patients who have not had parenteral opioids. This respiratory depression occurs acutely and therefore any patient receiving CSE must be appropriately monitored for signs of respiratory depression for a period of at least 20 minutes after administration of the subarachnoid opioid.

Inability to Achieve a Dural Tap Despite Presumed Proper Location of the Epidural Needle

Five explanations are possible when no CSF is noted despite "proper" epidural needle location:

- Epidural needle is not in midline;
- Spinal needle is not long enough;
- Spinal needle is tenting the dura;
- Epidural needle is not where you believe it is;
- Low CSF pressure may prevent spontaneous flow of CSF despite proper location of the spinal needle.

■ **KEY POINT:** The most common side effects following intrathecal administration of a lipid-soluble opioid are pruritus and nausea. Serious complications, including maternal respiratory depression and fetal bradycardia, have been reported but appear to be rare and treatable.

Figures 5–11, 5–12, and 5–13 demonstrate some of these problems.

Basic CSE Technique

The epidural space is identified in the usual fashion, using loss of resistance to air or saline or the hanging drop technique. The loss of resistance to saline technique, however,

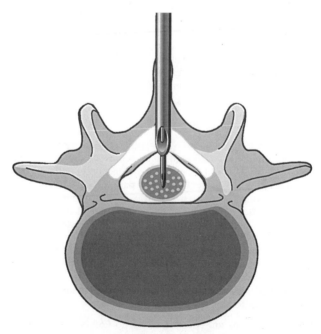

Figure 5–11 ■ Correct midline positioning of a combined spinal epidural.

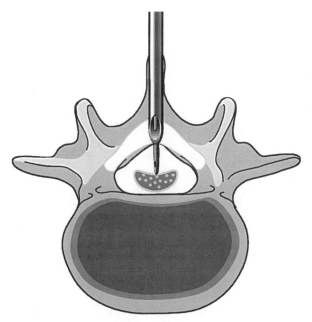

Figure 5–12 ■ Inability to obtain CSF due to tenting of the dura.

may cause confusion due to misinterpretation of the saline for CSF.

Once the epidural space is reached, a long spinal needle is advanced through the epidural needle until the dura is pierced and CSF is obtained. Although many combinations of epidural and spinal needles are now available, the spinal needle must protrude past the end of the epidural needle at least 12 mm (but optimally 14 to 16 mm). In addition, to decrease the risk of postdural puncture headache, many authors suggest that only atraumatic pencil-point spinal needles be used. Examples of atraumatic spinal needles that are available in long (CSE) lengths include Sprotte, Whitacre, Pencan, and Gertie Marx needles.

A syringe is attached to the spinal needle and the subarachnoid drug is administered. It is convenient to hold the hubs of the epidural and spinal needles together between two fingers to prevent needle movement.

The spinal needle is removed and a standard epidural catheter is inserted into the epidural space in the usual manner and then secured. The catheter can later be tested for an intravascular or intrathecal placement with the use of a test dose such as lidocaine plus epinephrine.

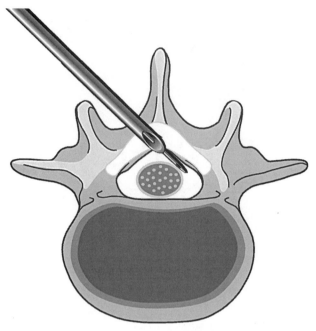

Figure 5–13 ■ Inability to obtain CSF due to malposition of the needle.

Protocol for Ambulation at St. Luke's–Roosevelt Hospital Center

- A patient must remain at bedrest for at least 30 minutes after initiation of CSE analgesia, during which time fetal heart rate and NIBP measurements will be monitored.
- Before ambulation, approval must be obtained from the labor nurse, obstetrician, and anesthesiologist. Fetal heart rate tracing must be within normal limits before ambulation.
- Ambulation is allowed only after the patient has been examined by the anesthesiologist to rule out motor block. This assessment includes the patient's ability to lift her legs while in the supine position, stand up, and perform a modified deep knee bend to verify motor strength.
- A blood pressure measurement taken immediately before ambulation while the patient is upright must be within normal limits.
- Patients may only ambulate in the labor and delivery suite. Patients may ambulate for no more than 15 minutes at a time before returning to the labor and delivery suite for blood pressure and fetal heart rate monitoring.
- Ambulating parturients must be supported on one side by a companion and by an IV pole (on wheels) for support on

their other side. Under no circumstances may a patient ambulate without an escort.

■ If a parturient does not wish to ambulate but wants to get out of bed (or for patients who need to have continuous fetal heart rate monitoring), she may be assisted out of bed into the rocking chair adjacent to the bed.

CONTINUOUS SPINAL ANESTHESIA

Continuous spinal anesthesia offers several advantages over either single-shot spinal or continuous epidural techniques. Interesting research involving the use of a microcatheter small enough to fit through a 22-gauge spinal needle was published in 1990.[17] Due to neurologic complications that were associated with the local anesthetic used (and were probably not directly related to the catheter), the U.S. Food and Drug Administration (FDA) withdrew approval for use of spinal microcatheters in the United States in 1992. The FDA has now allowed one multicenter trial to study the use of a spinal catheter[18] and, if the results are promising, will consider future approval for such a catheter. In the meantime, continuous spinal techniques can be used with a macrocatheter (standard epidural catheter). If an unintentional dural puncture occurs during attempted placement of an epidural, the epidural catheter can be safely threaded into the spinal space. After the administration of a bolus of opioid (sufentanil 5 to 10 μg, fentanyl 15 to 25 μg), the catheter can be used with a continuous infusion of dilute bupivacaine solution (0.1% bupivacaine with fentanyl 1 to 2 μg/mL at 1 to 3 mL/h).

Continuous spinal analgesia/anesthesia should also be considered in the management of the morbidly obese parturient.

REFERENCES

1. Bonica JJ: The nature of pain of parturition. Clin Obstet Gynaecol 2:500–511, 1975.
2. Hawkins JL, Koonin IM, Palmer SK, et al: Anesthesia-related deaths during obstetric delivery in the United States, 1979-1990. Anesthesiology 86:277–284, 1997.
3. Mendiola J, Grylack LJ, Scanlon JW: Effects of intrapartum maternal glucose infusion on the normal fetus and newborn. Anesth Analg 61:32-35, 1982.
4. Gibbs CP, Spohr L, Schmidt D: The effectiveness of sodium citrate as an antacid. Anesthesiology 57:44-46, 1982.
5. Reimann AE, Anson BJ: Vertebral level of termination of the spinal cord with a report of a case of sacral cord. Anat Rec 88:127-138, 1944.
6. Harrison GR, Clowes NWB: The depth of the lumbar epidural space from the skin. Anaesthesia 40:685-687, 1985.
7. Leighton BL, Gross JB: Air: an effective indicator of intravenously located epidural catheters. Anesthesiology 71:848-851, 1989.
8. Norris MC, Fogel ST, Dalman H, et al: Labor epidural analgesia without an intravenous "test dose." Anesthesiology 88:1495-1501, 1998.
9. Crawford JS: Some maternal complications of epidural analgesia for labour. Anaesthesia 40:1219-1225, 1985.

10. Hamilton CL, Riley ET, Cohen SE: Changes in position of epidural catheters associated with patient movement. Anesthesiology 86:778-784, 1997.
11. Paech MJ: Patient-controlled epidural analgesia in obstetrics. Int J Obstet Anesth 5:115-125, 1996.
12. Rawal N, Van Zundert A, Holmstrom B, et al: Combined spinal-epidural technique. Reg Anesth 22:406-423, 1997.
13. Collis RE, Davies DWL, Aveling W: Randomized comparison of combined spinal epidural and standard epidural analgesia in labour. Lancet 345:1413-1416, 1995.
14. Campbell DC, Camann WR, Datta S: The addition of bupivacaine to intrathecal sufentanil for labor analgesia. Anesth Analg 81:305-309, 1995.
15. Holmstrom B, Rawal N, Axelsson K, et al: Risk of catheter migration during combined spinal-epidural block: Percutaneous epiduroscopy study. Anesth Analg 80:747-753, 1995.
16. Leighton BL, Arkoosh VA, Huffnagle S, et al: The dermatomal spread of epidural bupivacaine with & without prior intrathecal sufentanil. Anesth Analg 83:526-529, 1996.
17. Hurley RJ, Lambert DH: Continuous spinal anesthesia with a microcatheter technique: preliminary experience. Anesth Analg 70:97-102, 1990.
18. Arkoosh VA, Palmer CM, Van Maren GA, et al: Continuous intrathecal labor analgesia: Safety and efficacy. Anesthesiology (suppl):A8, 1998.

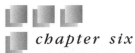

chapter six

REGIONAL ANESTHESIA FOR CESAREAN SECTION

Norah Naughton, MD

The frequency of delivery of an infant by cesarean section has increased significantly in recent years. Twenty years ago the incidence was 4 to 6%. This has risen to 9 to 30%, with rates of 25% common. The use of regional anesthesia has increased since 1981, from 16 to 84%.[1] Hawkins et al.[2] recently reviewed anesthesia-related deaths during obstetric delivery in the United States between 1979 and 1990 and reported the anesthesia-related maternal mortality rate decreased from 4.3 per million live births between 1979 and 1981 to 1.7 per million live births between 1988 and 1990. Between 1979 and 1990, death during cesarean section accounted for 82% of all deaths. Even though there has been a marked decrease in the use of general anesthesia for cesarean section, the number of deaths due to complications of general anesthesia has not decreased over time. In contrast, the number of regional anesthesia-related deaths has decreased since 1984 despite an increased use. Regional techniques allow for an awake parturient and avoidance of general anesthetic induction and intubation with its associated complications of failed intubation, hypoxemia, and aspiration.

The regional anesthetic techniques to be discussed in this chapter include spinal, epidural, and combined spinal-epidural. Advantages and disadvantages unique to each technique are listed in Tables 6-1 and 6-2, respectively. Contraindications to regional anesthesia are listed in Table 6-3.

SPINAL ANESTHESIA

The use of spinal anesthesia for cesarean section has dramatically increased and is now used in approximately 35% of cesarean sections nationwide. It is often the preferred choice because of the simplicity of the technique, rapid onset, and dense neural blockade. There is little risk of maternal exposure to local anesthetic toxicity and minimal transfer of drug to the fetus. Many anesthesiologists believe spinal anesthesia results in a higher quality of anesthesia compared with epidural anesthesia.

Complications

Hypotension

The incidence of hypotension after spinal anesthesia has been reported to be as high as 80% when no prophylactic

■ Table 6–1
ADVANTAGES OF SPINAL AND EPIDURAL ANESTHESIA

Spinal	Epidural
Simplicity	Lesser incidence and severity of hypotension
Speed of induction	Able to titrate desired cephalad level
Low failure rate	Used for longer operation
Low maternal/fetal drug exposure	Avoid dural puncture
	Continuous postoperative analgesia

Adapted from Datta S: Anesthesia for cesarean delivery. In: Datta S, ed. The Obstetric Anesthesia Handbook, 2nd ed. St. Louis: Mosby–Year Book, 1995:152, 161.

measures are taken.[3] This hypotension is produced primarily by the sympathetic blockade that is associated with the thoracic level required for surgery. Because a T2-4 sensory block is required for surgery, a complete sympathetic blockade occurs. The extensive venous dilation that occurs results in decreased venous return to the heart and, as a result, decreased cardiac output. This effect is further aggravated by aortocaval compression by the gravid uterus. Although there is no consensus, one definition of hypotension in obstetric patients is a decrease in systolic blood pressure of at least 30% from baseline or any systolic blood pressure less than 100 mm Hg.[4] The significance of hypotension in the pregnant patient is the subsequent fall in uteroplacental perfusion that may lead to fetal hypoxia and acidosis. Corke et al.[5] found that hypotension lasting less than 2 minutes was associated with significantly higher umbilical arterial and venous hydrogen ion concentrations but still within normal range. In addition, neonatal outcome, defined by Apgar scores and neurobehavioral testing at 2, 4, and 24 hours, was similar between the

■ Table 6–2
DISADVANTAGES OF SPINAL AND EPIDURAL ANESTHESIA

Spinal	Epidural
High incidence of hypotension	Increased complexity of technique
Nausea and vomiting	Higher failure rate
Dural puncture headache	Slower onset
Limited duration of action	Higher maternal/fetal drug exposure

Adapted from Datta S: Anesthesia for cesarean delivery. In: Datta S, ed. The Obstetric Anesthesia Handbook, 2nd ed. St. Louis: Mosby–Year Book, 1995:152, 161.

■ Table 6–3
CONTRAINDICATIONS TO REGIONAL ANESTHESIA

Patient refusal
Coagulation disorders
Severe maternal bleeding
Severe maternal hypotension
Some neurologic disorders
Technical problems
Sepsis, generalized or localized to site of needle insertion

Adapted from Datta S: Anesthesia for cesarean delivery. In: Datta S, ed. The Obstetric Anesthesiology Handbook, 2nd ed. St. Louis: Mosby–Year Book, 1995:161.

hypotensive and nonhypotensive groups. However, with prolonged periods of significant hypotension lasting greater than 4 minutes, fetal bradycardia, acidosis, and neurologic changes for up to 48 hours have been reported.[4] It is therefore essential that hypotension be detected early and promptly treated to avoid fetal compromise.

■ KEY POINT: Hypotension is common during spinal anesthesia for cesarean section. To ensure neonatal well-being, measures should be taken to prevent or immediately treat the hypotension.

One group of investigators reviewed the onset of hypotension after spinal anesthesia in 147 women and reported 51% were hypotensive in 3 minutes and 80% were hypotensive within 5 minutes.[6] Monitoring blood pressure every 3 to 5 minutes would have been inadequate to promptly detect and treat hypotension in most patients. Therefore, it is recommended that blood pressure be monitored every minute for at least 10 minutes after the induction of spinal anesthesia. Several techniques listed below have been recommended to prevent or minimize hypotension associated with spinal anesthesia.

■ KEY POINT: Hypotension occurs more frequently in women who are not in labor (e.g., elective cesarean section) than in women who have been in labor.

Left Uterine Displacement
When a parturient lies supine, the gravid uterus compresses the inferior vena cava and decreases venous return to

the heart. As a result, the supine parturient may not compensate for the hemodynamic changes that occur with the rapid blockade of sympathetic vasomotor activity after spinal anesthesia. Therefore, all parturients who undergo regional anesthesia must be positioned in left uterine displacement to avoid aortocaval compression (see Fig. 1-2). This can be accomplished by placing a wedge under the right hip, tilting the operating room table 15 to 30 degrees to the left, manually displacing the uterus, or using a mechanical uterine-displacing device. Left uterine displacement should be exaggerated if hypotension occurs.

Prehydration Before Spinal Anesthetic

Prophylactic intravenous fluid preload has become standard practice as part of the preparation of the elective patient for spinal anesthesia to decrease the incidence and severity of hypotension. Intravenous infusion of 1000 to 2000 mL of balanced non–dextrose-containing fluid should be administered within 15 to 30 minutes of the block. One thousand milliliters of crystalloid prehydration decreased the incidence of hypotension, but 2000 mL of crystalloid prehydration has been shown to be more effective.[3] Some investigators have compared prehydration with a combination of crystalloid and colloid. Because colloids stay in the vascular compartment longer than crystalloids, only one third to one fourth the volume of colloid is needed compared with crystalloid to expand the vascular compartment. Their use, however, does appear to decrease the incidence of hypotension. In addition, colloids are more expensive, have allergic potential, and may affect platelet function and therefore are not routinely used.

The value of crystalloid preload before spinal anesthesia has recently been challenged. One group of investigators studied the incidence of hypotension after spinal anesthesia for elective cesarean section in two groups of patients. One group received no preload and the other group received 20 mL/kg crystalloid preload. They found only a 16% reduction in the incidence of hypotension but no difference in the clinical or biochemical status of neonates between the preloaded and unpreloaded patients.[6] The authors suggested that the value of crystalloid preloading to prevent hypotension was in question and early detection and prompt treatment could counteract much of the effect of hypotension on uteroplacental blood flow. Although controversial, the data suggest that the use of spinal anesthesia should not be rejected because there has been inadequate time to administer prehydration. Fluid can often be rapidly administered via a pressure device while initiating the block.

Vasopressors

Hypotension unresponsive to left uterine displacement and fluid administration should be promptly treated with a vasopressor. The vasopressors of choice include ephedrine, mephentermine, or metaraminol. These drugs have only slight α-adrenergic activity and maintain or restore uterine blood flow when given to maintain or restore maternal blood pressure. Ephedrine is the most commonly used pressor and is usually administered in 5- to 10-mg increments. α-Adrenergic agonists (e.g., phenylephrine) have not been routinely used because these agents increase uterine vascular resistance and decrease uteroplacental perfusion in a dose-related fashion. Recently, however, investigators have studied the use of small doses of phenylephrine (50 to 100 μg) to treat hypotension in healthy patients at term undergoing spinal anesthesia for elective cesarean section. No difference in neonatal outcome was found when compared with patients who received ephedrine to treat hypotension.[7] An α-adrenergic agonist may be preferred in those patients unresponsive to ephedrine or those not tolerating the associated tachycardia. The use of α-agonists in the setting of the preterm fetus or in the face of fetal distress has not been explored. The prophylactic use of ephedrine to prevent hypotension is controversial. Recommendations include 35 to 50 mg IM before or 5 to 10 mg IV ephedrine immediately after injection of subarachnoid local anesthetic.[8] This has been shown to decrease the incidence of hypotension associated with spinal but not epidural anesthesia. However, one must consider the effects of prophylactic ephedrine on those patients who remained normotensive or in patients where spinal anesthesia was never obtained. In addition, there is no evidence to show that prophylactic treatment of hypotension with vasopressors is superior to immediate treatment with respect to maternal and neonatal outcome.

■ **KEY POINT:** Steps taken to avoid or minimize hypotension associated with spinal anesthesia include adequate uterine displacement, 1.0 to 2.0 L of crystalloid infusion before the block, and prompt recognition and treatment of any decrease in blood pressure with increased fluid administration and/or intravenous boluses of ephedrine.

High Spinal Anesthesia

High or total spinal anesthesia results from extensive rostral spread of local anesthetic. It is associated with complete sensory and motor blockade. Hawkins et al.[2] reported high spinal/epidural anesthesia accounted for 36% of anesthesia-related deaths during regional anesthesia for obstetric delivery between 1979 and 1990. The clinical presentation of a high spinal anesthesia is variable. The patient may remain conscious and normotensive with adequate ventilation and oxygenation but unable to protect her airway due to the inability to cough. In this situation, the patient is unable to speak or capable of only a whisper. Treatment includes administration of a hypnotic agent for amnesia, cricoid pressure, succinylcholine, 1 mg/kg, endotracheal intubation and positive pressure ventilation for airway protection. High spinal anesthesia can also present with hypotension, bradycardia, unconsciousness, and/or respiratory arrest. Respiratory insufficiency may be due to motor block of muscles of respiration or central nervous system hypoperfusion. Treatment is supportive and includes restoration of maternal circulation (adequate uterine displacement, intravenous fluid administration, elevation of legs, administration of ephedrine/epinephrine) and maintenance of adequate oxygenation, ventilation, and airway protection with endotracheal intubation and positive pressure ventilation. Caution must be exercised when administering small doses of induction agents in this setting for amnesia because this may lead to cardiovascular collapse.

■ **KEY POINT:** Prompt treatment of a high or total spinal anesthesia should prevent morbidity or mortality. Appropriate interventions include endotracheal intubation, positive pressure ventilation, and support of maternal hemodynamics.

Risk factors associated with sudden bradycardia during spinal anesthesia (in nonparturients) include age less than 50 years, cephalad level greater than T-6, and a PR interval greater than 0.20 seconds on the electrocardiogram. Bradycardia during a spinal anesthetic can be associated with high vagal tone.[9] This increase in vagal tone is due to a sudden severe drop in venous return to the heart, visceral stimulation, and/or emotional state. The blockade of myocardial sympathetic afferent fibers can lead to a small decrease in heart rate but is not considered a primary factor in sudden bradycardia. A closed claims analysis examined 14 cases of sudden cardiac arrest during spinal anesthesia.[10] The most common sign preceding the arrest was bradycardia followed by hypotension and cyanosis. The presentation of bradycardia and hypotension was consistent with inadequate venous return to the heart as a precipitating cause of the arrest. Resuscitation was successful only after the administration of epinephrine. The investigation highlighted the importance of adequate fluid preload before spinal anesthesia, vigilance for downward trends in heart rate, and the early use of subresuscitation doses of epinephrine when bradycardia occurs to prevent cardiac arrest.

Positioning the patient in reverse Trendelenburg to prevent the further cephalad spread of local anesthetic is discouraged.

This only accentuates the venous pooling and drop in venous return to the heart, leading to hypotension. Short stature, morbid obesity, and administration of spinal anesthesia immediately after a failed epidural anesthetic may be associated with a higher incidence of high spinal anesthesia. Increased vigilance for this complication should be exercised in these clinical situations.

Failed Spinal Anesthesia

Failed spinal anesthesia followed by general anesthesia is estimated to occur in 1% of planned spinal anesthesia cases. Causes include omitting local anesthetic from drug mixture injected, inappropriate dose of local anesthetic, administration of local anesthetic in a space other than the subarachnoid space, caudal pooling of hyperbaric drug with unsatisfactory cephalad spread, and low-potency drug lot.[8] Administration of a second spinal is appropriate if there is evidence of little to no block. However, care must be taken to evaluate the possibility of maldistribution of local anesthetic as the cause of the failed block. Recent case reports, using both the continuous and single-injection techniques, have implicated maldistribution of 5% hyperbaric lidocaine leading to persistent or transient neurologic deficits.[11] Before the second spinal anesthetic, evaluate evidence of a sacral blockade. If present, consider altering the patient's position during and after the repeat spinal anesthetic or switching to an isobaric preparation.

Dural Puncture Headache

Postdural puncture headache (PDPH) can be a very distressing complication for the patient. The reported incidence of PDPH in the obstetric population varies between 1 and 10%. The required clinical feature is the postural nature of the headache. Classically, it involves the frontal or occipital areas and may be associated with tinnitus, photophobia, or cranial nerve palsies. Onset is usually within 48 hours of the dural puncture, with an average duration of 4 days.

■ **KEY POINT:** Headaches after childbirth are multifactorial and do not necessarily signify PDPH, even after dural puncture. The classic sign of PDPH is that the headache is aggravated in the upright position and relieved by the supine position.

Several techniques have been suggested to reduce the incidence of a PDPH[12]:

1. Needle size: The smaller the needle, the less likely is a PDPH.

2. Direction of needle bevel: Insertion of the needle bevel parallel to the longitudinal fibers of the dura results in a lower incidence of PDPH. Parallel insertion minimizes the size of the dural hole and therefore cerebrospinal fluid (CSF) leak.

3. Type of needle: Needles with a pencil point spread rather than cut dural fibers are associated with a lower incidence of PDPH. Examples of pencil point needles are Whitacre, Sprotte, Gertie Marx, and Pencan needles. They differ by the shape of their conical tip and the size and position of the lateral eye and come in sizes ranging from 22 to 27 gauge. As with all spinal needles, the larger sizes may produce more headaches. However, a 22-gauge atraumatic spinal needle is associated with a lower incidence of PDPH compared with the 22-gauge Quincke. Currently, the 25- or 26-gauge atraumatic needle is popular and is associated with less than a 1% incidence of PDPH.

4. Angle of insertion: In vitro models have shown that dura mater punctured at an acute angle results in holes in the dura and arachnoid that are not opposed. This creates a flap valve and less CSF leak. However, results from clinical trials comparing paramedian to midline approach are conflicting and have failed to conclusively validate the in vitro model.

■ **K E Y P O I N T :**   Epidural blood patch is a safe and highly effective treatment for PDPH.

Nausea and Vomiting

Nausea and vomiting commonly occur with spinal anesthesia. Mechanisms likely include hypotension with decreased cerebral blood flow and peritoneal or visceral traction in the presence of an inadequate block. Early detection and prompt treatment of any drop in blood pressure with fluid and a vasopressor, typically ephedrine, will decrease the incidence of nausea and vomiting.

Manipulation of peritoneum or abdominal viscera (such as exteriorization of the uterus) will transmit afferent stimuli via the vagus nerve to the chemoreceptor trigger zone and produce nausea in the presence of an inadequate block. Adequate sensory anesthesia will minimize emetic symptoms. This can be achieved by administering appropriate doses of local anesthetics or adding intrathecal opioids to the spinal drug mixture. This will intensify the quality of sensory anesthesia.

Nausea and vomiting prophylaxis can be achieved by administering metoclopramide 10 mg or droperidol 0.625 to 1.25 mg preoperatively without adverse maternal or neonatal side effects.

Local Anesthetics

A T-4 sensory level is required for a cesarean section. Most of the time, hyperbaric mixtures are chosen. Table 6–4 lists local anesthetics commonly used in spinal anesthesia.

Lidocaine has a quick onset with dense sensory and motor blockade. It is ideal when the surgical duration is short. More often, bupivacaine or tetracaine is chosen, with bupivacaine becoming the local anesthetic of choice. Compared with tetracaine, bupivacaine has a more rapid onset, less motor block (usually associated with less maternal anxiety), fewer failed blocks, and greater patient satisfaction.[3]

Pregnant patients have been shown to be more sensitive to local anesthetics and require less amount of drug for the desired effect compared with the nonpregnant patient. The dose of local anesthesia necessary for a given cephalad level is 50 to 70% of the dose required for nonpregnant patients. Mechanisms include effect of progesterone on neural sensitivity, circulating endorphins, and mechanical effects of the gravid uterus on the subarachnoid space. Just how much local anesthetic to give any particular patient is the clinical question. Estimates based on height and weight may not be relevant. Norris[13, 14] using either 12 or 15 mg of hyperbaric bupivacaine, found spread did not correlate with the patient's age, height, weight, body mass index, or vertebral column length. All patients had adequate anesthesia for surgery. The higher dose produced up to T-2 levels with a few patients demonstrating analgesic levels up to C-2. It appears as though choosing a fixed dose of local anesthetic for most parturients is adequate. Suggested doses are 12.0 mg of bupivacaine, 60 mg of lidocaine, and 9 mg of tetracaine.

■ Table 6–4
LOCAL ANESTHETICS USED FOR SPINAL ANESTHESIA

Local Anesthetic	Dose (mg)	Duration (min)	Onset
5% Lidocaine/7.5% glucose	60–75	45–75	Rapid
0.75% Bupivacaine/8.25% glucose	7.5–15.0	90–120	Intermediate
0.5% Tetracaine/5% glucose	7.0–10.0	90–120	Slow
0.5% Bupivacaine/8.0% glucose	7.5–15.0	90–120 (not approved by Food and Drug Administration)	Intermediate

Adapted from Naulty JS, Becker RA: Neuraxial blockade for cesarean delivery. Anesth Clin North Am 10:121, 1992.

Adjuncts to Local Anesthetics

Table 6–5 lists adjuncts used to improve the quality and duration and/or to provide postoperative analgesia during spinal anesthesia for cesarean section.

Opioids

Fentanyl. Fentanyl[3] intensifies the quality and duration of anesthesia and may provide up to 4 hours of postoperative pain relief. Fentanyl 12.5 μg provided similar quality and duration of analgesia with fewer side effects compared with higher doses.

Sufentanil. Sufentanil increases the quality of analgesia, may provide up to 4 hours of postoperative pain relief, and had few side effects when administered with hyperbaric bupivacaine.

Morphine. Morphine, because of its hydrophilic properties, has a slower onset of action compared with fentanyl and sufentanil but a longer duration of action. It improves intraoperative anesthesia and is the opioid of choice when the desired effect is to provide up to 24 hours of postoperative analgesia.

Side effects are associated with the use of intrathecal opioids. They are pruritus, nausea and vomiting, urinary retention, and respiratory depression. Pruritus is the most common complication (up to 70% incidence) and is associated with all three opioids. The mechanism of action is not well understood. As a result, several approaches to treatment have reported success. These include administration of a pure mu antagonist (e.g., naloxone, naltrexone), combined agonist-antagonist (e.g., nalbuphine), and antihistamine (e.g., diphenylhydramine), and small doses of propofol (10 to 20 mg).

Respiratory depression from intrathecal narcotics results from rostal spread within the subarachnoid space. Hydrophilic narcotics (morphine) spread rostally, whereas lipophilic nar-

■ Table 6–5
ADJUVANTS TO LOCAL ANESTHETICS FOR SPINAL ANESTHESIA

	Dose (mg)	Duration (h)
Intrathecal opioids		
Fentanyl	0.00625–0.025	2–4
Sufentanil	0.005–0.010	2–4
Morphine	0.1–0.4	16–24
Adrenergic agents		
Epinephrine	0.2	—

Adapted from Reisner LS, Lin D: Anesthesia for cesarean section. In: Chestnut DH, ed. Obstetric Anesthesia Principles and Practice. St. Louis: Mosby–Year Book, 1994:468.

cotics (fentanyl, sufentanil) are not considered to undergo significant spread. However, recent case reports, especially with sufentanil, have reported patients with clinical symptoms suggestive of rostral spread within the first 30 minutes of administration.[15] The symptoms included altered mental status, respiratory depression, and inability to clear secretions. All resolved within 30 minutes. Delayed respiratory depression is associated with intrathecal morphine and occurs 6 to 8 hours after administration. Close monitoring of respiratory status is necessary throughout this time period.

Epinephrine. The effect of adding epinephrine to lidocaine and bupivacaine to prolong the duration of anesthesia is controversial. Some investigators find a higher quality longer duration block, whereas others do not.

Suggested technique for spinal anesthesia for cesarean section can be found in Table 6–6.

EPIDURAL ANESTHESIA FOR CESAREAN SECTION

Epidural anesthesia has numerous advantages. One is the ability to administer local anesthetic in fractionated doses and better control the ultimate cephalad level obtained. The slower onset of the block allows a greater time to compensate for the associated sympathetic block. As a result, the incidence and severity of hypotension are less compared with spinal anesthesia. Duration of anesthesia may be extended as needed by additional administration of local anesthesia, and the indwelling epidural catheter may be used for postoperative analgesia. Motor block is less intense compared with spinal anesthesia, and a PDPH is unlikely in the absence of an accidental dural puncture. However, there are complications associated with the technique.

Local Anesthetic Toxicity

Hawkins et al.[2] reported local anesthetic toxicity was the cause of 51% of anesthesia-related deaths during regional anesthesia for obstetric delivery between 1979 and 1990 in the United States. Local anesthetic toxicity is associated more with epidural than spinal anesthesia for several reasons. First, spread of anesthesia is volume dependent and not influenced by the specific gravity of CSF relative to the local anesthetic. A much larger volume is required for adequate spread compared with a spinal such that a 5 to 10 times greater absolute dose is required. Second, the epidural needle or catheter may inadvertently cannulate an epidural vein in up to 9% of cases. In addition, although original catheter placement may be uncomplicated, the catheter can migrate into a vessel at any time. Epidural venous engorgement occurs secondary to inferior vena caval obstruction with shunting of blood through

SUGGESTED TECHNIQUE FOR SPINAL ANESTHESIA FOR CESAREAN SECTION

Preoperative	Local Anesthetic/Narcotic Options
Nonparticulate antacid within 1 hr of anesthesia	Local anesthetic options
Metoclopramide 10 mg IV	1. 12–15 mg bupivacaine, 0.75% with 8.25% dextrose
Administer 1000–2000 mL dextrose-free balanced salt solution IV	2. 60–75 mg lidocaine, 5% with 7.5% glucose
	3. 7–10 mg tetracaine, 1% with equal volumes of 10% dextrose in water
Intraoperative	
	Intrathecal narcotic options
Apply monitors	1. Morphine, 0.1–0.25 mg preservative free for postoperative analgesia
Supplemental oxygen by face mask or nasal prongs	2. Fentanyl 10–25 µg to potentiate anesthesia
Lumbar puncture L2-L3 or L3-L4. Use smallest possible needle with noncutting point (such as Sprotte or Whitacre)	3. Both fentanyl and morphine in above doses
Left uterine displacement	Epinephrine option to above: add 0.1–0.2 mg for prolonged surgery
Monitor blood pressure every minute for first 10–15 min, then every 5 min	
Aggressive treatment of hypotension	

Adapted from Reisner LS, Lin D: Anesthesia for cesarean section. In: Chestnut DH, ed. Obstetric Anesthesia Principles and Practice. St. Louis: Mosby–Year Book, 1994:468; and Shnider SM, Levinson G: Anesthesia for cesarean section. In: Shnider SM, Levinson G, eds. Anesthesia for Obstetrics, 3rd ed. Baltimore, Williams & Wilkins, 1993:215.

the azygous system. Accidental injection of local anesthetic into an epidural vein results in rapid delivery of the drug to the heart. Third, the incidence of failed epidural block is 2 to 6%.[8] This can result in the clinical decision to administer more local anesthetic in an effort to improve the block.

The toxic effects are related to the central nervous system (CNS) and the cardiovascular system (CC). In general, the CNS is more sensitive than the CC to local anesthetics. CNS side effects usually occur first and range from dizziness, circumoral numbness, and tinnitus to convulsions and unconsciousness. Cardiac effects include ventricular arrhythmias and cardiovascular collapse. Comparison of toxicity between local anesthetics uses the CC/CNS toxicity ratio. Bupivacaine has the narrowest ratio compared with the other commonly used local anesthetics. As a result, cardiac effects may occur first or in association with CNS effects.

Several meaures are recommended to prevent local anesthetic toxicity. First, the desired anesthetic level should be obtained by delivery of fractionated doses that are below the recommended toxic dose. When using a continuous catheter technique, aspirate the catheter before each medication injection. Unfortunately, a negative aspiration does not totally eliminate the possibility of venous catheter cannulation. Therefore, an anesthetic test dose medication should be administered before the local anesthetic chosen for the block. The most common test dose used is local anesthetic with epinephrine, usually 3 mL of 1.5% lidocaine with 1:200,000 epinephrine. This amount of local anesthetic will produce a limited spinal block if injected subarachnoid. The 15 μg of epinephrine will produce a rise in heart rate of 20 to 30 beats/min within 20 to 30 seconds if injected intravascularly. However, maternal heart rate can increase within the test dose range during a uterine contraction. As a result, false positives are possible. It is important to administer the test dose in between contractions or repeat the test dose if needed. Low-dose epinephrine has been shown to transiently decrease uteroplacental perfusion but has not been clinically significant. Because this approach is not 100% reliable, alternative test dose medications have been suggested. They include chloroprocaine, isoproterenol, and air using a precordial Doppler probe. Each alternative has drawbacks and is currently not in widespread clinical use.

■ **KEY POINT:** No epidural test will exclude 100% of intravenous or intrathecal catheters; however, aspiration of multi-orificed epidural catheters will detect many of these. The combination of aspiration, use of a test dose, and fractionation of dose increases the safety of epidural anesthesia.

Bupivacaine and chloroprocaine each have potential toxic side effects unique for the drug. Several cases of maternal deaths were attributed to the rapid injection of large doses of 0.75% bupivacaine in the late 1970s. Subsequent animal experiments have shown bupivacaine is more cardiotoxic than lidocaine or chloroprocaine at equipotent doses[12] (bupivacaine CC/CNS is 3.7 ± 0.5; lidocaine CC/CNS is 7.1 ± 1.1). The mechanism is unclear but may be related to decreased protein binding in pregnancy or the effects of progesterone on sodium, potassium, and calcium channels. Resuscitation time may be prolonged. Although the U.S. Food and Drug Administration banned the use of 0.75% bupivacaine in obstetrics, it is important to remember cardiotoxicity is still possible with the lower concentrations currently in use. Therefore, when using bupivacaine, be aware of the potential cardiotoxicity and administer the drug in fractionated subtoxic doses. If maternal resuscitation is necessary, relieve aortocaval compression and promptly treat hypoxia and acidosis. Use bretylium to treat ventricular tachyarrhythmias, and high-dose epinephrine and atropine may be necessary for pulseless electrical activity and bradycardia.

Neurotoxicity has been associated with chloroprocaine. Original preparations of chloroprocaine included the antioxidant sodium metabisulfite. The combination of low pH and sodium metabisulfite was responsible for prolonged neurologic deficit when large doses of chloroprocaine were unintentionally administered in the subarachnoid space. Since that recognition, a newer preparation was released that replaced EDTA for the sodium metabisulfite. This preparation has been associated with severe lumbar back pain, usually when large volumes of the anesthetic were given. It was suggested that the EDTA was acting as a chelating agent and acutely lowering localized tissue calcium, leading to muscle spasm and back pain. Treatment is supportive. The most recent preparation does not contain EDTA and must be protected from ambient light. All three preparations are potentially available for use at the discretion of the practitioner.

Failed Epidural Anesthesia

Epidural anesthesia fails in 2 to 6% of cases.[8] Failure can manifest as complete absence of a block or an inadequate patchy block. In the former case, the catheter was most likely not in the epidural space during induction. Numerous explanations are postulated for a patchy incomplete block and include migration of the catheter within the epidural space, malposition of the catheter within the epidural space, anatomic compartmentalization of the epidural space preventing spread of local anesthetic to all spinal segments, and inadequate amount of local anesthetic administered. Options after a failed epidural include repeating the epidural, spinal, or general anesthesia. All options have their drawbacks. Local anesthetic toxicity with a second epidural is possible because it was preceded with a large volume of local anesthetic. Spinal anesthesia after a failed epidural may be associated with a higher incidence of high spinal anesthesia. General anesthesia is associated with greater maternal mortality secondary to complications associated with airway management.

Another reason for failure may be the sacral sparing property associated with epidural anesthesia. Significant pain may occur during traction of peritoneal structures and exteriorization of the uterus for repair. Some authors have suggested administering part of the dose of local anesthetic with the patient in the sitting or semisitting position to take advantage of gravity to influence sacral spread. Several authors have studied the effects of patient position on local anesthetic spread. Although some controversy may exist, it would appear as though the spread of neural blockade and sacral anesthesia are not affected by patient position when large volumes of higher concentrations of local anesthetics are administered.[16]

Accidental Dural Puncture

Accidental dural puncture occurs between 1 and 5%, with a higher incidence in training programs. It is complicated by a PDPH in up to 85% of cases using 17- or 18-gauge Touhy needles.[8] Advancement of the epidural needle toward the epidural space with the bevel parallel to the dura has been advocated to decrease the incidence of PDPH. However, this necessitates rotating the epidural needle 90 degrees to place the bevel cephalad or caudad before catheter placement. The rotation of the needle in the epidural space may increase the incidence of dural puncture or subdural placement of the catheter.

■ **KEY POINT:** An option for management of unintentional dural puncture with an epidural needle is the placement of the epidural catheter into the subarachnoid space to provide continuous spinal anesthesia. If, however, the epidural is re-positioned at the next interspace, the loss of resistance to air technique should not be used because of the risk of pneumocephalus and severe headache.

Subdural Injection of Local Anesthetic

The subdural space is a potential space between the dural and arachnoid membranes. It does not normally communicate with the subarachnoid space, and the dural and arachnoid membranes are separated by a thin layer of serous fluid. It is estimated that subdural placement of a catheter or medication occurs up to 0.82% of the time.[9] Injection of local anesthetic results in a greater block than expected for the volume administered. The block is characterized by slow onset time, up to 15 to 30 minutes; extensive patchy spread in the cephalad direction occasionally involving cranial nerves; and a sudden drop in blood pressure. Usually, the clinical diagnosis is one of exclusion. Maintenance of anesthesia with a subdural catheter is difficult and should be removed.

High Spinal Anesthesia Associated With Epidural Anesthesia

The unintentional injection of large volumes of local anesthetic into the subarachnoid space will result in high or total spinal anesthesia. Principles of management are similar to those previously described above under Spinal Anesthesia, Complications.

Shivering

Shivering after induction of epidural anesthesia has an incidence between 14 and 68%.[12] It is frequently the most distressing part of the birth experience described by pregnant patients. The mechanism of shivering is unknown, and some treatment options have been met with variable success, including administration of body temperature fluid for prehydration, use of warmed local anesthetic solutions, warming the operating room, or covering the patient with warm blankets. The administration of epidural fentanyl or sufentanil and the intravenous administration of 25 to 50 mg of meperidine after delivery has been observed to effectively treat shivering.

Local Anesthetics

Commonly used local anesthetics are listed in Table 6–7. Choice of local anesthetic will depend on the desired onset time, duration of the procedure, and maternal and fetal status. It is controversial if pregnancy reduces the amount of local anesthetic required for a given cephalad level with epidural anesthesia compared with the nonpregnant patient.

Lidocaine

Lidocaine (1.5 to 2%) has become increasingly popular as the local anesthetic of choice for epidural anesthesia. The addition of sodium bicarbonate (see Alkalinization of Local Anesthetics, below) decreases the onset time so that it becomes similar to 2-chloroprocaine. Some authors advocate its use over 2-chloroprocaine in extending existing epidural anesthesia for an urgent cesarean section.

Bupivacaine

Bupivacaine has a slow onset and may be appropriate in clinical settings that require a prolonged anesthetic induction,

■ Table 6–7
LOCAL ANESTHETICS COMMONLY USED FOR EPIDURAL ANESTHESIA

Local Anesthetics	Percent	Dosage Range (mg)	Duration (min)	Onset
Lidocaine	1.5–2	300–500	45–60	Intermediate
Lidocaine with epinephrine	1.5–2	300–500	75–90	Intermediate
Alkalinized lidocaine with epinephrine	1.5–2	300–500	75–90	Rapid
Bupivacaine	0.5	75–125	90–120	Slow
2-Chloroprocaine	3	450–750	30–45	Rapid
Ropivacaine	0.5	75–125	90–120	Intermediate

Adapted from Naulty JS, Becker RA: Neuraxial blockade for cesarean delivery. Anesth Clin North Am 10:108, 1992.

such as severe preeclampisa and certain maternal cardiac lesions. However, some authors believe that 0.5% does not provide a dense enough block.

2-Chloroprocaine

Chloroprocaine has a rapid onset of action, produces dense anesthesia, and has a short maternal and fetal half-life. It is considered by many to be the local anesthetic of choice in the face of "fetal distress" and the requirement for an urgent cesarean section. Chloroprocaine has two disadvantages: It is known to competitively antagonize the action of subsequently administered bupivacaine and it also decreases the quality and duration of analgesia from subsequently admnistered epidural narcotics. The mechanism is not entirely clear but may be due to the action of the metabolite of chloroprocaine, 2-chloro-4-aminobenzoic acid.

Ropivacaine

Ropivacaine is a new amide local anesthetic that is a homologue between mepivacaine and bupivacaine. Local anesthetics are chiral compounds because of the presence of an asymmetric carbon next to the amino group. As a result, the molecule can exist in the R or S stereoisomer. The S isomer has a longer duration of action and lower systemic toxicity than the R isomer. Unlike the other amide local anesthetics used clinically that exist as a racemic mixture, ropivacaine exists only in the S isomer form. Studies comparing ropivacaine to bupivacaine at equal concentrations highlight two major differences between the local anesthetics: Ropivacaine is associated with less myocardial toxicity in both pregnant and nonpregnant subjects and has less motor block. Recent studies have suggested that ropivacaine may be up to 40% less potent than bupivacaine.[17]

Adjuncts to Local Anesthetics

Table 6–8 lists adjuncts for epidural anesthesia for cesarean section.

Epinephrine

Epinephrine (1:400,000 to 1:200,000) may be added to local anesthetics for the following reasons: decreases systemic absorption of local anesthetic, prolongs the duration of the block, improves the density of the block, and increases the motor block obtained. The clinical profile of lidocaine is altered with use of epinephrine, providing a more satisfactory anesthetic. The effect on bupivacaine is less clear. The α effect from systemic absorption of epinephrine does not appear to have significant effect on uteroplacental perfusion. The β effect may decrease maternal diastolic pressure but has no effect on systolic pressure or uterine blood flow.[8]

Alkalinization of Local Anesthetics

Local anesthetics are weak bases, with pK_as ranging from 6.5 to 8.0. Adjustment of the pH of the mixture results in more of the molecule existing in the un-ionized form, thus making the drug more quickly available to the site of action. This results in a shorter onset time and more intense block. This technique has been shown to be effective with lidocaine. However, observations with chloroprocaine and bupivacaine are not as uniform. Recommended mixtures are listed in Table 6–8. Hypotension is a potential side effect due to the more rapid onset of epidural anesthesia. Hemodynamic effects of pH-adjusted lidocaine were similar to spinal anesthesia when compared with plain lidocaine.[3] It is also possible to form a precipitate of local anesthetic when excess bicarbonate has been added.

■ Table 6–8
**ADJUVANTS USED FOR EPIDURAL
ANESTHESIA FOR CESAREAN SECTION**

	Dosage Range	Duration (h)
Narcotics		
Morphine	3–5 mg	16–24
Fentanyl	50–100 µg	2–4
Adrenergic agents		
Epinephrine	1:200,000	—
Alkalizing agents		
8.4% Sodium bicarbonate	2 mL in 20 mL lidocaine or chloroprocaine	—
	0.1 mL in 20 mL bupivacaine	—

Narcotics

Opioids, when added to local anesthetics for cesarean section, improve the quality of intraoperative anesthesia and provide postoperative analgesia. Common narcotics used are listed in Table 6–8. The lipophilic narcotics fentanyl and sufentanil are characterized by rapid onset and short duration, whereas the hydrophilic narcotic morphine has a slow onset and a long duration of action.

Fentanyl

Fentanyl is usually administered in a dose of 50 to 100 μg. Administration before delivery of the infant is not associated with adverse neonatal effects. Fentanyl should be given in a minimum volume of 10 mL to gain the maximal effects. Postoperative analgesia is of short duration, ranging between 2 and 4 hours.

Sufentanil

Sufentanil is usually administered in a dose of 20 to 30 μg, which is equivalent to 100 μg of fentanyl. Its use has not been associated with adverse maternal or neonatal side effects. Postoperative analgesia duration ranges between 2 and 4 hours.

Morphine

Morphine is most commonly used to provide a long duration of postoperative analgesia. The administration of a single dose of 3 to 5 mg will provide 12 to 24 hours of postoperative analgesia. When 5 mg of epidural morphine was administered to 1000 women, 85% reported good to excellent postoperative pain relief lasting 23 hours.[3] Side effects occur and include pruritus, nausea and vomiting, urinary retention, and severe respiratory depression. The incidence of the latter is considered to be 0.1% with similar morbidity associated with intramuscular or patient controlled analgesia (PCA) administration. Its use is considered safe when basic postoperative maternal monitoring criteria are exercised.

COMBINED SPINAL–EPIDURAL

A combined spinal–epidural takes advantage of the rapid onset and density of spinal anesthesia while at the same time having the capability to extend the duration of the blockade or provide postoperative analgesia using the epidural catheter. One approach to the technique is to locate the epidural space with a Touhy needle, pass a long spinal needle through the epidural needle into the CSF, inject local anesthetic, and then thread the epidural catheter into the epidural space and use the catheter, if needed, to reinforce or extend the anesthesia.

The suggested technique for epidural anesthesia for cesarean section can be found in Table 6–9.

ADDITIONAL CONSIDERATIONS

Supplementary Oxygen

Patients should be given supplementary oxygen by nasal prongs or face masks. Increasing maternal inspired oxygen concentration from room air to 100% resulted in an increase in umbilical venous Po_2 from 28 to 47 torr and umbilical artery Po_2 from 15 to 25 torr.[3]

Supplementary Drugs for Anxiety or Analgesia

Generally, one avoids the intravenous administration of anxiolytics or analgesics before delivery of the neonate. However, certain clinical situations may necessitate the use of these drugs. Small doses of a benzodiazepine (midazolam 0.5 to 2 mg or diazepam 2 to 5 mg) or narcotic (fentanyl 25 to 50 μg) should have little effect on the neonate. Supplementation of a sensory block with 30 to 40% nitrous oxide, low-dose ketamine, 0.25 mg/kg, or fentanyl, 1 μg/kg, does not adversely affect the neonate. General anesthesia with endotracheal intubation should be administered in the face of an obvious inadequate regional block.[3]

Electrocardiographic Changes

ST segment changes during cesarean section have been reported. They predominately occur at the time of delivery and are associated with tachycardia. They may or may not be associated with chest pain. These changes do not appear to be associated with myocardial ischemia or impaired function and most likely represent a hyperdynamic circulation.[1]

EFFECTS OF REGIONAL ANESTHESIA ON THE NEONATE

Standard measures of neonatal well-being include Apgar scores, umbilical cord blood pH measurements, and neurobehavioral scores typically assessed at 2, 4, 24, and 48 hours after birth.

Fluid loading before regional anesthesia should use non–dextrose-containing fluid. The administration of a glucose load can result in maternal and fetal hyperglycemia and hyperinsulinemia. The neonate may experience reactive hypoglycemia after delivery because the insulin has a longer half-life than the glucose. In addition, jaundice is more common in neonates born to mothers who received a glucose load before a cesarean section.

■ Table 6-9

SUGGESTED TECHNIQUE FOR EPIDURAL ANESTHESIA FOR CESAREAN SECTION

Preoperative	Local Anesthetic/Narcotic/Adjunct Options
Nonparticulate antacid within 1 hr of anesthesia Metoclopramide 10 mg IV Administer 1500–2000 mL dextrose-free balanced salt solution IV	Local anesthetic options 1. 1.5–2.0% lidocaine 2. 0.5% bupivacaine 3. 3.0% chloroprocaine 4. 0.5% ropivacaine
Intraoperative	
Apply monitors Supplemental oxygen by face mask or nasal prongs Epidural catheter at L2-L3 or L3-L4 Test dose: 3 mL local anesthetic containing epinephrine 1:200,000 (15 μg), observe for heart rate increase within 60 s or spinal blockade within 3–5 min Administer up to 20 mL local anesthetic in fractionated 5-mL increments up to T-4 sensory block Left uterine displacement Monitor blood pressure every minute for first 10–15 min then every 5 min Aggressive treatment of hypotension	Epinephrine option to above: maximum concentration of 1:200,000 pH adjustment option 1. Add 2 mL sodium bicarbonate (8.4%) to 20 mL lidocaine *or* 2. 0.1 mL sodium bicarbonate (8.4%) to 20 mL bupivacaine Epidural narcotic options 1. Fentanyl 50–100 μg or sufentanil 10–20 μg before delivery to potentiate anesthesia 2. Morphine 3–5 mg after delivery for postoperative analgesia 3. Either fentanyl/sufentanil plus morphine in above doses

Adapted from Reisner LS, Lin D: Anesthesia for cesarean section. In: Chestnut DH, ed. Obstetric Anesthesia Principles and Practice. St. Louis: Mosby-Year Book, 1994:470; and Shnider SM, Levinson G: Anesthesia for cesarean section. In: Shnider SM, Levinson G, eds. Anesthesia for Obstetrics, 3rd ed. Baltimore, Williams & Wilkins, 1993:215.

> ■ **KEY POINT:** An acute increase in maternal glucose concentration after the administration of a dextrose-containing intravenous solution can cause reactive neonatal hypoglycemia. Therefore, acute volume administration before delivery should be accomplished with a non–dextrose-containing solution.

In the absence of hypotension, spinal and epidural anesthesia are not associated with adverse neonatal outcome. Severe or uncorrected hypotension can be associated with lower umbilical cord blood pH measurements and Apgar scores. Evidence suggests that hypotension successfully treated within 2 minutes does not affect Apgar or neurobehavioral scores.[5] Uncorrected hypotension for greater than 4 minutes has been associated with fetal bradycardia, acidosis, and neurobehavioral changes for up to 48 hours.[4]

The placental transfer of local anesthetics and effects on the neonate are negligible. The infant is exposed to a very low concentration of drug during spinal anesthesia, and no adverse effects have been observed. Administration of epidural bupivacaine and 2-chloroprocaine does not alter neurobehavioral scores. The effects of lidocaine are somewhat controversial. Most investigators have not demonstrated effects on neurobehavioral scores, but there are isolated reports that suggest subtle changes in neurobehavioral scoring in neonates born to mothers who received lidocaine.

REFERENCES

1. Hawkins JL, Gibbs CP, Orleans M, Schmid K: Obstetric anesthesia work force survey: 1992 versus 1981 [abstract]. Anesthesiology 81:A1128, 1994.
2. Hawkins JL, Koonin LM, Palmer SK, et al: Anesthesia related deaths during obstetric delivery in the United States 1979-1990. Anesthesiology 86:277–284, 1997.
3. Shnider SM, Levinson G: Anesthesia for cesarean section. In: Shnider SM, Levinson G, eds. Anesthesia for Obstetrics, 3rd ed. Baltimore: Williams & Wilkins, 1993:211-246.
4. Shnider SM, Levinson G: Hypotension and regional anesthesia in obstetrics. In: Shnider SM, Levinson G, eds. Anesthesia for Obstetrics, 3rd ed. Baltimore: Williams & Wilkins, 1993:397-406.
5. Corke BC, Datta S, Ostheimer GW, et al: Spinal anesthesia for cesarean section: the influence of hypotension on neonatal outcome. Anesthesiology 37:658-662, 1982.
6. Rout CC, Rocke DA: Prevention of hypotension following spinal anesthesia for cesarean section. In: Rocke DA, ed. International Anesthesiology Clinics Shaping Future Obstetric Anesthesia Practice. Vol. 32. Boston: Little, Brown and Company, 1994:117-135.
7. Moran DH, Perillo M, LaPorta RF, et al: Phenylephrine in the prevention of hypotension following spinal anesthesia for cesarean delivery. J Clin Anesth 3:301-305, 1991.
8. Reisner LS, Lin D: Anesthesia for cesarean section. In: Chestnut DH, ed. Obstetric Anesthesia Principles and Practice. St. Louis: Mosby-Year Book Inc., 1994:459-486.

9. Fielder MA: AANA journal course: update for nurse anesthetists—improving the safety of subarachnoid and epidural blocks. Part A. J Am Asso Nurse Anesth 65:371-381, 1997.
10. Caplan RA, Ward RJ, Posner K, et al: Unexpected cardiac arrest during spinal anesthesia: a closed claims analysis of predisposing factors. Anesthesiology 68:5-11, 1988.
11. Ross BK, Coda B, Heath CH: Local anesthetic distribution in a spinal model: a possible mechanism of neurologic injury after continuous spinal anesthesia. Reg Anesth 17:69-77, 1992.
12. Datta S: Anesthesia for cesarean delivery. In: Datta S, ed. The Obstetric Anesthesia Handbook, 2nd ed. St. Louis: Mosby-Year Book, Inc., 1995:151-186.
13. Norris MC: Height, weight, and the spread of hyperbaric bupivacaine in the term parturient. Anesth Analg 67:555-558, 1988.
14. Norris MC: Patient variables and the subarachnoid spread of hyperbaric bupivacaine in the term parturient. Anesthesiology 72:478-482, 1990.
15. Cohen SE, Cherry CM, Holbrook H, et al: Intrathecal sufentanil for labor analgesia-sensory changes, side effects and fetal heart rate changes. Anesth Analg 77:1155-1160, 1993.
16. Naulty SJ, Becker RA: Neuraxial blockade for cesarean delivery. Anesth Clin North Am 10:102-127, 1992.
17. Polley LS, Columb MO, Naughton NN, et al: Relative analgesic potencies of ropivacaine and bupivacaine for epidural analgesia in labor: implications for therapeutic indexes. Anesthesiology 90:944-950, 1999.

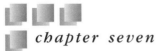

chapter seven

GENERAL ANESTHESIA FOR CESAREAN SECTION

Glenn Shopper, MD

INDICATIONS

The use of general anesthesia for cesarean section has declined in recent decades, partly due to increased awareness of its risks and to improvements in regional anesthesia. Nevertheless, general anesthesia is still the method of choice for specific indications (Table 7-1). The ability to achieve surgical anesthesia expeditiously makes general anesthesia appropriate in cases of extreme fetal "distress." General anesthesia is also appropriate in instances when regional anesthesia is contraindicated or has failed. Although there are no specific contraindications to general anesthesia, certain conditions (e.g., allergies to agents, malignant hyperthermia, maternal morbidity, or potentially difficult airway) may require modification of the usual anesthetic technique.

> ■ **KEY POINT:** Although general anesthesia is not routinely used for elective cesarean sections, it continues to have a place in current practice—primarily in cases in which regional anesthesia is contraindicated.

RISKS

A recent study[1] found anesthesia-related maternal mortality to be declining over the past decade. However, most of this improvement was secondary to a decrease in deaths involving regional anesthesia despite an increase in its utilization. The absolute number of deaths involving general anesthesia has remained relatively constant, with airway-related problems accounting for approximately three fourths of these deaths. It is disconcerting that these mortality figures do not reflect recent improvements in monitoring (pulse oximetry, capnography) and appreciation of the risks of airway mishaps. Perhaps with the multitude of airway appliances (e.g., laryngeal mask airway, combitube) and anesthesiologists' and obstetricians' increasing awareness of the hazards of general anesthesia, we will see a reduction of maternal mortality in this arena.

> ■ **K E Y   P O I N T :** General anesthesia for cesarean section continues to be associated with failed intubation and pulmonary aspiration of gastric contents. When administering general anesthesia to the parturient, steps should be taken to minimize these risks.

FETAL EFFECTS

General anesthesia is comparable with spinal and epidural anesthesia with respect to fetal acid-base status. Differences in the administration of anesthesia have more consequence than choice of anesthetic. Fetal hypoxia or acidosis is usually secondary to maternal hypotension, hyperventilation, aortocaval compression, or a prolonged uterine incision to delivery time. Apgar scores at 1 minute are lower in infants born to mothers undergoing general anesthesia. At 5 minutes, however, the incidence of neonatal depression is no different from that of infants born after regional anesthesia. The degree of neonatal depression mirrors the duration of general anesthesia. Thus, anesthesia is usually not induced until the mother has been prepped and draped so that skin incision can occur as soon as airway control has been attained.

PREPARATION FOR GENERAL ANESTHESIA

All operating rooms where cesarean sections are performed should be checked daily and after each case. The anesthesiologist should be prepared to induce general anesthesia, knowing that all anesthetic and resuscitative drugs and equipment are present and intact (Table 7-2). Although few operating rooms and airway carts will have every item, it is wise for the anesthesiologist to have a wide variety of airway appliances and to be skilled at the use of each.

The technique of general anesthesia for cesarean section is

■ Table 7–1
INDICATIONS FOR GENERAL ANESTHESIA

Fetal asphyxia
Failed regional anesthetic
Contraindications to regional anesthesia
    Maternal refusal
    Coagulopathy
    Infection
    Hemorrhage/volume depletion
    Progressive neurologic disease
    Cardiac disease that would not tolerate acute sympathectomy
        Aortic stenosis
        Right to left shunt

▪ Table 7–2
SETUP FOR GENERAL ANESTHESIA

In addition to the usual preanesthetic room check, the following should
be available:

Operating rooms
  Sodium citrate
  Pressure bags/blood warmers
  Wedge for left uterine displacement
  Blankets/pillows for positioning
  Nitroglycerine (for uterine relaxation)
  Short laryngoscope handle
  Assortment of Miller and MacIntosh blades
  Assortment of styletted smaller tubes (5.0-7.0 mm)
  Oral and nasal airways
  Assortment of face masks
  Jet ventilator
  Oxygen source with flowmeter
Difficult airway cart
  Fiberoptic bronchoscope with light source
  Intubating airways (Ovassapian, etc.)
  Patil facemask
  Eschmann stylet (gum-elastic bougie)
  LMAs in assorted sizes
  Esophageal-tracheal combitube
  Percutaneous dilational cricothyrotomy kit
  Retrograde wire kit
  Illuminating intubating stylet ("light wand")
  Special laryngoscope blades (Belscope, WuScope, Bullard, Augustine,
    etc.)
  Local anesthetic for topical airway anesthesia (spray, gel, viscous,
    nerve block)
  Nasal vasoconstrictor (oxymetazoline, phenylephrine)
  Magill forceps
  Tongue depressors, gauze

---

illustrated in Table 7-3. As with all anesthetics, a history and
physical examination must be performed before induction.
Occasionally, the urgency of the situation may dictate that
a focused workup is performed, with attention directed at
concurrent obstetric or medical conditions, medications, allergies, anesthetic history, and potential airway difficulties. Ongoing bleeding, venous access, the availability of compatible
blood, and maternal volume status should also be noted. The
urgency of operative indications should be reviewed with
the obstetric team, because a calm realistic appraisal of fetal
condition may lead to the conclusion that there is adequate
time for the performance of a regional anesthetic.

Premedication

The parturient is at risk for aspiration because gastric emptying is delayed, acid secretion is increased, lower esophageal

■ Table 7–3
TECHNIQUE OF GENERAL ANESTHESIA FOR CESAREAN SECTION

1. Administer sodium citrate 30 mL orally within 30 min of induction; additional agents for gastric preparation as time for onset permits.
2. Evaluate patient directed with respect to difficult intubation, contraindications to rapid-sequence induction, venous access, fetal asphyxia.
3. Apply usual monitors (electrocardiogram, blood pressure cuff, pulse oxymeter); ensure left uterine displacement and optimal "sniff" positioning.
4. Denitrogenate with high-flow oxygen (3 min or 4 vital capacity breaths) as time permits during abdominal preparation and draping.
5. Administer thiopental 4 mg/kg (or ketamine 1 mg/kg) and succinylcholine 1–1.5 mg/kg. Apply cricoid pressure as patient loses consciousness. Intubate; do not release cricoid pressure until tracheal tube position is verified and cuff is inflated.
6. Ventilate with 50% oxygen, 50% nitrous oxide, isoflurane 2/3 MAC. Maintain normocarbia (usually 10 mL/kg tidal volume, 10 breaths/min).
7. If needed, relaxation can be provided with succinylcholine infusion or nondepolarizing agent.
8. After delivery, administer narcotic, increase nitrous oxide to 70%; discontinue or reduce isoflurane (discontinue and administer benzodiazepine if uterine atony is present). Add oxytocin 20 U/L of intravenous fluids. Administer antibiotics if requested.
9. Decompress stomach with orogastric tube.
10. Extubate when awake and following commands.

tone is decreased, and obstetric emergencies frequently make an 8-hour fast unachievable. Historically, a gastric volume greater than 0.4 mL/kg and pH less than 2.5 were considered determinants of aspiration risk. Although there is little evidence that the avoidance of these conditions will protect the parturient from aspiration, most premedication regimens have been directed toward these ends. Nonparticulate antacids (sodium citrate/citric acid), metoclopramide, H_2 blockers, and omeprazole are all currently in common use alone and in combinations. Ranitidine 50 mg or omeprazole 40 mg intravenously at least 30 minutes before surgery is effective in reducing gastric acidity and volume. An additional dose given by mouth the evening before elective cesarean section will increase the efficacy of gastric preparation. Although metoclopramide has had variable success decreasing gastric volume, it increases lower esophageal sphincter tone, is an effective antiemetic, and is frequently given before induction. Particulate antacids can cause pneumonitis if aspirated; therefore, 15 to 30 mL of a nonparticulate antacid is given immediately before induction, with a duration of action of approximately 30 minutes.

> ■ **KEY POINT:** There is no need to administer a defasciculating dose of nondepolarizing muscle relaxant before the administration of succinylcholine. At term gestation, the incidence of fasciculations is low and pretreatment does not further reduce this incidence.

Positioning

A wedge or roll must be placed under the parturient's right hip to ensure left uterine displacement. Trendelenburg positioning should be avoided where possible, because small venous air emboli can occur during cesarean section. Although usually of little clinical significance, their incidence can be decreased with head-up positioning. The head should be elevated to a "sniff" position, with attention paid to avoiding the possibility of the patient's enlarged breasts impinging on the laryngoscope handle. A short handle is useful in this situation. In the case of the obese parturient, a "ramp" can be created on the bed to elevate the thorax and head and improve intubating conditions. It cannot be overemphasized that a few seconds spent in optimizing the initial intubating conditions are preferable to attempting to reposition the patient when intubation and ventilation attempts are hampered by poor positioning. Cricoid pressure must be applied by a skilled designated person who will be available to hold it throughout the entire case if intubation is impossible and surgery takes place while the patient is ventilated by mask.

Monitoring

It is unfortunate that the oldest and most obsolescent equipment occasionally winds up in the obstetric suites—the parturient should be entitled to the same standards of intraoperative monitoring that nonobstetric patients enjoy. Pulse oximetry and capnography are mandatory. Capnography can aid in avoidance of hyper- and hypocarbia, because both can lead to decreased uterine blood flow. End-tidal nitrogen monitoring can determine adequacy of denitrogenation. Fetal monitoring should continue as long into the perioperative period as practical, because a change in fetal heart rate patterns in the operating room occasionally decreases (or increases) the urgency of cesarean.

Preoxygenation

Pregnancy increases maternal oxygen consumption and decreases functional residual capacity, a measure of oxygen stores during periods of apnea. Therefore, it is imperative that denitrogenation with 100% oxygen at high flow rates is performed before induction. Although denitrogenation attained after 3 minutes of tidal breathing is superior to four vital capacity breaths, the time constraints imposed by the urgency of delivery usually dictate more rapid denitrogenation.

INDUCTION OF ANESTHESIA

In the parturient, the requirements for induction agents are decreased by 30 to 40%. Thiopental and most other induction agents readily cross the placenta and can be found in fetal blood by the time the fetus is delivered. Fetal hepatic metabolism and dilution of umbilical venous blood in the fetal vena cava contribute to awake vigorous infants being born to anesthetized mothers.

Thiopental

Thiopental's long record of safety has made it the most commonly used induction agent in the United States. In doses of 4 to 7 mg/kg pregnant body weight (PBW), general anesthesia is produced with minimal effects on the fetus delivered within 10 minutes. Thiopental is a negative inotrope and causes vasodilation; this effect is minimal in the healthy euvolemic patient, but significant hypotension can result if hypovolemia or ventricular dysfunction is present.

Ketamine

Although ketamine's potential for psychomimetic effects has made many clinicians hesitant to use it, when narcotics and benzodiazepines are given concurrently, these risks are minimized. Ketamine given 1 mg/kg PBW produces no more fetal depression than thiopental; at higher doses, low Apgar scores and even neonatal hypertonus interfering with ventilation have been reported. Administration results in release of endogenous catecholamines that can support the maternal circulation in the face of hemorrhage and also make ketamine beneficial in asthmatic patients. Because of the potential for an exaggerated hypertensive response to laryngoscopy and intubation, it should be avoided in hypertensive patients. An interesting benefit of ketamine is the reduction in the incidence of awareness and recall under anesthesia compared with thiopental.

■ **KEY POINT:** Ketamine is the induction agent of choice for a parturient with either significant hemorrhage or acute asthma symptoms.

Etomidate

Etomidate is used infrequently for cesarean section. It has the disadvantages of causing pain and myoclonus on injection and has been associated with neonatal depression and the potential for postoperative adrenal suppression. However, etomidate produces minimal cardiovascular depression and has found a role for obstetric patients with impaired cardiac function.

Propofol

Propofol is enjoying increasing popularity in the nonobstetric population, because it provides a rapid awakening after unconsciousness. It causes pain upon injection in a significant portion of patients, and there have been reports of bradycardia when used with succinylcholine for induction. Propofol has fetal effects similar to pentothal, although lower Apgar and neurobehavioral scores have been reported.

Muscle Relaxants

All commonly used neuromuscular blocking agents are lipid soluble and highly ionized at physiologic pH and therefore have limited placental transfer to the fetus. Succinylcholine is the relaxant of choice for rapid-sequence inductions; however, a short-acting nondepolarizing agent (e.g., raparcuronium, *cis*-atracurium) can be substituted when succinylcholine is contraindicated. The risks of a slower onset and a longer duration of action (in the face of a potentially difficult airway) must be considered. A defasciculating dose of a nondepolarizing agent is usually not given before succinylcholine, because pregnant patients are at decreased risk of myalgias. Additionally, an occasional complication of defasciculation is an exaggerated response to the relaxant (especially if the patient is receiving magnesium), causing the patient to be unable to maintain a patent airway and necessitating emergent induction of anesthesia. After induction, if relaxation is desired, a nondepolarizing agent or succinylcholine infusion can be used, although the abdominal musculature is usually sufficiently stretched by the previously gravid uterus that muscle relaxation is frequently unnecessary.

Maintenance of Anesthesia

Nitrous oxide is usually administered along with a volatile agent immediately after induction. To avoid unnecessary fetal drug exposure, we routinely withhold opioids until after delivery. Although inhalational agents cross the placenta, neonatal uptake is not significant unless induction to delivery time is prolonged. Nitrous oxide is usually administered in concentrations of 50% until delivery and then increased to 70%. Increasing maternal inspired oxygen concentration to 100% is associated with minimal, if any, improvement in fetal oxygenation.

The choice of volatile anesthetic has little effect on outcome; isoflurane has the longest history of maternal and fetal safety. Although the halogenated agents can produce uterine atony at high concentrations, this risk is usually a theoretical one at concentrations less than ⅔ MAC, a concentration that should provide adequate anesthesia with the coadministration of narcotics and nitrous oxide. After delivery, oxytocin (20 units/ liter) is added to the intravenous fluids. If uterine atony unresponsive to oxytocin were to occur, the volatile agent can easily be discontinued and a benzodiazepine administered for amnesia. Most anesthesiologists reduce or discontinue the volatile agent after delivery in order to minimize the risk of uterine atony and postpartum hemorrhage.

THE DIFFICULT AIRWAY

Much attention has been paid to the problem of the difficult airway in obstetrics, because airway misadventures account for most anesthesia-related maternal mortality. The most commonly occurring adverse respiratory events are failure to ventilate, failure to recognize esophageal intubation, and failure to intubate the trachea. Although these are very different events, they all share the cornerstone of difficult tracheal intubation, because the airway of pregnant patients is associated with an eightfold increase in the incidence of difficult intubation. Many theories have been proposed to account for this phenomenon. Increases in body water during pregnancy will result in glossal edema, making the tongue larger and less mobile. Pharyngeal and laryngeal edema also occur, necessitating smaller tracheal tubes. Pregnancy causes nasal capillary engorgement, making nasal intubations and placement of nasal airways relatively contraindicated, as epistaxis can easily result. Increased breast size and difficulty in positioning secondary to left uterine displacement can hamper intubation attempts. Finally, inadequate airway evaluation in emergent situations and inexperienced, fatigued, inadequately trained, and poorly supervised providers rendering obstetric anesthetic coverage will result in poor management decisions.

> ■ KEY POINT: Most airway misadventures occur when airway difficulty is not recognized prior to induction of general anesthesia. Careful airway evaluation, although imperfect, should be performed on all parturients and should identify the majority of these patients.

The pregnant patient is also prone to complications resulting from delays in intubation. The physiologic changes of pregnancy and the resultant decreases in lung volumes and increases in oxygen consumption will result in a precipitous decline in oxygen saturation if ventilation is interrupted during multiple intubation attempts. The parturient is at risk for aspiration, and the occurrence of aspiration is increased in difficult airways that are unprotected during multiple intubation attempts.

The incidence of difficult intubation varies with its definition. Although airways that require more than one attempt to intubate are relatively frequent, the incidence of patients who cannot be intubated (but on whom mask ventilation is possible) is 0.35 to 0.5%. Airways that can be neither intubated nor ventilated are rare: approximately 2 per 10,000 patients. Although this may appear comforting, it is a mixed blessing because most anesthesiologists will have had limited experience in this situation. For this reason, failed intubation drills must be learned and practiced before the event, so that one can act calmly and confidently in the face of a dire situation.

Despite the development and widespread adoption of fiberoptic bronchoscopy, the number of airway-related maternal deaths has not changed significantly in the past decade. This is surprising, because difficult airways can now be managed relatively safely, easily, and expeditiously when they are recognized before induction. If airway-related deaths are related to underutilization of awake fiberoptic bronchoscopy, then their continued prevalence would suggest a deficiency in the preoperative evaluation of the difficult airway.

RECOGNITION OF THE DIFFICULT AIRWAY

Numerous risk factors have been elucidated for difficult intubations (Table 7–4); evaluating the presence or absence of these characteristics has formed the foundation for most preoperative airway evaluations. The most commonly used evaluations center around the size of the tongue relative to the

■ Table 7–4

ANATOMIC FACTORS ASSOCIATED WITH DIFFICULT INTUBATION

Inability to visualize oropharyngeal structures
Receding mandible
Short muscular neck
Full dentition
Protruding incisors
Decreased thyromental distance
Decreased mandibular range of motion
Decreased cervical range of motion
Obesity
Long, high, arched palate

oropharynx and the presence of a receding mandible, buck teeth, obesity, decreased incisor gap, and decreased cervical range of motion.

Problems with Airway Examinations

There are many interpretations of what constitutes a difficult airway, with definitions including difficult but successful intubation, inability to intubate but success in mask ventilation, and complete inability to intubate or ventilate. Although the anticipated difficulty may vary along a continuum, all subsequent management centers around one decision: whether to induce anesthesia before or after intubation has been achieved. Therefore, the ideal airway exam, if it existed, would tell the anesthesiologist simply whether intubation attempts will be successful or not. It would be specific, identifying only the truly difficult airways; it would also be sensitive, missing no difficult airways.

All airway exams in common use fail to achieve these goals. They do not predict success of intubation but rather how much of the vocal cords will be seen during laryngoscopy. They do not even tell which view will be seen but rather the probability of a particular view. All commonly used airway exams were developed using nonpregnant patients. Because pregnancy can change airway anatomy, difficulties in extrapolating the results to a pregnant population are to be expected. Airway exams changing during pregnancy have been documented, as have changing scores during labor and delivery.

Difficult airways can be the result of a multitude of factors. No airway examination, however, addresses more than just a few of these. Airway exams are difficult to perform correctly. Improvements on older exams, changing definitions in the literature, and variable methods of performing the exams (sitting vs. supine, head position) add to the confusion. When visualizing pharyngeal structures, phonation can elevate the uvula, making a difficult airway appear easy. Many variables are subjective (e.g., small chin, buck teeth, etc.). Even among experienced anesthesiologists using rigid criteria, interobserver variability is common.[2]

Most importantly, airway exams are neither sensitive nor specific. False negatives (difficult airways that look easy) and false positives (easy airways that look difficult) abound. Although a false-positive test will result in the inconvenience and fetal risks of delayed delivery during awake intubation, the risks to the mother are minimal. Conversely, a false-negative result will cause general anesthesia to be induced in a patient who may not be able to be intubated or ventilated. Although the relative importance of fetal versus maternal safety is a personal judgment, the maternal risks of airway mishaps generally outweigh the fetal risks of minimally delayed delivery.

Current airway exams have attempted to correlate external airway anatomy with the degree of laryngeal exposure obtained during direct laryngoscopy.[3] The most commonly used measure of laryngeal exposure recognizes four grades (Fig. 7-1). These range from complete visualization of the vocal cords (grade I) to a partial view of the vocal cords (grade II), epiglottis only (grade III), and the inability to view even epiglottis (grade IV).

Specific Tests

The Mallampati test[4] evaluates the size of the tongue in relation to the oropharynx. The patient is asked to sit up, open her mouth with the head in a neutral position, and stick out her tongue without phonating. Subsequent investigation[5] found greater accuracy when head extension and phonation were performed. The airway is rated by the ability to visualize certain oropharyngeal structures (Fig. 7-2). Mallampati et al.

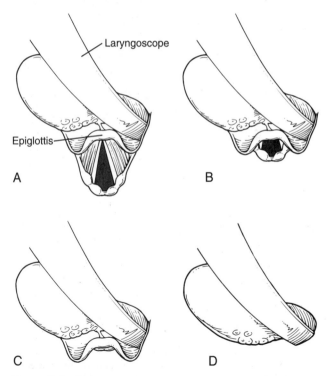

Figure 7-1 ■ The four grades of the most commonly used measure of laryngeal exposure. (From Cormack RS, Lehane J: Difficult tracheal intubation: a retrospective study. Anesthesia 39:1105-1111, 1984.)

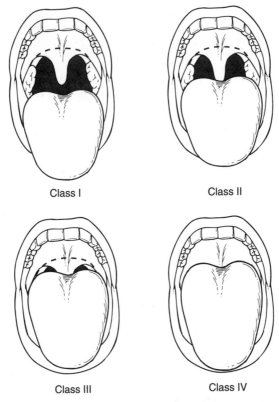

Figure 7–2 ■ The external airway anatomy is rated by the ability to visualize certain oropharyngeal structures. (From Samsoon G, Young J: Difficult tracheal intubation: a retrospective study. Anesthesia 42:487–490, 1987.)

described three classes; class IV was added by Samsoon and Young[6]:

- Class I: faucial pillars, soft palate, and entire uvula;
- Class II: faucial pillars, soft palate, and base of the uvula;
- Class III: soft palate only;
- Class IV: hard palate only.

The Wilson risk sum test[7] identifies five risk factors for difficult intubation. Weight, head and neck movement, jaw movement, receding mandible, and buck teeth are evaluated on a scale of 0 to 2 and total score summed. Tongue size and oropharyngeal visualization are not evaluated. A score greater than 2 is considered predictive of a difficult intubation.

A study of 1500 parturients having cesarean section under general anesthesia prospectively evaluated potential risk fac-

■ Table 7–5
RELATIVE RISK OF FACTORS ASSOCIATED WITH DIFFICULTY AT TRACHEAL INTUBATION COMPARED WITH UNCOMPLICATED MALLAMPATI CLASS I

Risk Factor	Relative Risk
Mallampati class	
II	3.23
III	7.58
IV	11.30
Short neck	5.01
Receding mandible	9.71
Protruding maxillary incisors	8.0

Adapted from Rocke DA, Murray WB, Rout CC, et al: Relative risk analysis of factors associated with difficult intubation in obstetric anesthesia. Anesthesiology 77:67-73, 1992.

tors for difficult intubation.[8] Mallampati class, obesity, short neck, missing or protruding maxillary incisors, receding mandible, facial edema, and swollen tongue were noted. Although facial and lingual edema were not found to be risk factors, high Mallampati class, short neck, receding mandible, and protruding maxillary incisors increased the relative risk of difficult intubation (Table 7-5). The contribution these risk factors made are summated in Figure 7-3.

A recently described test[9] uses laryngeal view during indirect laryngoscopy to predict difficult intubation. Although obstetric patients were excluded from the study, indirect laryngoscopy was superior to both Mallampati and Wilson risk sum evaluations with respect to sensitivity, specificity, and positive predictive value (Table 7-6). Although sensitivity was increased (69.2%), almost one third of all difficult intubations

■ Table 7–6
POSITIVE PREDICTIVE VALUE (PPV), SENSITIVITY, AND SPECIFICITY OF THREE PREDICTIVE METHODS

	PPV (%)	Sensitivity (%)	Specificity (%)
Prediction with Wilson risk sum score	5.9	55.4	86.1
Prediction with modified Mallampati score	2.2	67.9	52.5
Prediction with indirect laryngoscopy	31.0*	69.2†	98.4*

*$p < 0.01$ vs. Wilson risk sum and modified Mallampati score.
†$p < 0.01$ vs. Wilson risk sum score.

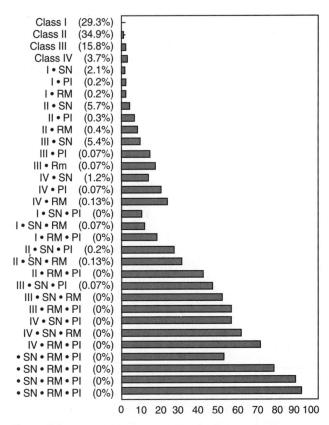

Figure 7–3 ■ The probability of experiencing a difficult intubation for the varying combinations of risk factors and the observed incidence of these combinations. (From Rock D, Murray W, Rout C, et al: Relative risk factors associated with difficult intubation in obstetric anesthesia. Anesthesiology 77:67–73, 1992.)

still were not predicted to be difficult. Positive predictive value was dramatically increased but still would identify over twice as many false positives as true positives. Use of Mallampati or Wilson criteria would yield less useful results.

Recommendations

Airway evaluation is, at best, an imperfect science. Approximately one half to one third of difficult airways will be missed, and when an airway is predicted to be difficult, the chance of a false positive is so great that it is easy to discount this usually erroneous prediction. How can we safely care for patients when the best test will frequently be wrong? Should all patients be intubated awake so that no unanticipated difficult airways are encountered? Although it is difficult to find fault with this argument, difficult airways are relatively rare, and the overwhelming majority of patients will experience an unnecessary awake intubation. Should we tolerate lesser degrees of caution and subject a small number of our patients to the risks of airway misadventures? Personal thresholds and practice patterns will vary widely based on experience, concern for fetal well-being, and tolerance for false-negative and false-positive errors. However, the following recommendations should be applicable to most situations.

Because unanticipated difficult airways are an unfortunate reality of obstetric practice, preparation for them is essential. A difficult intubation drill must be developed and regularly reviewed. All resuscitative and emergency equipment must be maintained, clearly labeled, and rapidly obtainable. When inducing general anesthesia, if there is any doubt about the parturient's airway, gentle mask ventilation with cricoid pressure may be attempted while awaiting intubating conditions. Maintaining low inspiratory pressures should minimize gastric dilation, and knowing whether mask ventilation is possible will help to plan one's next move if intubation attempts fail. Additionally, we occasionally mark the cricothyroid membrane before induction in anticipation of possible cricothyrotomy.

Early identification of the patient with a difficult airway is crucial. When a difficult airway is anticipated, then communication with the patient and obstetric team is essential if airway concerns will take precedence over fetal indications for an expeditious delivery and an awake intubation will be necessary. This is a topic that is much easier to discuss early in labor rather than in the face of fetal asphyxia. If a "crash" induction will be denied, then other options for delivery must be explored.

Elective Cesarean Delivery

Although many options can provide reasonably rapid and sure anesthesia for most obstetric emergencies, it is always possible that the anesthetic may be inadequate, delaying operative delivery. It is reasonable for the obstetrician to choose to perform an elective cesarean section rather than risk the possibility of fetal asphyxia occurring without a means to perform an immediate general anesthetic.

Regional Anesthesia

The decision to perform regional anesthesia on a patient with a questionable airway is a controversial one. Although a successful regional anesthetic will usually obviate the need for airway management, complications such as maternal hemorrhage, intravascular catheters, high spinals, total spinals, and failed blocks can and do occur. In the event of any of these complications, one may need to manage a difficult airway emergently while simultaneously resuscitating the patient. Because of this, a few practitioners prefer to avoid this possibility and perform a general anesthetic, managing the difficult airway electively and definitively with an awake intubation followed by a general anesthetic.

Nevertheless, a functioning epidural or spinal catheter can provide surgical anesthesia for most obstetric emergencies, and early placement of an epidural catheter has been advocated for difficult airways. In the event of fetal asphyxia, if the epidural is dosed with local anesthetic in the labor room at the time of the decision for emergent cesarean section, adequate anesthesia can usually be achieved by the time the patient is in the operating room and prepped for surgery. Although effective and frequently practiced, this technique is fraught with risk. Large volumes of local anesthetic will be given rapidly, making testing of catheter location difficult. Monitoring of the patient during transport may be impractical, and ephedrine may be needed to treat presumed hypotension when unable to monitor. Titration of the block is not practical with the initial bolus, and inappropriate levels can occur.

A continuous spinal anesthetic will avoid some of these risks when an "epidural" catheter is placed into the subarachnoid space. Aspiration of cerebrospinal fluid will confirm correct position of the catheter. The rapid onset of a spinal block will make titration easier and allow dosing in the operating room after adequate monitoring has been achieved. One disadvantage is the need to create a large dural puncture with an epidural needle. Although a postdural-puncture headache will likely result from this technique, it is preferable to the risk of losing an airway. One patient population in which subarachnoid catheters may be especially useful is morbidly obese patients. The benefits of maintaining a natural airway are obvious, and the incidence of postdural-puncture headache in these patients is low.

■ **KEY POINT:** If a parturient with a known "difficult airway" is to undergo a nonemergent cesarean section, regional anesthesia with a catheter technique or general anesthesia via awake fiberoptic intubation should be considered. Continuous spinal anesthesia using a "macrocatheter" offers many advantages in this patient population.

Local Anesthesia

Before widespread improvements in regional and general anesthesia, many obstetricians performed cesarean section under local anesthesia. This technique allows a patient to maintain her airway, causes minimal hemodynamic derangements, and can be performed without waiting for an awake intubation or regional anesthetic. Patient discomfort can be expected, often requiring generous sedation. Large volumes of local anesthetic are required, and the anesthesiologist will need to monitor total amount. Dilute lidocaine (0.5%) with epinephrine should allow an adequate volume; if this is insufficient, additional 2-chloroprocaine, because of its rapid plasma hydrolysis, can be offered. Most obstetricians, however, are inexperienced in this technique. It is unfortunate that this technique is infrequently taught, because it should be considered when fetal asphyxia occurs in a parturient with an unintubatable airway.

Awake Direct Laryngoscopy

When it is unclear if the patient will be difficult to intubate, an "awake look" can provide the answer. With a gentle hand, a frank discussion with the patient, and good airway anesthesia, direct laryngoscopy can be performed atraumatically. Glossopharyngeal block will reduce the gag reflex more effectively than topical oropharyngeal anesthesia. In an emergency situation, laryngoscopy can be performed rapidly, especially if awaiting a fiberoptic bronchoscope or additional help. If vocal cords can be seen, then the patient may be intubated at that point or after induction of general anesthesia. If, however, adequate exposure of the larynx is not obtained, then the anesthesiologist can stand firm, knowing that the patient is not a candidate for a rapid-sequence induction, and other anesthetic strategies should be pursued.

MANAGEMENT OF THE DIFFICULT AIRWAY

The goals for the management of the difficult airway fall into two categories depending on whether the airway was diagnosed to be difficult before or after induction of anesthesia. The American Society of Anesthesiologists' difficult airway algorithm, illustrated in Figure 7–4, consists of two arms, each with different objectives. If the patient is anticipated to be difficult to intubate, then management centers around preserving spontaneous ventilation and inducing anesthesia only after the airway is secured. If the patient is found to be difficult to intubate after induction of anesthesia, then management centers around delivering oxygen to the alveoli until spontaneous respirations return or definitive airway control is achieved.

Anticipated Difficult Airway

Although there are many reasonable alternatives to performing a general anesthetic, if general anesthesia is planned, then the patient should be intubated before induction of anesthesia. Exceptions may need to be made for the uncooperative pa-

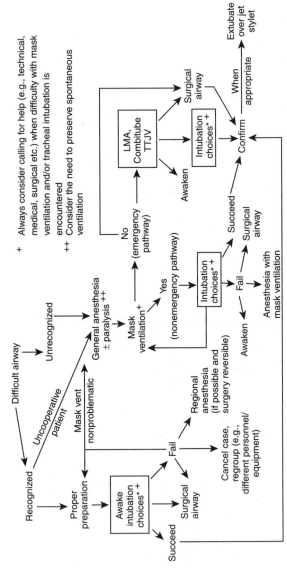

Figure 7–4 ■ The ASA difficult airway algorithm. (From Benumof J: Laryngeal mask airway and the ASA difficult airway algorithm. Anesthesiology 84:(686–699, 1996.)

tient who will not tolerate either awake intubation or creation of a surgical airway. There are numerous methods for managing the patient with a difficult airway:

- Fiberoptic bronchoscopy;
- Retrograde wire intubation;
- Illuminating intubating stylet;
- Intubation through a laryngeal mask airway (blind or via fiberoptic guidance);
- Special intubating laryngoscopes (Bullard, Belscope, etc.);
- Blind nasal intubation (relatively contraindicated);
- Awake cricothyrotomy or tracheostomy under local anesthesia.

Preparation of the patient involves a discussion of the importance of awake intubation and the need for patient cooperation. Glycopyrrolate will assist in drying secretions and allow better application of topical anesthetics. Although respiratory depressant drugs are generally not administered until delivery of the infant, judicious use of sedation will often facilitate awake intubation. Fentanyl can be used, although midazolam, droperidol, and ketamine will cause less respiratory depression.

Airway anesthesia can be obtained through topical local anesthesia, glossopharyngeal and superior laryngeal nerve blocks, and translaryngeal injection through the cricothyroid membrane. Controversy exists regarding whether there is an increased risk of aspiration after airway anesthesia. Although aspiration is a possibility, it will be minimized in the awake, alert, and cooperative patient.

Unanticipated Difficult Airway

For the patient whose trachea is found difficult to intubate after the induction of anesthesia, an additional attempt at tracheal intubation is warranted, but hypoxia will soon ensue, limiting the number of opportunities for laryngoscopy. If the initial attempt to intubate is unsuccessful, then subsequent attempts must differ from the failed one. New blades, head position, laryngoscopes, or use of adjuncts (external laryngeal pressure, Eschmann stylet) may be tried. Repeating an unsuccessful technique will only waste time and traumatize the airway, hindering subsequent attempts to intubate or mask ventilate.

If intubation is still unsuccessful, then the primary objective is to deliver oxygen to the alveoli. Usually this can be accomplished via mask ventilation, although this may require additional maneuvers such as jaw thrust and chin elevation, oral (and possibly nasal) airways, and two-person mask ventilation. Cricoid pressure should be maintained unless it interferes with mask ventilation.

CANNOT INTUBATE; CAN VENTILATE

If intubation is unsuccessful but mask ventilation can be accomplished, then the patient is not in immediate danger of hypoxia, but management dilemmas arise. In the absence of fetal asphyxia, the patient should be allowed to awaken. However, if "fetal distress" or maternal hemorrhage is present, then should the obstetrician be allowed to begin surgery on a patient whose airway is not adequately controlled? Although it might be tenable to defer delivery until a definitive airway (or regional anesthetic) has been established, the cost to the fetus may be enormous. If merited by maternal or fetal indications, most clinicians would consider allowing surgery to proceed while continuing to mask ventilate the patient with cricoid pressure. Communication with the obstetrician is necessary to discuss indications for surgery and to attempt to reduce aspiration risks by minimizing abdominal compression and increases in intragastric pressure with delivery.

If mask ventilation can be performed without difficulty, then we would not place a laryngeal mask airway (LMA) as a primary airway, because this might place the patient at increased risk of aspiration. An exception could be made, however, to place an LMA if it were to be used to facilitate fiberoptic tracheal intubation.

CANNOT INTUBATE; CANNOT VENTILATE

If neither intubation nor ventilation is possible, then a bad outcome is likely if oxygenation is not restored rapidly. Options are limited and include performing a cricothyrotomy, inserting a combitube, or placing an LMA. Help should be sought early so that one can obtain both a skilled assistant and also a surgeon capable of obtaining a surgical airway.

Cricothyrotomy

The cricothyroid membrane should be a familiar landmark for all anesthesiologists. It is relatively avascular, easily identified, and located below the vocal cords. Additionally, most anesthesiologists are comfortable performing cricothyroid puncture. Three airway techniques exploit these qualities to gain access to the trachea via cricothyrotomy.

Transtracheal Jet Ventilation

A large-gauge intravenous catheter is inserted through the cricothyroid membrane and directed caudad; aspiration of air will confirm tracheal placement. The needle is withdrawn, leaving the cannula that can be attached to a transtracheal jet ventilation (TTJV) source. Oxygen under pressure can be injected into the trachea to maintain oxygenation and, frequently, ventilation. Although this technique is lifesaving, rapid, and relatively atraumatic, the following precautions must be considered. First, a route for egress of the exhaled gasses must be present, or intrathoracic pressure will rise dramatically. Second, although gastric contents refluxed into the pharynx may be blown away from the trachea, TTJV does not offer a high degree of protection from aspiration; cricoid pressure must be interrupted to perform cricothyroid puncture. Finally, although TTJV can forestall hypoxia, it is not a definitive airway. The possibility of barotruma or migration of the cannula increases with time, and in the case of cesarean section for fetal asphyxia, it does not provide a means to continue the anesthetic. TTJV would be of greatest utility in nonemergent situations when it is acceptable to awaken the mother or when a temporary means of oxygenation must be instituted while attempts to establish a definitive airway continue.

Percutaneous Dilational Cricothyrotomy

Numerous commercially available kits for percutaneous dilational cricothyrotomy (PDC) can be obtained with both cuffed and uncuffed tracheal tubes. All use a variant of the Seldinger technique for placing a wire through the cricothyroid membrane and then a dilator followed by a tracheal tube over the wire. Although more invasive and time consuming than TTJV, PDC provides protection from aspiration and a means to continue the anesthetic.

Open Surgical Cricothyrotomy

This procedure has become a technique of last resort for establishing an emergency airway. An incision is made through the cricothyroid membrane, the incision is spread, the distal edge is elevated with a clamp or skin hook, and a small cuffed tracheal tube is inserted. Ideally, this procedure should be performed by a surgeon with experience in surgical airways. Occasionally, surgeons (and obstetricians) may offer to perform an emergency tracheostomy. This procedure is rarely appropriate in this situation, because it takes longer to perform than a cricothyrotomy and the overlying thyroid can cause brisk bleeding in the absence of meticulous dissection.

Combitube

The esophageal–tracheal combitube is a double-lumen tube inserted blindly into either the esophagus or trachea (Fig. 7-5). A 100-mL pharyngeal cuff creates a seal against the base of the tongue and the soft palate. A smaller cuff seals the distal lumen against the trachea or esophagus. When the combitube is inserted into the esophagus, the patient will be ventilated via perforations in the proximal lumen; these perforations are located just distal to the pharyngeal cuff and usually face the glottis. The distal lumen in the esophagus can

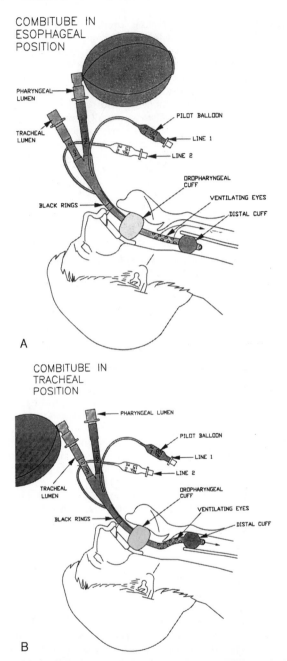

Figure 7–5 ■ The esophageal-tracheal combitube is a double-lumen tube, which is inserted blindly into either the esophagus or trachea. (Courtesy of Kendall, Mansfield MA.)

be used to suction gastric contents, with the inflated esopha-geal cuff affording some protection against aspiration. Occa-sionally, the combitube will be inserted into the trachea, and the distal lumen can be used as a tracheal tube to ventilate the patient. As the combitube is more likely to enter the esophagus after a blind insertion, the proximal lumen will therefore be used to ventilate via its pharyngeal perforations, and the connector to this lumen is made longer for easier identification.

Although the combitube has been used successfully in a variety of clinical situations, it has not gained widespread acceptance in the United States. Success rates for insertion range from 69 to 100%, with most failures secondary to poor retention of training and inappropriate insertion angle. The combitube is intended for single-patient use, making training, routine use, and continued familiarity with the technique relatively expensive and impractical. An additional concern with the combitube involves the possibility of glottic edema, limiting the inflow into the trachea when the combitube is placed into the esophagus.

Laryngeal Mask Airway

The introduction of the LMA (Fig. 7-6) must be considered a milestone in the history of emergency airway management. Originally developed as an alternative to the face mask, it has enjoyed widespread popularity as an airway device intermedi-ate in function between a tracheal tube and a face mask. The LMA creates a low-pressure seal against the hypopharynx and therefore is not suited for patients who will require high inspiratory pressures. Furthermore, the LMA can provide a patent airway in the face of supraglottic obstruction but will be unable to overcome periglottic (e.g., laryngospasm, edema, hematoma) and infraglottic obstructions. Although the elec-tive use of an LMA is contraindicated in the patient at risk for aspiration, the LMA has a definite place in obstetric anesthesia as an emergency airway, because it can be inserted easily and rapidly and can allow ventilation even when it is grossly malpositioned. In addition to its role as an emergency airway, the LMA has found utility as a guide for tracheal intubation. A small tracheal tube can be inserted down the LMA, out the apertures, and through the vocal cords, either blindly or via fiberoptic guidance. Thus, the LMA can be used to achieve tracheal intubation both in the awake patient and in the patient who has an LMA placed emergently.

Although most reports of the LMA as an emergency airway device are anecdotal, a growing number of anesthesiologists are favoring the LMA as an alternative to cricothyrotomy. Adequate ventilation and oxygenation were obtained in over 90% of a nonobstetric population when an LMA was placed by inexperienced personnel. Insertion times averaged 20 sec-

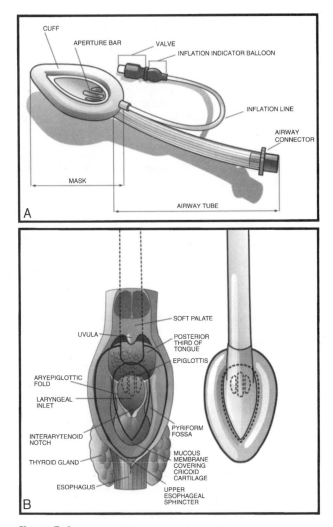

Figure 7–6 ■ *A,* The LMA consists of three main components: an airway tube, mask, and mask inflation line. *B,* The LMA is designed to be a minimally stimulating and invasive device.

onds. After 15 insertions, one study found a success rate of 100%. Whereas numerous methods of insertion have been reported, none has improved upon the method originally described by the inventor, using the LMA fully deflated, midline approach, and no rotation of the LMA. An explanation for this high degree of success is that exact positioning is not essential for adequate function. The position of the LMA with

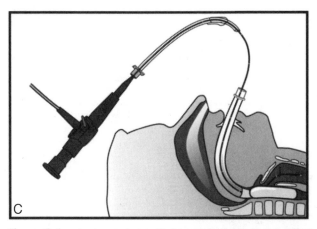

Figure 7–6 ▪ *Continued.* *C,* A well-lubricated fully deflated endotracheal tube is threaded over the fiberoptic bronchoscope. (Courtesy of LMA North America Inc.)

respect to laryngeal structures can be evaluated by fiberoptic inspection; a correctly positioned LMA requires visualization of the laryngeal inlet through the aperture, with the esophagus and epiglottis not seen within the bowl of the LMA. This is achieved in approximately half of all placements. Although visualization of the esophagus is relatively infrequent, the epiglottis is frequently downfolded against the aperture bars, obstructing the view of the laryngeal inlet.

The correct positioning of the LMA is in the hypopharynx, with the tip resting in the upper esophageal sphincter. The application of cricoid pressure before insertion can impede the placement of the LMA. By compressing the hypopharynx and the esophagus, the distal portion of the mask may be prevented from occupying its usual space in the hypopharynx. Although one report found no impediment from cricoid pressure, numerous other investigators have reported failure rates up to 86%. Such wide variability has been ascribed to differences in insertion technique, cricoid pressure, neck support, and head position.

Cricoid pressure can also interfere with the use of the LMA as an intubating guide. It is likely that the LMA will be positioned too high in the pharynx, resulting in the apertures being positioned cephalad to the laryngeal inlet. Additionally, the inflated LMA will function as a fulcrum when cricoid pressure forces the larynx posteriorly, causing the glottis to tilt in an anterior and caudad direction around the tip of the LMA. If a stylet or tracheal tube were advanced from the LMA, then cricoid pressure would have the effect of angulating the glottic inlet away from the tracheal tube, increasing the probability of both failed intubation and glottic trauma from the advancing tube or stylet.

■ **KEY POINT:** The application of cricoid pressure before insertion of an LMA can sometimes prevent proper placement. If that occurs, release cricoid pressure during placement and resume it following correct LMA placement.

Because the LMA is directed toward the esophagus, it would appear that correct placement of the LMA would be easier in patients who were difficult to intubate; however, this speculation is without merit. Attempts to find a correlation between Mallampati class and LMA insertion (and positioning) found either no relationship or that all failures of insertion occurred in only the higher grade Mallampati group. Additionally, this group required more attempts than class I patients.

The use of the LMA in patients at risk for aspiration is controversial. Reports can be found of aspiration during elective use of the LMA and also of no aspiration occurring when the LMA was used in high-risk patients. The tip of the LMA in the esophageal inlet may form a seal against reflux, although LMA insertion has been reported to decrease lower esophageal sphincter pressure, thus increasing the probability of reflux. Fiberoptic visualization of the esophagus within the bowl of the LMA occurs in up to 10% of placements and occurs more frequently when cricoid pressure is applied during LMA insertion. In these instances, gastric contents that reflux into the LMA would likely be directed toward the trachea. Dye studies using methylene blue capsules ingested before anesthesia and ventilation with a face mask versus LMA have shown a higher incidence of staining in the LMA group, even when the esophagus was not visible within the LMA. These investigations were performed without cricoid pressure, however. A correctly placed LMA does not compromise the effectiveness of cricoid pressure in preventing reflux of gastric contents.

The LMA has been used with great success as a conduit for tracheal intubation. In addition to intubating through an LMA placed emergently, the LMA can be placed in an awake patient and used as an intubating guide. An intubating LMA has been developed that has a shorter tube, a grill that can fold forward, and can accommodate a 8.0-mm tracheal tube. The LMA is well tolerated by awake patients after topical pharyngeal anesthesia; instructing the patient to swallow during insertion may facilitate placement. Techniques for intubating through the LMA include blind passage of a lubricated tracheal tube (6.0 mm for a no. 3 or no. 4 LMA, 7.0 mm for a no. 5 LMA), intubating stylet, or fiberoptic bronchoscope through the apertures and into the trachea. Although variable success rates have been reported for blind intubation through the LMA, almost all attempts using fiberoptic bronchoscopy have been successful. Because variability in insertion techniques, aperture location, and glottic angulation with cricoid pressure can confound blind intubation attempts, we recommend fiberoptic visualization when available. As an adjunct to fiberoptic intubations, the LMA was found superior to the Williams airway intubator, with lower mean intubating times. Other potential benefits of the LMA include successful intubation when secretions, blood, or anterior glottic positioning have made conventional fiberoptic intubation impossible, and the LMA can also be used to provide a higher oxygen concentration during fiberoptic intubation. The availability of a new "intubating LMA" should increase the success of securing the airway with an endotracheal tube in a parturient who has experienced a failed intubation.

SUMMARY: THE FAILED INTUBATION

If initial attempts to intubate fail, then mask ventilation with cricoid pressure should be attempted. If attempts to ventilate fail, then cricoid pressure should be relaxed briefly, because tracheal obstruction secondary to cricoid pressure has been reported. If mask ventilation was not achieved, then an LMA should be attempted. Cricoid pressure should be momentarily released while advancing the tip into the hypopharynx. Alternately, an initial attempt could be made with cricoid pressure; if correct positioning is not achieved, then replacing it without cricoid pressure would be appropriate. If ventilation was successful, then, in the absence of fetal or maternal distress, the patient would be allowed to awaken. If fetal asphyxia was present, then allowing surgery to begin would be considered while intubating through the LMA under fiberoptic guidance. If intubation, ventilation, and LMA placement are all unsuccessful, then either a combitube or a cricothyrotomy should be attempted, with fetal condition determining whether TTJV should be instituted or a PDC should be performed.

REFERENCES

1. Hawkins JL, Koonin LM, Palmer SK, et al: Anesthesia-related deaths during obstetric delivery in the United States, 1979–1990. Anesthesiology 86:277–284, 1997.
2. Oates JDL, Macleod AD, Oates PD, et al: Comparison of two methods for predicting difficult intubation. Br J Anaesth 66:305–309, 1991.
3. Cormack RS, Lehane J: Difficult tracheal intubation in obstetrics. Anaesthesia, 39:1105–1111, 1984.
4. Mallampati SR, Gatt SP, Gugino LD, et al: A clinical sign to predict difficult

tracheal intubation: a prospective study. Can Anaesth Soc J 32:429–434, 1985.

5. Lewis ML, Keramati S, Benumof JL, et al: What is the best way to determine oropharyngeal classification and mandibular space length to predict difficult laryngoscopy? Anesthesiology 81:69–75, 1994.

6. Samsoon GLT, Young JRB: Difficult tracheal intubation: a retrospective study. Anaesthesia 42:487–490, 1987.

7. Wilson ME, Spiegelhalter D, Robertson JA, et al: Predicting difficult intubation. Br J Anaesth 61:211–216, 1988.

8. Rocke DA, Murray WB, Rout CC, et al: Relative risk analysis of factors associated with difficult intubation in obstetric anesthesia. Anesthesiology 77:67–73, 1992.

9. Yamamoto K, Tsubokawa T, Shibata K, et al: Predicting difficult intubation with indirect laryngoscopy. Anesthesiology 86:316–321, 1997.

10. Benum of JL: Laryngeal mask airway and the ASA difficult airway algorithm. Anesthesiology 84:686–699, 1996.

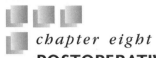

chapter eight

POSTOPERATIVE PAIN MANAGEMENT AFTER CESAREAN DELIVERY

Ferne B. Sevarino, MD

Physiologic responses to surgical injury result in changes to pulmonary, gastrointestinal, and cardiovascular systems.[1] In the parturient, these derangements are superimposed on the normal physiologic changes occurring with pregnancy and delivery. The high-risk parturient with coexisting cardiac or pulmonary disease or pregnancy-induced hypertension is at significant risk for postoperative complications if postoperative pain is not adequately controlled. For these patients, aggressive analgesia through the use of intravenous or neuraxial opioids alone or as part of a multimodal approach is essential to decrease or eliminate the physiologic perturbations associated with poorly controlled postoperative pain.[2]

Most parturients are healthy, without comorbid disease, and can tolerate the changes associated with operative delivery without significant morbidity. The provision of optimal analgesia in these patients presents a different challenge because pain relief must balance with patient satisfaction, which means providing analgesia that has minimal impact on the new mother's ability to bond with her infant.

Intraoperative anesthetic management will have a direct impact on postoperative analgesia. Most nonemergency cesarean deliveries in the United States are performed under regional anesthesia. This provides the opportunity to extend its use into the postoperative period, providing some or all postoperative analgesic therapy. Obstetric postoperative practice also has an impact on postcesarean analgesia. Most parturients remain *non per os* (NPO) only until the first postoperative morning and thus are candidates for early use of oral analgesics to treat pain.

> **■ KEY POINT:** Poorly controlled pain following cesarean section interferes with ambulation, breast feeding, and early maternal-infant bonding.

INTRATHECAL OPIOIDS

As discussed above, the choice of postoperative analgesia is influenced by the intraoperative technique chosen. Intraoperative use of spinal anesthesia permits the use of a single dose of intrathecal opioid or opioid combination, which, depending on the duration of analgesia, would be followed by either parenteral or oral analgesic therapy.

Neuraxial administration of opioids, whether administered intrathecally or epidurally, penetrate spinal tissue in amounts proportional to the agent's lipid solubility. Nociceptive input is blunted effectively as the opioid binds with opioid receptors in the spinal cord. Drugs administered intrathecally are administered in very small amounts, directly into the cerebral spinal fluid, and thus vascular uptake is minimal. Epidural administration is at higher doses and often results in significant vascular uptake, producing plasma levels comparable with those achieved with intramuscular injection.

Morphine

Several studies have attempted to define the optimal dose of intrathecal morphine for postcesarean analgesia. Abboud et al.[3] obtained 18.6 and 27.7 hours of analgesia with 0.1 and 0.25 mg of morphine, respectively. The onset of analgesia with morphine requires 45 to 60 minutes, so coadministration with a more lipophilic agent should be considered for a preemptive effect. Experience with doses less than 0.5 mg intrathecal morphine show reduced respiratory effects, making respiratory monitoring other than routine vital signs unnecessary in the healthy "progesterone-driven" parturient. Neuraxial morphine administration is associated with nonrespiratory side effects, inducing pruritus (40 to 60% incidence) and nausea and vomiting (20 to 60% incidence).[4] Table 8-1 summarizes recommended treatment/prophylaxis for these common side effects.

Lipophilic Opioids

Fentanyl in doses of 12.5 to 25 μg may provide up to 2 to 3 hours of analgesia. Because the effect resolves in the immedi-

■ Table 8–1
**PROPHYLAXIS/TREATMENT OF
OPIOID-RELATED SIDE EFFECTS**

Side Effect	Therapy
Nausea/vomiting	Metoclopramide 10 mg IV q 6 hr
	Droperidol 0.625 mg IV q 6 hr
	Ondansetron 4 mg IV q 6 hr or 8 mg PO q 6 hr
Pruritus	Naloxone 40 μg IV with or without further therapy with 400 μg/L infused in maintenance intravenous fluid.
	Diphenhydramine 25–50 mg IV or PO
Respiratory depression	Naloxone 40–80 μg IV, repeat as needed

ate postoperative period, its advantage is primarily to improve intraoperative anesthesia and to ease the transition to parenteral therapy. Sufentanil, the only opioid approved by the U.S. Food and Drug Administration (FDA) for neuraxial use in obstetrics, also provides approximately 2 to 3 hours of analgesia in doses of 5 to 7.5 μg. Both of these opioids may be associated with pruritus and nausea.

> ■ **KEY POINT:** Lipophilic opioids penetrate spinal tissues rapidly but are also absorbed systemically. Although the onset is rapid, the duration of action of these drugs is relatively short and of little use as a sole agent for postoperative pain management.

Other Opioids and Opioid Combinations

Intrathecal meperidine provides effective postoperative analgesia of intermediate duration (4 to 6 hours) and thus also facilitates the transition to parenteral therapy. Feldman et al.[5] evaluated two doses of meperidine, 10 and 20 mg, both of which provided effective analgesia; however, the higher dose was associated with a high incidence of nausea. Buprenorphine 45 μg has been shown to provide approximately 7 hours of analgesia; however, excessive sedation and a high incidence of nausea and vomiting do not make it an acceptable choice.

Intrathecal administration of morphine in combination with a lipophilic opioid (fentanyl 5 μg + morphine 0.1 mg) offers the advantage of better intraoperative anesthesia with postoperative analgesia comparable with morphine 0.2 mg, with fewer side effects.[6] The combination of 10 mg meperidine with morphine 0.15 mg provided better analgesia and greater patient satisfaction than either drug alone. Table 8–2 provides dosages of commonly administered neuraxial opioids.

> ■ **KEY POINT:** Intrathecal opioid administration provides the most efficient method of activating spinal opioid receptors and the greatest gain in analgesic potency.

EPIDURAL OPIOIDS

Epidural analgesia after cesarean delivery can be used in those patients who had epidural labor analgesia followed by epidural anesthesia for cesarean delivery. These patients usually receive a single dose of epidural opioid, and thereafter oral or parenteral analgesia is used. This approach maximizes analgesia and

■ Table 8–2
POSTCESAREAN ANALGESIC THERAPY

Route	Drug	Dose	Duration
Epidural	Morphine	SD: 3–5 mg	16–24 hr
		CI: 50 μg/mL at 8–10 mL/hr	—
	Meperidine	SD: 50 mg	5–6 hr
		CI: 10 μg/mL at 8–10 mL/hr	—
	Fentanyl	SD: 50–100 μg	2–3 hr
		CI: 4 μg/mL at 10 mL/hr	—
	Sufentanil	SD: 25–50 μg	2–3 hr
		CI: 1 μg/mL at 10 mL/hr	—
	Hydromor-phone	SD: 0.2–0.5 mg	17 hr
		CI: 10 μg/min at 8–10 mL/hr	—
Subarachnoid	Morphine	0.1–0.5 mg	16–24 hr
	Meperidine	10 mg	5–6 hr
	Fentanyl	12.5–25 μg	2–3 hr
	Sufentanil	5–7.5 μg	2–3 hr
IV-PCA	Morphine	Dose: 1–1.5 mg	—
		Interval: 6 min	
		4-hr maximum: 30 mg	
	Meperidine	Dose: 10–15 mg	—
		Interval: 6 min	
		4-hr maximum: 300 mg	
Oral	Meperidine	100–150 mg every 3–4 hr	—
	Ibuprofen	400–800 mg every 3–4 hr	—
	Percocet	1–2 tablets every 3–4 hr	—

SD, single dose; CI, continuous infusion.

patient satisfaction without significantly increasing the side effects of therapy. In the low-risk patient, intravenous patient-controlled analgesia (IV-PCA) opioid therapy, when compared with epidural opioid therapy, was shown to provide the greatest patient satisfaction with the least side effects.[7] Thus, in the uncomplicated patient, lower patient satisfaction combined with the added complexity associated with continuous epidural opioid therapy precludes its use.

Individuals who receive epidural anesthesia due to comorbid disease or the potential for extensive surgery might benefit from continuous postoperative epidural analgesia. The advantages of continuous postoperative epidural analgesia in these patients include superior analgesia, earlier return of bowel function, and less respiratory embarrassment than in patients receiving parenteral analgesia.

The epidural route of administration is complicated by drug penetration of the dura mater, absorption of drug by epidural fat, and by the consequences of vascular uptake and redistribution. In addition to the side effects also seen with intrathecal administration—nausea, vomiting, pruritus—side effects of epidural opioid administration include respiratory depression related to vascular uptake and delayed respiratory depression in patients receiving doses of greater than 5 mg of morphine. This is due to circulation of drug in the cerebrospinal fluid (CSF) to the medullary respiratory center.

Morphine

A single dose of epidural morphine provides effective analgesia for 20 to 24 hours. The optimal dose for postcesarean pain is that which maximizes analgesia while minimizing side effects. Based on information from many investigators, there appears to be no benefit to increasing the dose above 3.75 mg. Continuous epidural infusion (see Table 8–2) of morphine is a reasonable analgesic choice in the high-risk parturient. Again, side effects preclude its use in the low-risk parturient.

Lipophilic Opioids

Lipid-soluble agents leave the CSF rapidly and so are not associated with the delayed respiratory depression seen with the rostral spread of hydrophilic morphine. A bolus dose of epidural fentanyl 50 to 100 μg provides 2 to 3 hours of analgesia. Continuous epidural infusion of fentanyl 4 μg/mL administered at 10 mL/hr provides excellent analgesia with little or no need for supplemental patient-controlled doses.

Sufentanil 25 to 50 μg provides 2 to 3 hours of analgesia. Continuous infusion provides rapid sustained analgesia. Vascular uptake of both fentanyl and sufentanil results in a progressive increase in plasma levels. For this reason, therapy with these opioids should be discontinued at 32 to 36 hours. Early-onset, but not delayed-onset, respiratory depression may occur with epidural fentanyl and sufentanil administration. Side effects of therapy include pruritus (33%), nausea, and vomiting. Unlike with neuraxial morphine, pruritus and nausea with fentanyl and sufentanil are mild and rarely require therapy.

Other Opioids and Opioid Combinations

Meperidine, in a bolus dose of 50 mg, provides 5 to 6 hours of analgesia with few side effects. This immediate duration of action allows a smooth transition to parenteral therapy. It is also efficacious in a continuous infusion; however, the local anesthetic effects associated with its neuraxial use necessitate strict assessment of motor function before allowing the patient out of bed. Buprenorphine, a highly lipid-soluble agent, provides good quality analgesia in doses of 0.15 to 0.2 mg. A high incidence of sedation and respiratory depression limits its use. Butorphanol and nalbuphine, mixed agonists–antagonists, have been administered epidurally with varying degrees of success. Both are associated with an unacceptable degree of maternal sedation.

Hydromorphone has a lipid solubility intermediate between morphine and meperidine. Available in preservative-free solutions, it provides effective analgesia in patients recovering from cesarean delivery. The quality of analgesia experienced with hydromorphine is similar to that seen with morphine, although the onset is faster and the duration is less prolonged. As is the case with all neuraxial opioids used in the parturient, pruritus and nausea are common side effects. Given as a single dose of 0.5 mg, hydromorphone provides analgesia for 12 to 18 hours, after which oral analgesics can be administered. Continuous infusion of 3- to 5-μg/mL solutions at a rate of 10 mL/hr provides excellent postoperative analgesia.

Morphine–fentanyl or morphine–sufentanil combinations provide rapid onset and prolonged duration of analgesia. Patients receiving 50 μg of fentanyl with small doses (1 to 3 mg) of morphine displayed analgesia similar to those receiving 5 mg of morphine alone. Similar effects are seen with morphine (2 mg) and sufentanil (25 μg).

■ KEY POINT: Epidural or intrathecal opioids provide excellent analgesia, a decrease in total opioid administered, decreased sedation, and minimal accumulation in the breast milk.

Patient-Controlled Epidural Analgesia

In those patients in whom continuous epidural infusions are warranted after cesarean delivery, patient-controlled epidural analgesia may allow patients to tailor their analgesic dosing to minimize opioid-related side effects and improve analgesia with movement. The self-administration regimen also allows the patient the psychological benefits of a PCA technique.

INTRAVENOUS PATIENT-CONTROLLED ANALGESIA

IV-PCA is an effective flexible method of pain control after cesarean delivery. In patients in whom regional anesthesia for cesarean delivery is not used, it can be initiated immediately postoperatively. In these cases, the patient is "loaded" with boluses of opioid to establish an analgesic plasma level and then IV-PCA is instituted. Patients who receive neuraxial opioids and who remain NPO when the effects of the administered neuraxial opioid wear off may also safely and effectively use IV-PCA. These patients do not require intravenous loading because they are analgesic from the neuraxial opioid. Timing and dosage of IV-PCA therapy after a bolus dose of neuraxial opioid should be individualized to the neuroaxial medication administered and the patient's response to that therapy.

Advantages of IV-PCA over traditional intramuscular on-demand therapy include the elimination of delays in treatment related to nursing assessment and drug preparation, the rapid absorption and distribution of opioid administered intravenously, and less variability of plasma opioid levels over time.

As referred to earlier in this chapter, healthy patients receiving IV-PCA are more satisfied with their therapy than those receiving epidural morphine. These patients do not report superior analgesia, but they have a lower incidence of opioid-related side effects, which translates into a greater satisfaction with therapy. Parturients seem willing to accept greater discomfort to be more alert, have less nausea, and thus feel better able to interact with their infant.

Maternal use of IV-PCA carries the potential risk of neonatal neurobehavioral changes secondary to opioid distribution via the breast milk and its subsequent distribution and metabolism in the infant. Wittels et al.[8] compared the neonatal effects on maternal IV-PCA morphine and meperidine and concluded that infants exposed to morphine were more alert than those exposed to meperidine. This is likely due to the presence of normeperidine, an active metabolite of meperdine that depends on renal excretion. These behavioral effects resolve over time, and in most infants studied were detectable only with assessment by trained observers.

Commonly used medications for IV-PCA therapy include morphine and meperidine and hydromorphone, fentanyl, and oxymorphone (see Table 8–2).

■ **K E Y   P O I N T :**   Intravenous PCA allows the mother to titrate pain medication in amounts suitable to control excessive discomfort while not causing undue sedation.

ORAL ANALGESIC THERAPY

Postcesarean patients often are given a clear liquid diet on the evening of their operative day or on the morning of the first postoperative day. Patients who received neuraxial opioids with durations of greater than 10 to 12 hours may then transition directly to oral analgesics, eliminating the need and expense of instituting IV-PCA therapy. Patients who initially received IV-PCA therapy may also begin oral analgesic therapy on the first postoperative day, giving them easier mobility because they do not need an intravenous pump. Oral therapy may be with oral opioids or nonsteroidal anti-inflammatory drugs (NSAIDs). If an NSAID is the chosen therapy for your patient, the FDA contraindicates ketorolac tromethamine (Toradol) in nursing mothers. This contraindication does not extend to other NSAIDs. Table 8-2 summarizes the recommended doses for oral medication.

SUMMARY

Analgesia after cesarean delivery requires attention not only to the need for satisfactory pain relief but also to the maternal desire to interact with the newborn infant. Because cesarean delivery often occurs under regional anesthesia, neuraxial opioid therapy should be provided for postoperative analgesia, followed either by intravenous or oral analgesic therapy when additional medication becomes necessary. In those patients who do not receive regional anesthesia, IV-PCA therapy should be initiated in the early postoperative period, followed by oral analgesics when oral therapy is appropriate. The high-risk parturient may benefit from continuous epidural analgesia in the postoperative period. Intraoperative anesthetic choice should encompass this potential benefit.

REFERENCES

1. Blunnie WP, McIlroy PDA, Merrett JD, et al: Cardiovascular and biochemical evidence of stress during major surgery associated with different techniques of anesthesia. Br J Anaesth 55:611-618, 1983.
2. Breslow MJ, Jordan DA, Christopher R, et al: Epidural morphine decreases hypertension by attenuating sympathetic nervous system hyperactivity. JAMA 261:3577-3581, 1989.
3. Abboud TK, Dror A, Mosaad P, et al: Minidose intrathecal morphine for the relief of postcesarean section pain: safety, efficacy, and ventilatory responses to carbon dioxide. Anesth Analg 67:137-141, 1988.
4. Chadwick HS, Ready LB: Intrathecal and epidural morphine sulfate for post cesarean analgesia: a clinical comparison. Anesthesiology 68:925-929, 1988.
5. Feldman JM, Griffin F, Fermo L, et al: Intrathecal meperidine for pain after cesarean delivery: efficacy and dose-response. Anesthesiology 77:A1011, 1992.
6. Naulty JS: The combination of intrathecal morphine and fentanyl for postcesarean analgesia. Anesthesiology 71:A864, 1989.
7. Harrison DM, Sinatra R, Morgese L, et al: Epidural narcotic and patient-controlled analgesia for post cesarean section pain relief. Anesthesiology 68:454-457, 1988.
8. Wittels B, Glosten B, Faure EA, et al: Postcesarean with both epidural morphine and intravenous patient-controlled analgesia: neurobehavioral outcomes among nursing neonates. Anesth Analg 85:600-606, 1997.

Key References

Parker RO: Postoperative analgesia: system techniques. In: Chestnut DH, ed. Obstetrical Anesthesia Principles and Practice. New York: Mosby, 1994:501-512.
Sinatra RS: Postoperative analgesia: epidural and spinal techniques. In: Chestnut DH, ed. Obstetrical Anesthesia Principles and Practice. New York: Mosby, 1994:513-547.

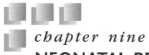

chapter nine
NEONATAL RESUSCITATION
Angela M. Bader, MD

A variety of personnel is available in the delivery room and may be responsible for participating in resuscitation of the newborn. Ideally, this should be accomplished by the most skilled person available, preferably someone other than the obstetrician and anesthesiologist, who are caring for the mother.

■ **KEY POINT:** The American Society of Anesthesiologists Guidelines for Regional Anesthesia in Obstetrics state that qualified personnel *other than the anesthesiologist attending to the mother* should be immediately available to assume responsibility for resuscitation of the newborn.

The availability of pediatricians and neonatal nurses at delivery varies greatly with the institution. It is inherent upon the anesthesiologist to determine the standards at his or her own institution and the personnel designated responsible for immediate neonatal care.

Effective resuscitation demands a knowledge of fetal and neonatal physiology, an understanding of the effects of specific maternal medical conditions on the fetal well-being, and competency regarding the technical skills involved.

Identification of the fetus at risk for requiring significant resuscitation as early during labor as possible is necessary so that appropriate personnel can be prepared. A number of maternal conditions may put the infant at risk; familiarity with these conditions is essential to adequately prepare for the neonate requiring resuscitation.

FETAL PHYSIOLOGY

Cardiovascular Changes

Transition from intrauterine to extrauterine circulatory flow is essential for successful adaptation to extrauterine life. Briefly, the umbilical vein carries the most highly saturated blood from the placenta to the fetus. About half of this blood flow enters the inferior vena cava via the ductus venosus; the other half enters the liver and passes through the hepatic vein before reaching the inferior vena cava. Venous blood from the lower portion of the body joins with the oxygenated blood from the placenta to enter the right atrium. The majority of flow is then shunted via the foramen ovale into the left ventricle and aorta. The intense pulmonary vasoconstriction present in utero results in the majority of blood in the pulmonary artery passing directly through the ductus arteriosus into the descending aorta.

Immediately after delivery, cardiorespiratory changes occur that facilitate the transition to normal extrauterine circulation. Expansion of the lungs with the onset of respiration results in an increase in fetal Po_2 and subsequent decrease in pulmonary vascular resistance and closure of the ductus arteriosus. An increase in pH is also seen as the mixed acidosis present in utero improves. The absence of placental circulation after delivery results in an increase in fetal systemic vascular resistance, leading to closure of the foramen ovale.

Immediate initiation of respiration is therefore essential, because persistence of hypoxia and acidosis will prevent pulmonary vascular resistance from decreasing, prevent closure of the foramen ovale and ductus arteriosus, and result in continued shunting and worsening hypoxemia and acidosis.

Respiratory Changes

After approximately 25 weeks of gestation, pulmonary capillaries have developed to the extent that oxygen and carbon dioxide exchange are possible. Surfactant is present in sufficient quantity on the alveolar surface slightly later. Maternally administered steroids, particularly when given between 28 and 32 weeks of gestation, will facilitate fetal surfactant production. Intratracheal administration of animal and synthetic surfactant at delivery has also been shown to reduce morbidity and mortality from respiratory distress syndrome.

In utero, the tracheobronchial tree is fluid filled. Pressure exerted during vaginal delivery expels a large portion of this fluid from the lungs; the remaining fluid is carried away by lymphatics and capillaries. The lungs of infants born by cesarean delivery will therefore contain more fluid at delivery.

Stimuli to the initiation of respiration include rebound of the thoracic cage from vaginal pressure during delivery, tactile stimulation, umbilical cord clamping, hypoxia, and hypercarbia. High pressures in the range of 40 to 100 cm H_2O are required for initial lung expansion with the first breath to overcome surface tension of the collapsed alveoli. After sustained respiration is established within the first few minutes of life, a tidal volume of 10 to 30 mL with a respiratory rate of 30 to 60/min is maintained.

Thermoregulation

Evaporation of fluids from the skin surface of the neonate and exposure to the cold temperature of the delivery room can result in enormous heat loss and increased oxygen consumption. Minimizing heat loss immediately after delivery is necessary to maintain neonatal temperature; significant decreases in body temperature may result in pulmonary vasoconstriction and increased right to left shunt. Neonates do not shiver when exposed to cold; they maintain heat via nonshivering thermogenesis. In response to a cold environment, the neonate releases norepinephrine that activates an adipose tissue lipase capable of breaking down brown fat. Brown fat is adipose tissue with a rich vascular supply present in several sites in the neonate. Metabolism of brown fat produces heat.

▪ **KEY POINT:** Nonshivering thermogenesis is the primary method of temperature regulation in the newborn. Minimizing heat loss immediately after delivery is essential.

MATERNAL AND FETAL FACTORS ASSOCIATED WITH NEONATAL DEPRESSION

The anesthesiologist needs to be aware of which maternal and fetal conditions can be associated with neonatal depression requiring resuscitation. This requires identification of high-risk patients early in labor so that adequate preparations can be made for the time of delivery. Ideally, in high-risk cases both the anesthesiologist and the pediatrician should perform pre-delivery consultations with the parents so that all are aware of the specific problems that can occur and possible therapeutic options.

The following maternal conditions may put the neonate at increased risk:

1. Hypertensive disorders of pregnancy
2. Cardiac problems resulting in decreased maternal oxygen saturation
   a. Conditions resulting in significant intracardiac shunts
   b. Pulmonary hypertension
3. Diabetes mellitus
4. History of maternal drug or alcohol abuse
5. Maternal infection
6. Placenta previa
7. Abruptio placenta

The following fetal conditions may put the neonate at increased risk:

1. Known congenital anomalies
2. Prematurity (<36 weeks)
3. Postmaturity (>42 weeks)
4. Significant meconium present in amniotic fluid

5. Small-for-gestational-age fetus
6. Macrosomic fetus
7. Abnormal fetal presentation
8. Multiple gestation
9. Evidence of nonreassuring fetal heart rate tracing during labor and delivery
10. Difficult delivery (breech extraction or forceps delivery)

PREPARATION FOR RESUSCITATION

The following recommendations are made by the Joint Program in Neonatology for the labor and delivery rooms at the Brigham and Women's Hospital[1]:

1. Radiant heat warmers; these should be turned on in anticipation of delivery to allow time for warming.
2. Humidified oxygen source with adjustable flowmeter capable of providing 100% oxygen; the flow should be adjusted to between 5 and 8 L/min.
3. Appropriately sized face masks.
4. Flow-through anesthesia bag with adjustable pop-off valve; this should be tested for pop-off control and flow immediately before use.
5. Bulb syringe.
6. Infant stethoscope.
7. Emergency box equipped with
   a. Laryngoscope with no. 0 (for premature infants) and no. 1 (for full-term infants) blades;
   b. 2.5-, 3.0-, and 3.5-mm internal diameter endotracheal tubes. In general, a 3.5-mm tube is used for full-term infants, a 3.0-mm tube for premature infants greater than 1250 g, and a 2.5-mm tube for smaller preterm infants;
   c. Drugs (to be discussed below);
   d. Umbilical catheterization tray with no. 3.5 and no. 5 French catheters;
   e. Syringes, connectors, and stopcocks.
8. Transport incubator with portable heat and oxygen source.

PERFORMING NEONATAL RESUSCITATION

Published algorithms for neonatal resuscitation include the three major steps of evaluation, decision making, and action.[2, 3]

Neonatal Evaluation

The tactile stimulation of the neonate inherent in the delivery process should result in immediate initiation of motor, circulatory, and respiratory activity. The Apgar score is widely used

■ Table 9–1
APGAR SCORING SYSTEM

Sign	Score		
	0	1	2
Heart rate	Absent	Under 100 beats/min	Over 100 beats/min
Respiratory effort	Absent	Slow	Good crying
Tone	Limp	Some flexion	Active motion
Reflex irritability	None	Grimace	Cough or sneeze
Color	Blue, pale	Pink body, blue extremities	All pink

From Apgar V: A proposal for a new method of evaluation of the newborn infant. Anesth Analg 32:260, 1953.

to assess this initial response as a guide upon which to base further intervention (Table 9–1).[4]

Resuscitation of the Normal Neonate

In the healthy newborn with a high Apgar score, the following measures should be performed:

1. The neonate should be immediately placed under a radiant heat source and dried thoroughly.
2. The nose and mouth should be aspirated with a bulb syringe. In most cases, onset of spontaneous respiration will occur simultaneously with clearing of the oral cavity and tactile stimulation. Care should be taken not to stimulate the posterior pharynx with the bulb syringe because this may lead to a reflex bradycardia. Mild nasal flaring and retractions, especially in infants born by cesarean delivery, can be seen initially even in normal healthy newborns but should resolve quickly within the first hour of birth.
3. Standard ophthalmic prophylaxis is given if required.
4. Identification procedures standard for your institution should be performed.

■ **KEY POINT:** Vigorous nasal suctioning should be avoided in the newborn with a normal heart rate, respiratory pattern, and color. Acrocyanosis is common and if the infant has a normal heart rate and respiratory effort, therapy is not necessary. If the Apgar score is less than 8, supplemental oxygen should be considered.

Resuscitation of the Depressed Neonate

The American Heart Association has provided algorithms for delivery room resuscitation.[2] Although the Apgar score can be used as a guide, resuscitative efforts should begin immediately after delivery and should not wait for assignment of the 1-minute score.

Airway Management

In the depressed neonate, adequacy of ventilation should be assessed immediately while administering tactile stimulation. In the syndrome of primary apnea, the infant does not breathe spontaneously but rapidly responds to tactile stimulation with establishment of a normal respiratory pattern. Blow by oxygen can be administered during this period. Secondary apnea involves the persistence of apnea despite tactile stimulation and suctioning and requires immediate bag and mask ventilation.

To achieve adequate bag and mask ventilation, proper positioning of the neonate is essential. The infant's head is relatively larger than that of the adult and a caput may be present. Care should be taken to adequately extend the neck without excessive flexion or hyperextension that may interfere with establishment of adequate ventilation. In some cases, placement of a small roll under the shoulders may facilitate this. Ventilation should be maintained at a rate of about 40/min and a pressure that does not exceed 30 to 35 cm H_2O; normally, 15 to 20 cm H_2O is sufficient. Higher pressures may be required for the initial breath as described above. A built-in pressure release valve with adjustable setting can be extremely helpful. Adequacy of ventilation can be assessed by observation of chest movement and auscultation of breath sounds at the axilla. In most cases, successful bag and mask ventilation can be readily achieved; if there is difficulty, immediate endotracheal intubation may be necessary.

Endotracheal intubation is indicated if bag and mask ventilation is ineffective or in the presence of specific congenital anomalies such as diaphragmatic hernia. After proper positioning, the endotracheal tube inserted under direct visualization and ventilation confirmed as described above.

Circulation

The neonatal heart rate can be assessed immediately after delivery by either direct ausculation of the heart via stethoscope or by palpation of the cord at the umbilicus. If the heart rate is greater than 100 beats/min, ventilation can then be supported if necessary. If the heart rate is less than 100 beats/min, immediate bag and mask ventilation with 100% oxygen is begun. The great majority of these infants will respond with an improvement in heart rate and color after adequate ventilation is established.

Neonatal blood pressure is rarely taken during an acute resuscitation; the adequacy of pulse is felt at the umbilical cord. In the infant, cardiac output is heart rate dependent. Therefore, bradycardia has significant hemodynamic implications. Neonatal blood volume is approximately 90 mL/kg.

■ **KEY POINT:** The newborn's cardiac output depends on the heart rate. Epinephrine is considered to be the drug of choice for treatment of bradycardia.

If the heart rate fails to increase in the presence of bag and mask ventilation, further resuscitative measures are necessary. First, adequacy of ventilation should be ensured by rechecking head position mask seal and oxygen flow. Intubation may be required if bag and mask ventilation is ineffective. Anatomic differences between the neonate and adult need to be considered when respiratory support of the infant is performed.

1. The neonatal head is large relative to the body.
2. The neonatal neck is relatively short.
3. The neonate is an obligate nasal breather; nasal passages are narrow and may be easily blocked by secretions.
4. The cricoid cartilage is the narrowest portion of the airway.
5. The length of the trachea is about 4 cm.
6. The chest is relatively small with ribs more horizontal and the intercostal musculature is more poorly developed.

If the heart rate remains in the range of 60 to 80 beats/min or less in the presence of adequate ventilation with 100% oxygen, chest compressions should be instituted. The most commonly recommended technique involves encircling the infant's chest with the thumbs lying over the middle and lower third of the sternum. The neonate should be lying on a rigid surface while these maneuvers are performed. The sternum is then compressed a distance of 1 to 2 cm at a rate of about 90 to 100 compressions per minute. Ventilation should be continued by a second resuscitator at a ratio of about 1 breath per three compressions. The umbilical cord can be palpated to determine effectiveness of compressions.

After 15 to 30 seconds, the spontaneous heart rate should be assessed and compression and ventilation continued if no improvement is noted. Markedly depressed infants may require medication administration.

Drug Therapy

If the initial heart rate is zero or if no improvement is seen after several minutes of compression and ventilation, the resuscitator should prepare to administer drug therapy. Drug therapy and dosages recommended by the Joint Program of Neonatology at Brigham and Women's Hospital are described below.[1] Several routes of access are available.

Routes of Access for Drug Therapy

1. Generally, the most easily accessible intravenous access in the neonate involves catheterization of the umbilical vein. A 3.5 or 5 French catheter is attached to a syringe and flushed with heparinized saline solution to avoid accidental introduction of air into the vessel. An umbilical tie is placed around the base of the cord, and after a sterile prep the cord is cut horizontally; a length of a least 1 to 1.5 cm should be left. The two smaller thicker walled umbilical arteries and single umbilical vein are identified. The catheter is inserted into the vein with gentle pressure just far enough to establish a good return of blood flow; this usually requires a distance of about 2 to 4 cm of insertion. Inserting the catheter too far risks liver damage from injected medications. Once adequate blood return is established, the umbilical tie can be tightened and the catheter secured with tape.

2. The endotracheal tube can be used to administer certain drugs such as epinephrine and naloxone.

Medications

1. As in an adult resuscitation, the first drug to be administered once access is achieved is epinephrine in a dose of 0.01 to 0.03 mg/kg via the venous catheter. This translates to a dose of about 0.2 mL/kg intravenously or 0.5 mL/kg via the endotracheal tube. The dilution normally used is 1:10,000 (0.1 mg/mL). The dose may be repeated every 5 minutes as needed. For administration via the endotracheal tube, the epinephrine in a dose two to three times the intravenous dose can be diluted to a total volume of 1 to 2 mL and given.

2. Sodium bicarbonate is given only in cases of significant metabolic acidosis and should be given slowly. A dilution of 0.5 mEq/mL is used; the dose is 2 mEq/kg IV given over several minutes. This can be repeated in 5 to 10 minutes as needed.

3. If depression secondary to maternal administration of narcotics is suspected, naloxone can be given in a dose of 0.1 to 0.2 mg/kg. The standard dilution is 0.4 mg/mL, so that the dose given is about 0.25 mL/kg. This dose can be repeated up to three times. Remember to avoid this drug in cases of maternal narcotic addiction because it may precipitate symptoms of withdrawal in the neonate.

Volume Expansion

In the setting of acute bleeding or if the infant's response is still poor despite all efforts described above, volume expansion with albumin or blood can be considered. Acute hypovolemia can be seen in the setting of placental abruption, uterine rupture, fetal–maternal hemorrhage, placenta previa, or twin-twin transfusion. Normal saline, O-negative packed red cells, or 5% albumin can be used. Generally, a volume of 10 mL/kg is administered slowly via the umbilical venous catheter.

■ **KEY POINT:** If intravenous access is not possible, the endotracheal tube can be used to administer resuscitative drugs. Interosseous access can also be utilized, by inserting a 20-gauge needle into the proximal tibia.

SPECIFIC CAUSES OF NEONATAL DEPRESSION

Transient Tachypnea of the Newborn

Transient tachypnea of the newborn is usually a mild disorder of term infants. These infants may exhibit tachypnea, mild retractions, and mild cyanosis. This disorder results from delayed removal of fetal lung fluid. This is more commonly seen in infants delivered by cesarean section in which the vaginal squeeze does not occur. The excess lung fluid results in decreases in pulmonary compliance, fluid filled alveoli, and difficulties with ventilation. In this disorder, symptoms can persist for 12 to 24 hours, and usually only administration of supplemental oxygen by hood or nasal cannula is required. If oxygen requirements are significant, other causes of neonatal respiratory distress should be considered, such as respiratory distress syndrome, pneumonia, or congenital cardiac disease.

Meconium Aspiration

Meconium staining of amniotic fluid is reported to occur in about 10 to 15% of all deliveries. Although historically meconium has been considered a sign of fetal distress, management of the newborn with meconium-stained fluid has been controversial. The concern has been that a small percentage of these infants will develop meconium aspiration syndrome, often associated with air leaks, difficulty with ventilation, and persistence of fetal circulation.[5, 6] The mortality of this syndrome has been reported to be as high as 50%.

Initially, tracheal intubation was recommended regardless of the level of vigor of the infant and the thickness of the meconium. Recently, evidence suggests that changes resulting in persistent pulmonary hypertension may have been present chronically in utero and not a result of aspiration at birth; however, suctioning may decrease the severity of symptoms in infants predisposed to develop the syndrome. Routine suctioning of the vigorous infant with thin meconium may be associated with increased morbidity from airway trauma; how-ever, some authors believe that infants who develop meco-nium aspiration syndrome but were not initially suctioned may be at higher risk for complications.

Current recommendations include the following. Initial management should be done by the obstetrician with suc-tioning of the mouth and pharynx via bulb syringe after the head is delivered and before the onset of sustained respiration. If the meconium is thin and the infant vigorous, the infant should be carefully assessed, but generally no special treat-ment is required. If the meconium is thick or particulate, the infant should be immediately evaluated by the pediatrician and tracheal aspiration of the meconium performed, prefera-bly before the onset of respiration. Tracheal suctioning should be repeated until no further meconium can be removed. Gastric emptying should be also done to remove meconium in the stomach that could potentially be aspirated.

■ **KEY POINT:** Prevention of meconium aspiration should be attempted by use of nasopharyngeal and oropharyn-geal suctioning before delivery of the shoulders of meconium-exposed neonates. Endotracheal intubation and suctioning should be performed in those newborns exposed to thick or particulate meconium.

Infants with severe meconium aspiration syndrome may experience complications of air leaks and persistent pulmo-nary hypertension, with failure of the fetal circulation to con-vert to the typical extrauterine pattern, high pulmonary pres-sures, and persistent hypoxemia.

Pneumothorax

In the infant who fails to improve despite establishment of adequate ventilation, the presence of an air leak should be considered. Tachypnea, cyanosis, and chest asymmetry with decreased breath sounds and overexpansion on the side with the pneumothorax may be seen. Bradycardia and hypotension are frequent. Diagnostic thoracentesis can be performed with a butterfly needle connected to a syringe and inserted at the second intercostal space in the midclavicular line. If a pneumothorax is present, air will flow rapidly into the syringe when the needle enters the pleural space. Spontaneous pneu-mothoraces occur in a small percentage of all newborns. Most are small and will not require treatment.

Prematurity

The premature infant requires special considerations in the delivery room.[7] The Apgar score is not designed to be accurate in the presence of prematurity and is less reliable for assessment. Equipment appropriately sized for the anticipated gestational age should be available as described above. Extremely premature infants will frequently require intubation in the delivery room and may require higher ventilatory pressures to adequately support respiration in lungs that are deficient of surfactant. Warming is especially critical because these infants have decreased subcutaneous tissue and fat stores. These infants may experience complications of intraventricular hemorrhage, necrotizing enterocolitis, and retinopathy of prematurity and respiratory complications and chronic lung disease.

Respiratory distress syndrome is associated with surfactant deficiency in the premature infant.[8] These infants exhibit diffuse atelectasis with resultant ventilatory inadequacy and need for respiratory support. Maternal glucocorticoid therapy is recommended for infants with gestational ages of less than 34 weeks to accelerate fetal lung maturation. Improvement in neonatal outcome is seen after 24 hours of treatment and will last for about 7 days.

Surfactant replacement therapy given through the endotracheal tube may decrease the morbidity from this disorder. Ideally, this should be given as soon as the diagnosis of respiratory distress syndrome is made and initial resuscitative efforts have been performed. In extremely premature infants, prophylactic therapy may be warranted.

Choanal Atresia

The neonate is an obligate nasal breather; therefore, anatomic obstruction of the nasal passage can result in the cyanosis at rest that improves when crying and the mouth is open. Treatment involves establishment of an oral airway and definitive evaluation and therapy performed in the neonatal nursery. Swallowing may be difficult, necessitating intravenous hydration until the disorder can be corrected.

Diaphragmatic Hernia

Diaphragmatic hernia is a rare condition occurring in between 1:3000 and 1:10,000 live births. In this condition, formation of the musculature of the diaphragm is incorrect and a portion of the abdominal contents herniate through the opening into the chest.[9] Herniation is more commonly seen on the left side, with hypoplasia on the lung resulting from compression and inability to achieve appropriate lung development of the affected side.

With the advent of more routine prenatal ultrasonography, most of these infants are diagnosed antenatally so that appropriate plans for resuscitation and therapy can be made. These infants are usually tachypneic and cyanotic immediately after delivery. The abdomen is scaphoid and the heart is usually displaced to the side opposite the hernia. This infant may rapidly deteriorate if bag and mask ventilation is applied because of expansion of the abdominal contents that are in the chest, resulting in further lung compression.

Therapy is therefore as follows. Bag and mask ventilation should not be used and the infant should be immediately intubated and 100% oxygen administered. Excessive pressures (<25 cm) should not be used to avoid producing a pneumothorax. Relatively lower peak pressures and a rapid rate of 60 to 80 breaths/min should be used. Placing the infant with the head slightly up may prevent the hernia from enlarging. A nasogastric tube should be placed as well. Arrangements should be made for immediate transportation to an intensive care nursery. Mortality from this disorder is in the range of 40%.

Tracheoesophageal Fistula

In this disorder, the esophagus has developed abnormally. There is typically an atresia of the upper esophagus and a fistula between the trachea and lower esophagus (about 85% of cases). These infants will present with drooling, coughing, and cyanosis. Aspiration results in bronchospasm and respiratory distress. Abdominal distention can be seen from air traveling from the fistula into the lower esophagus. A significant percentage of these infants will have associated congenital cardiac disease.

Inability to pass a catheter into the stomach will help diagnose this disorder. A multiple-hole suction catheter should be placed in the proximal pouch and put to suction to remove secretions and decrease aspiration. Definitive surgical therapy is warranted.[9]

■ **K E Y   P O I N T :**   If a tracheoesophageal fistula is suspected, bag and mask ventilation should not be used. If mechanical ventilation is necessary, an endotracheal tube should be inserted.

Maternal Substance Abuse

Maternal substance abuse is being recognized with increasing frequency, and specific inquiries in this regard need to be a part of every maternal medical history. The most commonly abused drugs currently include cannabinoids, heroin, and cocaine.[10]

Cocaine abuse during pregnancy has been associated with an increased risk of premature labor, spontaneous abortion, and placental abruption. Uterine contractility is increased; maternal hypertension and abnormalities of uteroplacental blood flow can be seen. The fetus is therefore at risk from the complications resulting from any of these conditions.

Infants of cocaine-addicted mothers rarely require pharmacologic treatment unless other drugs have been abused as well. These infants may exhibit neurologic abnormalities at birth.

Maternal narcotic addiction can result in symptoms of acute narcotic withdrawal in the neonate. The onset of symptoms can vary from shortly after birth to 2 weeks of age. Severity of symptoms depends on the amount of drug used and may be exhibited as irritability, vomiting and diarrhea, tremors, and, in severe cases, seizures. These infants should be transferred to the neonatal nursery for evaluation and treatment planning. Neonatal morphine solution can be used if symptomatic treatment is ineffective.

REFERENCES

1. Ringer SA: Resuscitation in the delivery room. In: Cloherty JP, Start AR, ed. Manual of Neonatal Care, 4th ed. Philadelphia: Lippincott-Raven, 1998:53-64.
2. Bloom RS, Cropley C: Textbok of Neonatal Resuscitation. Dallas: American Heart Association, 1994:1-36.
3. Ringer SA, Stark AS: Management of neonatal emergencies in the delivery room. Clin Perinatol 16:23-41, 1989.
4. Apgar V: A proposal for a new method of evaluation of the new born infant. Anesth Analg 32:260-267, 1953.
5. Wiswell TE, Henley MA: Intratracheal suctioning, systemic infection and the mecomium aspiration syndrome. Pediatrics 9:203-206, 1992.
6. Wiswell TE, Tussle JM, Turner BS: Meconiumn aspiration syndrome: have we made a difference? Pediatrics 85:715-721, 1990.
7. Allen MC, Donohue PK, Dusman AE: The limit of viability-neonatal outcome of infants born at 22 to 25 weeks gestation. N Engl J Med 329:1597-1601, 1993.
8. Jobe AH: Pulmonary surfactant therapy. N Engl J Med 328:861-868, 1993.
9. Dillon PW, Cilley RE: Newborn surgical emergencies. Pediatr Clin North Am 40:1289-1314, 1993.
10. Schechner S: Drug abuse and withdrawal. In: Cloherty JP, Start AR, eds. Manual of Neonatal Care, 4th ed. Philadelphia: Lippincott-Raven, 1998:211-224.

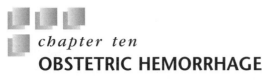

chapter ten
OBSTETRIC HEMORRHAGE
Maya S. Suresh, MD

INCIDENCE AND ETIOLOGY OF OBSTETRIC HEMORRHAGE

The most common causes of third-trimester bleeding are placenta previa (22%) and abruptio placenta (31%). In the remaining 47% of cases, uterine rupture, local genital tract lesions, and marginal placental sinus bleeding may be responsible for bleeding. Given the potential for loss of both mother and fetus, all antepartum bleeding should be immediately assessed and, as far as is possible, a definite diagnosis should be made.

CLINICAL STAGING AND CLASSIFICATION OF HEMORRHAGE IN THE PREGNANT PATIENT

Average blood loss for single and twin vaginal deliveries is 500 and 900 mL, respectively. Blood loss typically measures 1000 mL for repeat cesarean section. The average 60-kg pregnant woman's blood volume is 6000 mL at 30 weeks gestation. Blood loss of 1000 mL leads to vasoconstriction in both arterial and venous compartments to preserve essential vital organ blood flow. With blood loss that has occurred 4 hours earlier, the phenomenon of transcapillary refill leads to significant fluid shifts from interstitial space into intravascular space to partially correct the volume deficit. Traditional signs of hypovolemic shock in the nonpregnant person become evident after 15 to 20% of total blood volume is lost. Hemorrhage in the parturient is classified into one of four classes, depending on the degree of blood loss.[1, 2] The clinical findings and manifestations are shown in Table 10–1.

■ KEY POINT: The hematocrit alone is not a good indicator of blood loss. Significant changes in hematocrit after an acute blood loss may take 4 hours; complete compensation may not occur until 48 hours. Urine output is a superior indicator, and adequate urine production is a positive indication of adequate perfusion posthemorrhage.

■ Table 10–1
**CLASSIFICATION AND CLINICAL STAGING
OF HEMORRHAGIC SHOCK IN
THE PREGNANT WOMAN**

Class	Acute Blood Loss (mL)	Percent Lost	Clinical Findings	Severity of Shock
I	900	15	None	None
II	1200–1500	20–25	Tachycardia (100 ± beats/min) Mild hypotension, peripheral vasoconstriction (VC)	Mild
III	1800–2100	30–35	Tachycardia (100–120) Hypotension (80–100 mm Hg) Restlessness, oliguria	Moderate
IV	2400	40	Tachycardia (>120 beats/min) Hypotension (<60 mm Hg) Altered consciousness Anuria	Severe

Modified from Gonik B: Intensive cardiac monitoring of the critically ill pregnant patient. In Creasky RK, Resnik P (eds), Maternal Fetal Medicine, 2nd ed. Philadelphia: W.B. Saunders, 1989; and Baker RN: Hemorrhage in obstetrics. Obstet Gynecol Annu 6:295, 1977.

ASSESSMENT, MONITORING, AND MANAGEMENT OF HEMORRHAGIC SHOCK

The two basic goals in the management of hemorrhagic shock are restoration of blood volume with adequate oxygen-carrying capacity and definitive treatment of the underlying disorder. The degree of obstetric hemorrhage encountered may not allow full resuscitation to occur, especially with ongoing extensive blood loss. An algorithm for management of hemorrhagic shock is shown in Figure 10–1.

Rapid-infusion devices using mechanical pumps may be necessary to force fluid through low-resistance tubing. Warming of intravenous fluids and keeping the parturient warm are extremely important, especially if the parturient requires several exchanges of blood volume, because hypothermia decreases the effectiveness of hemorrhagic shock resuscitation.

The priorities in hemodynamic resuscitation of obstetric hemorrhage in decreasing order of importance include restoring blood volume, hemoglobin concentration, and coagulation. Proponents of crystalloid use claim that such solutions replace extracellular water more effectively than colloidal solu-

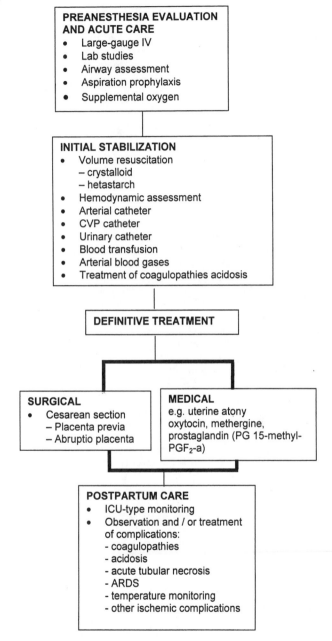

PREANESTHESIA EVALUATION AND ACUTE CARE
- Large-gauge IV
- Lab studies
- Airway assessment
- Aspiration prophylaxis
- Supplemental oxygen

INITIAL STABILIZATION
- Volume resuscitation
  - crystalloid
  - hetastarch
- Hemodynamic assessment
- Arterial catheter
- CVP catheter
- Urinary catheter
- Blood transfusion
- Arterial blood gases
- Treatment of coagulopathies acidosis

DEFINITIVE TREATMENT

SURGICAL
- Cesarean section
  - Placenta previa
  - Abruptio placenta

MEDICAL
e.g. uterine atony
oxytocin, methergine,
prostaglandin (PG 15-methyl-
$PG F_2$-a)

POSTPARTUM CARE
- ICU-type monitoring
- Observation and / or treatment of complications:
  - coagulopathies
  - acidosis
  - acute tubular necrosis
  - ARDS
  - temperature monitoring
  - other ischemic complications

Figure 10–1 ■ Algorithm for management of hemorrhagic shock. CVP, central venous pressure; ARDS, adult respiratory distress syndrome. (From Suresh MS, Belfort MA: Antepartum hemorrhage. In: Datta S (ed): Anesthetic and Obstetric Management of High-Risk Pregnancy, 2nd ed. St. Louis: Mosby Yearbook, 1996.)

tion. Studies in nonpregnant patients show that colloid solutions such as hydroxyethyl starch preserve intravascular volume and microcirculatory blood flow more efficiently than crystalloids, and they increase cardiac output and oxygen delivery and blood pressure at much lower infused volumes than do crystalloid solutions. Generally accepted replacement is 3 mL of crystalloid solution per 1 mL of blood lost. Crystalloid solutions may merely restore blood pressure without increasing cardiac output. A reasonable approach is to use a balanced crystalloid/colloid regimen until the point at which blood component therapy becomes necessary.

For blood loss ≤ 30% of pregnant blood volume, crystalloid replacement of three times the volume of shed blood volume will provide adequate resuscitation as long as hemorrhage is controlled. Patients with 30% of blood volume or with continuing hemorrhage not only require colloid replacement but also require 100% oxygen to maximize oxygen delivery to the tissues until hemoglobin can be replaced.

Patients with hemorrhage > 35% of blood volume require immediate red blood cell (RBC) transfusion along with colloid or crystalloid resuscitation fluids. Type O-negative packed cells can be safely administered to these patients without typing or crossmatch. Significant coagulopathy should be corrected with appropriate blood component therapy (Table 10-2).

Shock is usually accompanied by some degree of metabolic acidosis. Usually, enhancing perfusion to vital organs and peripheral tissues will correct the acidosis. However, severe acidosis (pH < 7.2) may be corrected with sodium bicarbonate. Care must be taken to avoid hypercapnia, hypokalemia, fluid overload, and overcorrection of acidosis during administration of bicarbonate.

The type of definitive treatment (medical or surgical) necessary varies with the etiology, severity, and therapeutic re-

■ Table 10–2
GUIDELINES FOR BLOOD PRODUCT ADMINISTRATION TO CORRECT COAGULOPATHY

Fresh Frozen Plasma	Platelets	Cryoprecipitate
Generalized bleeding	One platelet concentrate usually produces an ↑ of 7000–10,000 platelets in a 70-kg adult	1.4 bag per 10 kg ↑ fibrinogen level is ~100 mg/dL
Partial thromboplastin time > 1.5 times		70-kg patient requires 10 bags of cryoprecipitate
↓ Factors V, VIII	Ten units of platelet concentrate required to ↑ platelet count by 100,000	100 mg/dL—hemostasis 200 mg/dL—prevents further bleeding

sponse of hemorrhagic shock. Despite surgical intervention to treat the etiology of obstetric hemorrhage, blood and blood product replacement, management of ongoing hemorrhage involves uterine or hypogastric artery ligation, thus preserving fertility. However, in cases of refractory hemorrhage, a hysterectomy may be the definitive treatment.

Management and treatment of hemorrhagic shock are gauged by resolution of clinical symptoms and signs of shock, stabilization of vital signs, normalization of hemodynamic assessment, and restoration of urine output. Subsequent management is directed toward the detection and treatment of the complications of shock.

ABRUPTIO PLACENTAE

Abruptio placentae is defined as the premature separation of a normally situated placenta from its attachment to the decidua basalis before the birth of the fetus. It is also called placental abruption, accidental hemorrhage, or placental separation and is estimated to occur in 0.5 to 1.8% of all pregnancies. The placental separation may be complete, partial, or may involve only the placental margin. Complete detachment of placenta with either concealed or torrential hemorrhage can be fatal to the mother and fetus (Fig. 10-2). Maternal mortality ranges from 0 to 3.1% depending on the facilities available for treating the patients. Fifty percent of perinatal deaths from abruption are the result of stillbirths. Abruption associated with hypertension increases fetal mortality threefold.

Pathophysiology

Normal delivery is followed by myometrium contraction, muscle retraction, and compression of the open vascular channels. This mechanism is important for the control of blood loss from the uterus. In an abruption, rupture of a spiral artery

**Partial
separation**

**Marginal
separation**

**Complete
separation
with concealed
hemorrhage**

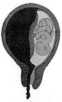
**Complete
separation
with heavy
vaginal bleeding**

Figure 10–2 ■ Various degrees of separation of normally implanted placenta. (Drawn by Carl Clingman, Baylor College of Medicine.)

results in retroplacental clot formation. Hemorrhage occurs into the decidua basalis, and blood, which would normally have perfused the placenta, is pumped into the uterine cavity at a rate that can potentially empty the maternal vascular system within minutes. A retroplacental hematoma then forms and may expand, separating further placenta and involving more vessels. The uterus, distended by products of conception, cannot contract to effectively compress the torn vessels, and persistent retroplacental bleeding results. This process continues, leading to an ever-enlarging retroplacental hematoma and progressive loss of placental function. The presence of fetus and blood clot within the uterine cavity leads to ineffective myometrial contraction and retraction, thus impairing hemostasis at the separation site. In some cases, the maternal blood escapes into the amniotic cavity, but more frequently it tracks between the membranes and the uterine wall, ultimately escaping via the cervix.

Extensive concealed intrauterine hemorrhage results in misdiagnosis, especially if the assessment of the severity of the case is based on the amount of visible vaginal bleeding. Increased intrauterine pressure forces tissue thromboplastin and amniotic debris through open venous sinuses into the maternal circulation. The sudden entry of thromboplastin into maternal circulation seen in conjunction with placental abruption may lead to amniotic fluid embolism and disseminated intravascular coagulation (DIC).

Clinical Diagnosis

The classic signs and symptoms of abruptio placentae include abdominal pain, hemorrhage (revealed, 20 to 35%, or concealed, 65 to 80%), uterine irritability/tetany and tenderness, coagulopathy, and "fetal distress"/death.

Characteristics of bleeding from placental separation is dark and nonclotting: however, sudden separation is arterial looking, massive, and life threatening. The shed blood is almost always a mixture of fetal and maternal blood, and for this reason the fetal condition frequently mirrors the degree of blood loss whether it is revealed or concealed. The different grades and severity of placental abruption and its implications are shown in Table 10-3.

■ **KEY POINT:** Fetal death associated with placental abruption indicates significant hemorrhage (usually >2.5 L), and coagulopathy is a real risk (35%). Coagulopathy and maternal hypovolemic shock should be anticipated and prepared for whenever fetal demise occurs in association with abruption.

■ Table 10–3

SEVERITY OF PLACENTAL ABRUPTION AND ITS IMPLICATIONS

Grade	Severity	Proportion of Placenta Separated	Estimated Blood Loss	Fetal Distress	Hypotension Coagulopathy
I	Mild	Less than ⅙	<250 mL	None	None
II	Moderate	⅙ to ½	250–1000 mL	Common	Unlikely
III	Severe	More than ½	>1000 mL	Usual or intrauterine death occurs	Common

From Gatt SP: Anaesthetic management of the obstetric patient with antepartum or intrapartum haemorrhage. Clin Anaesth 4:373–387, 1986.

Risk Factors

The associated risk factors in abruptio placentae include hypertensive disorders, low-lying placenta or placenta previa, fibroids, trauma, cocaine abuse, cigarette smoking, increased parity and age, physical work and stress, and a history of a previous abruption.

Hypertension

Parturients with chronic hypertension and superimposed preeclampsia (10%) or those with severe preeclampsia (2.3%) or eclampsia (23.6%) have an increased incidence of retroplacental abruption.

Trauma

Blunt trauma, particularly as a result of automobile accidents, is a definite risk for placental abruption. This risk may be exacerbated by lap seat belts. Auto deceleration after collision flattens the uterus against the abdominal wall, which produces an opposite tearing force between the elastic uterine muscle and the unelastic placenta. The placenta separates from the uterine wall, resulting in placental abruption, pain, and bleeding.

Recreational Cocaine Use

Cocaine abuse during pregnancy causes placental vasoconstriction, decreased blood flow to the fetus, increased uterine contractility, and is a risk factor for abruption.

Cigarette Smoking

Cigarette smoking has been shown to increase the incidence of placental abruption, usually in the form of marginal abruption.

■ **KEY POINT:** A pregnant women presenting with acute abdominal pain, vaginal bleeding, or fetal compromise and an associated history of preeclampsia, cocaine abuse, or trauma/automobile accident should be evaluated and have an ultrasound to rule out placental abruption.

Obstetric Management

Major factors in the obstetric management of abruptio placentae are the severity of the abruption as determined by the presence or absence of hypotension and coagulopathy, the gestational age, and the condition of the fetus (Table 10–4).

The decision to proceed with vaginal delivery or cesarean section is based on maternal hemodynamic and coagulation status, the well-being of the fetus, and whether the patient is at term or remote from delivery. Vaginal delivery can be

■ Table 10–4
MANAGEMENT OF PARTURIENTS WITH PLACENTAL SEPARATION

Grade I	Grade II	Grade III
No fetal distress	Fetal distress, but fetus salvageable	Intrauterine death
Cervix more than half dilated	Cervix not dilated ↓ ↓ ↓ ↓	Irrespective of dilatation ↓ ↓
Rupture membranes, start oxytocin	Immediate cesarean section	Vaginal delivery if possible.
Vaginal delivery	Cesarean section	Cesarean if bleeding continues or progress of labor obstructed

From Gatt SP: Anaesthetic management of the obstetric patient with antepartum or intrapartum haemorrhage. Clin Anaesth 4:373-387, 1986.

pursued in the presence of stable maternal hemodynamics coupled with active labor and no fetal distress. Continuous electronic fetal heart rate and intrauterine pressure catheter monitoring are essential. Oxytocin augmentation is not contraindicated if the patient is not already in strong labor. Labor frequently progresses more rapidly in patients with abruption. Blood and blood products should be readily available with preparations for emergency cesarean section should it be necessary. Operative vaginal delivery with forceps or vacuum extractor is not contraindicated and should be used to shorten the second stage of labor.

Occasionally, vaginal delivery can be attempted in cases of severe abruption associated with fetal demise and coagulopathy after appropriate component replacement and oxytocin augmentation as required. Major resuscitation measures for the patient with a dead fetus and DIC are often necessary.

Cesarean section is reserved for usual obstetric indications and for severe hemorrhage or worsening coagulopathy developing at a time remote from expected delivery.

Anesthetic Management

Anesthetic management in abruptio placentae is influenced by maternal hemodynamics and volume status of the mother.

Evaluation

Overt hypotension and tachycardia are signs of dangerous hypovolemia that cannot be ignored. Normal or even hypertensive blood pressure does not preclude imminently dangerous hypovolemia. Hypertension, either pregnancy induced or chronic, is associated with abruption of the placenta. Serious hemorrhage and hypovolemia result in blood pressure drop to normotensive levels. Therefore, normal vital signs in a hypertensive patient can be misleading.

Some parturients who bleed appreciably have normal blood pressure and pulse rate when recumbent. If sitting, they are hypotensive and/or develop tachycardia. In parturients with an epidural who subsequently develop abruption, a sympathetic blockade exaggerates the hypotension in the sitting position. Monitoring and management of hemorrhage is as outlined previously.

■ **KEY POINT:** A normotensive blood pressure reading in a preeclamptic patient creates false security and delays identification of compromised vital organs. The pulse rate may be equally misleading.

Anesthesia for Vaginal/Cesarean Delivery

With mild abruption and absence of fetal compromise, uteroplacental insufficiency, hypovolemia, or coagulopathy, a vaginal delivery is allowed. In these patients, avoid anesthetic drugs or techniques that exaggerate hypotension, thus protecting maternal and fetal safety. Thus, regional anesthesia is relatively contraindicated in a hypovolemic, coagulopathic, or severely compromised fetus. Without these complications, a continuous epidural analgesia technique is used for labor, vaginal, or cesarean delivery in patients with mild abruption. Close attention to hemodynamics and fetal effects is mandatory.

Most cases of severe abruption with acute fetal compromise require abdominal delivery. General endotracheal anesthesia with rapid sequence induction and cricoid pressure is recommended. Ketamine (0.75 to 1 mg/kg) is the optimum induction agent if uterine tone is normal or decreased. Theoretically, larger doses of ketamine in abruption increase uterine tone and further compromise the stressed fetus. Ketamine 2 mg/kg increased uterine tone only in the first trimester. There were no effects on uterine tone at term. Etomidate (0.3 mg/kg) can be used if uterine tone is increased or if hemodynamic instability exists.[3] Uterine relaxation with inhalation anesthetics helps increase placental perfusion. Low doses of inhalational anesthetics also maintain circulatory hemostasis and allows for administration of high inspired oxygen. Halogenated agents, by causing uterine relaxation, potentially increase the risk for blood loss. Although under normal clinical circumstances this is not significant, it may be pertinent in a bleeding parturient.

Complications

The most important sequelae of severe abruption in the post-partum period are uterine atony, postpartum hemorrhage, coagulopathy with DIC, acute renal failure, pituitary necrosis or Sheehan's syndrome, anemia, rhesus sensitization and infection, in utero fetal death, and newborn depression.

Uterine Atony

If excessive bleeding occurs per vagina after vaginal delivery without vaginal or cervical laceration, the uterine fundus is poorly contracted. Exploring the uterine cavity eliminates retained placenta, retained blood clot, and disruption of the uterine wall. Initial management includes bimanual fundal massage and administration of oxytocin 20 to 30 U/L by rapid intravenous rate or via direct intramyometrial injection, methergine or prostaglandin. Intramuscular injection of methergine 0.2 mg is ineffective in a poorly perfused hemorrhagic patient.

■ **KEY POINT:** Methergine should be avoided in patients with antepartum hypertension, preeclampsia, or connective tissue disorders. In these patients, it may precipitate a hypertensive crisis with severe vasospasm.

Prostaglandin derivatives are effective in treating postpartum uterine atony if other modalities fail. Intramyometrial administration of $PGF_{2\alpha}$ is superior to both intravenous or intramuscular injection, especially in patients in shock. Drugs, dosages, and side effects of various pharmacologic agents useful for controlling uterine atony are shown in Table 10–5.

Consumptive Coagulopathy

Placental abruption is the most common cause of consumptive coagulopathy in pregnancy. DIC complicates approximately 10% of all abruptions but is more common in those where fetal death has occurred.

Retroplacental consumption of clotting factors also causes DIC by deposition of substantial fibrin in the uterine cavity. This process stimulates the secondary activation of circulating plasminogen to plasmin, which enzymatically destroys circulating fibrinogen. Thromboplastin release into the maternal circulation from a retroplacental clot is a possible cause of consumption of coagulation factors and platelets. Laboratory evidence of prolonged prothrombin time and partial thromboplastin time, hypofibrinogenemia, thrombocytopenia, and elevated fibrin degradation products confirms DIC.

■ Table 10–5
PHARMACOLOGIC AGENTS USEFUL FOR CONTROLLING UTERINE ATONY

Agent	Dose	Route	Side Effects
Oxytocin (Pitocin)	0–20 units	IV drip, IM, intramyometral (multiple sites)	Hypotension, ↑ heart rate, Water intoxication Uterine hypertonicity: uterine rupture
Ergonovine (Ergotrate) and methylergonovine (Methergine)	0.2 mg	IM	Hypertension, pulmonary/cerebral edema, intracerebral hemorrhage, cardiac arrest
Prostaglandin 15 Methyl $F_{2\alpha}$ Hemabate	0.25 mg 0.25 mg diluted in 10 mL saline	IM Intramyometrial (multiple sites)	↓ Systemic vascular resistance (SVR), ↓ MAP: ↑ Cardiac output, ↑ heart rate, bronchospasm

From Suresh MS, Belfort MA: Antepartum Hemorrhage—Anesthetic and Obstetric Management of High-Risk Pregnancy, 2nd ed. New York: Mosby Yearbook, 1996.

■ **KEY POINT:** A simple observation test in the delivery or emergency room gives immediate clotting assessment for acute situations. This test requires 5 mL maternal venous blood drawn into a clean glass tube, shaken gently, and allowed to stand. If a clot does not form within 6 minutes or the clot is lysed within 1 hour, a clotting defect is present. The fibrinogen level is <100 mg/100 dL when clots fail to form in 30 minutes. Severe hypofibrinogenemia is also noted in abruptio placentae associated with fetal death. Cryoprecipitate is indicated if fibrinogen levels decrease below 100 mg/dL (normally 100 mg/dL is required for adequate hemostasis) and if active bleeding is present.

Dilutional Coagulopathy

Massive transfusion can be defined as the transfusion of 10 or more units of blood or an amount greater than one blood volume. Dilutional coagulopathy causes hemorrhagic diathesis in patients receiving multiple units of blood. Storage temperatures of 4°C damage platelets. They are trapped and absorbed by the reticuloendothelial system. Total platelet activity lessens to 50 to 70% of original in vivo activity after 6 hours. After 24 or 48 hours, platelet activity reduces to 10 or 5% of normal. Infusions of multiple units of stored blood (>24 hours) dilute the patient's available platelet pool.

Prophylactic platelet administration during massive transfusion has no benefit. The practice of giving platelets to treat laboratory evidence should be discouraged. Platelet therapy is needed when the platelet count is below 50,000 to 75,000/mm^3. Each platelet concentrate increases platelet count 10,000 to 12,000/mm^3 in a 70-kg patient.

Fresh frozen plasma contains all the clotting factors except platelets. Most factors are stable in stored blood with two exceptions, factors V and VIII. Factors V and VIII are not stable in stored blood and decrease to 15 and 50% of normal, after 21 days. Packed RBCs have even fewer coagulation factors; consequently, FFP is recommended if generalized bleeding cannot be controlled with surgical hemostasis or cautery, 2 partial thromboplastin time is at least 1.5 times control, and factors V and VIII are deficient based on laboratory evidence. Two to three units of fresh frozen plasma will generally increase factors II, VII, IX, and X to levels adequate for proper coagulation.

Intraoperative Monitoring of Coagulopathy

If a coagulopathy is suspected, the diagnosis should be confirmed with laboratory data, including prothrombin time, activated partial thromboplastin time, platelet counts, fibrin split products, and thromboelastography, if available. The bleeding time evaluates the integrity of the whole blood hemostatic system and although controversial, according to some authors it may be useful for determining the adequacy of platelet function. Most anesthesiologists have abandoned the bleeding time.

■ **KEY POINT:** In anesthetized patients, the bleeding time is difficult to perform, and hypothermia can affect its accuracy. Recently, several reviews have pointed out that the bleeding time is unreliable as a preoperative screening test.

The thromboelastogram (TEG) is a whole blood viscoelastic test and gives information on the platelet function. The maximum amplitude of the tracing is affected by the quality and quantity of platelets; hence, a decreased maximum amplitude suggests a functional platelet disorder. Variables measured by the TEG and the common abnormalities that can be distinguished by means of TEG are shown in Figure 10-3 and Table 10-6.

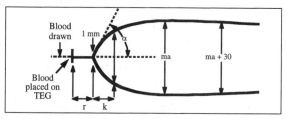

r time (min) = reaction time to initial fibrin formation
k time (min) = rapid fibrin build-up and crosslinking
ma (mm) = maximum amplitude of the TEG trace -- a measure of maximum clot strength and
    dependent on the concentration of fibrinogen, platelet numbers and function
α = angle of divergence -- rate of clot formation
ma + 30 = clot retraction after 30 minutes

Figure 10–3 ■ Typical TEG curve and variables measured. (From Faust RJ: Functional platelet disorders. In: Faust RJ (ed): Anesthesiology Review, 2nd ed. New York: Churchill Livingstone, 1994:481.)

Acute Renal Failure

The overall incidence of renal failure in abruptio placentae is 1.2 to 8.9%. Acute renal failure occurs in severe abruption with and without DIC. It is believed to be secondary to hypotension and hemorrhagic shock (prerenal), microvascular clotting and fibrin deposition in periglomerular arterioles, and myoglobinuria alone or in combination. With acute blood loss, renal blood flow reduces and glomerular filtration decreases. Sodium and water absorption increase, urine sodium content decreases, and urine osmolality rises. Urine sodium concentration of 20 mEq/L and urine/serum osmolar ratio > 2 with urine osmolality > 500 indicate reduced renal perfusion and prerenal failure. Some degree of renal ischemia occurs in 10% of patients with severe hemorrhage. Renal failure may manifest as transient oliguria or anuria accompanied by renal tubular or cortical necrosis. Renal cortical necrosis has been reported in cases of placental abruption; the probable cause is severe intrarenal vasospasm from massive hemorrhage. Renal failure is reversible in most cases (acute tubular necrosis) but may be associated with varying degrees of long-term failure if cortical necrosis exists.

■ **KEY POINT:** To prevent renal ischemia and acute renal failure, aggressive blood, fluid, and volume resuscitation is required to treat hypovolemic shock.

Urine output should be monitored closely postoperatively. Persistently low urine output even after hypovolemia is corrected may signal the onset of renal failure. If oliguria persists despite a central venous pressure (CVP) reading of 7 cm H$_2$O,

■ Table 10–6
TYPICAL TEG PATTERN AND VARIABLES MEASURED, NORMAL VALUES, AND EXAMPLES

Variable	Measures		Abnormality	Example
r; reaction time	Thromboplastin generation via the intrinsic pathway	$\uparrow r$	Factor deficiency Heparin Severe thrombocytopenia	Factor deficiency
α; angle of divergence	Rate of clot formation	$\downarrow \alpha$	Hypofibrinogenemia Thrombocytopenia Thrombocytopathy	Hypofibrinogenemia
m_a; maximum amplitude	Maximum clot strength/elasticity	$\downarrow m_a$	Thrombocytopenia Thrombocytopathy Hypofibrinogenemia Factor XIII deficiency	Thrombocytopenia
$m_a + 30$	Clot retraction after 30 min	$\downarrow m_a + 30$	Fibrinolysis	Fibrinolysis

r = 21–30 mm (normal; 3–6 min); α = 50–60 degrees; m_a = 50–60 mm; $m_a + 30$ = minimal reduction.
From Faust RJ: Functional platelet disorders. In: Faust RJ, ed. Anesthesiology Review, 2nd ed. New York: Churchill Livingstone, 1994:481.

then placement of a pulmonary artery (PA) catheter may be considered, especially in a patient who has severe preeclampsia with placental abruption. A pulmonary artery catheter allows preload and afterload assessment along with cardiac output and other variables. These patients may require inotropic support or the administration of low-dose (2.5 μg/kg/min) dopamine.

Fetal Considerations

Hypoxia and anemia are major risks to the fetus. The infant often needs aggressive, effective, and immediate resuscitation at delivery. Administering blood from the fetal surface of the placenta with a heparinized syringe corrects neonatal hypovolemia.

PLACENTA PREVIA

Definition and Incidence

Placenta previa is defined as implantation of the placenta in the lower uterine segment in advance of the fetal presenting part. The placenta is normally placed in the body of the uterus and away from the cervical internal os. If the placenta obstructs the descent of the fetus, there is the potential for maternal hemorrhage as the fetus impacts it and separates it from the decidual plate. The four variations and classification of placenta previa are shown in Figure 10-4 and Table 10-7. The incidence of placenta previa varies from 0.1 to 1.0% of third-trimester pregnancies, and maternal mortality can reach 0.9%.

Etiology

Multiparity and the mother's advancing age are risk factors for placenta previa. A strong factor in the development of placenta previa is defective vascularization of the decidua caused

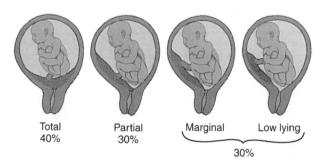

| Total | Partial | Marginal | Low lying |
| 40% | 30% | 30% | |

Figure 10–4 ■ Four variations of placenta previa. (Drawn by Carl Clingman, Baylor College of Medicine.)

■ Table 10–7
CLASSIFICATION OF PLACENTA PREVIA

Complete Total	Partial	Marginal	Low Lying
40%	30%	30%	30%
Placenta completely covers internal cervical os	Placenta partially covers internal cervical os	The internal cervical os is just encroached by placenta	Placenta is implanted in lower uterine segment but not encroaching on the cervical os

From Gatt SP: Anaesthetic management of the obstetric patient with ante-partum or intrapartum haemorrhage. Clin Anaesth 4:373-387, 1986.

by previous inflammatory or atrophic changes. The association between increasing parity and placenta previa suggests that damage of the endometrium by a prior pregnancy may be an etiologic factor. The endometrium underlying the implantation site may be rendered less available for subsequent implantation, causing future pregnancies to implant in the lower uterine segment by a process of elimination.

Clark et al.[4] assessed the relationship between increasing numbers of previous cesarean sections and the subsequent development of placenta previa and placenta accreta. The risk of placenta previa was 0.26% with an unscarred uterus, and the incidence increased linearly with the number of prior cesarean sections up to 10% with four or more cesarean sections. The risk of recurrent placenta previa is between 4 and 8%. Poorly developed decidua in the lower uterine segment results in an abnormally firm attachment of the placenta and an increased risk of placenta accreta.

■ **KEY POINT:** The risk of placenta accreta with placenta previa and one previous cesarean section is 24% and increases to 67% with placenta previa and four or more previous cesarean sections (Fig. 10–5).

Signs and Symptoms

The most characteristic event in placenta previa—painless bleeding—does not usually appear until near the end of the second trimester or during the third trimester. Patients with vaginal bleeding in the third trimester are assumed to have placenta previa until diagnosed otherwise. The distinction of painless bleeding in some cases may be confusing because

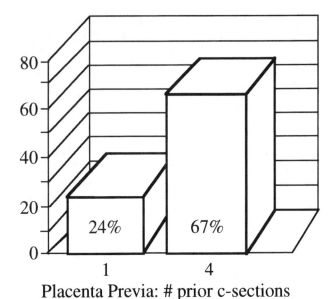

Placenta Previa: # prior c-sections

Figure 10–5 ■ Placenta accreta after prior cesarean sections. (From Suresh MS, Belfort MA: Antepartum hemorrhage. In: Datta S (ed): Anesthetic and Obstetric Management of High-Risk Pregnancy, 2nd ed. St. Louis: Mosby Year-book, 1996.)

approximately 10% of cases of placenta previa are associated with placental separation and symptoms and signs suggestive of abruption. In as many as 25% of cases there are signs of labor, with or without rupture of the membranes. Bleeding results from tearing of the placenta and its attachments to the decidua. The lower uterine segment contracts very poorly and therefore is unable to compress the spiral arteries. Bleeding thus continues unabated and may persist despite delivery of the fetus and removal of the placenta.

Diagnosis

Clinically, the diagnosis of placenta previa is supported by palpation of a relaxed uterus. The presenting part is usually in the upper uterine segment, due to the presence of the placenta in the lower uterine segment. An abnormal presentation is very common, with the fetus being in breech or transverse position in 33% of cases. In those fetuses with a cephalic presentation, the presenting part is frequently high above the pelvic brim and difficult to palpate, especially when there is an anterior placenta previa.

Although clinical findings are important, the definitive diagnosis is currently made by ultrasound examination. With trans-abdominal ultrasound and a full maternal urinary bladder, the accuracy of the diagnosis approaches 97%. Transvaginal ultrasound has recently become popular and has been shown to be safe in the diagnosis and management of patients with placenta previa despite the theoretic risk of probe-induced trauma. The transvaginal approach allows superior definition of the lower uterine segment and placental anatomic relationship and has been reported to be 100% sensitive.

Magnetic resonance imaging (MRI) has been used to diagnose placenta previa and provides excellent magnetic resolution of the soft tissues and in particular the cervical placental interface. The cost of the MRI study does not justify its routine use and should be reserved for only those cases where ultrasound is nondiagnostic.

Only in rare circumstances is a definitive diagnosis made using a "double-setup" examination. The only indication for such an examination is when ultrasound and/or MRI studies are inconclusive or when a patient presents with ongoing, but not life-threatening, bleeding in labor. Under these circumstances, a digital vaginal examination in an operating room may be indicated with very specific precautions (see Double Setup under Anesthesia Management, below). Using a double setup, with all prerequisites accomplished, the vaginal fornices should be initially explored very gently (using the ultrasound information, if available, to further direct the examining finger to the regions of interest). If the fetal presenting part can be clearly felt in all four quadrants, vaginal delivery is usually feasible and the membranes can be ruptured. If there is any bogginess suggestive of placenta previa, the procedure is usually abandoned and abdominal delivery performed.

Obstetric Management

The initial management of any life-threatening bleeding in a patient with placenta previa should be directed toward stabilizing the patient. Therefore, patients with active vaginal bleeding should be hospitalized immediately and appropriate resuscitative efforts begun. Fetal heart rate monitoring is also important during this phase. Once the mother has been stabilized, more detailed ultrasound examination can be used to confirm the diagnosis.

■ **KEY POINT:** Until such time as placenta previa is excluded, vaginal examination should be avoided. Digital exploration of the cervical canal can precipitate life-threatening hemorrhage in the presence of placenta previa.

Elective cesarean delivery is preferred because emergency surgery has an adverse effect on the perinatal outcome, independent of gestational age. In cases of complete placenta previa with the gestational age ≤ 37 weeks, an amniocentesis is indicated before elective cesarean section. Corticosteroids are recommended to enhance fetal lung maturity, such as betamethasone, 12 mg every 24 hours for the first two doses, followed by weekly steroid injection up to 34 weeks gestation.

The management of placenta previa in the last four decades has changed dramatically. Expectant management with the goal of prolonging pregnancy is no longer believed to be contraindicated. Cases in which there has been heavy vaginal bleeding, even to the point of maternal hypovolemia requiring blood transfusion, have been managed expectantly, with good maternal and fetal outcome.[5] As a general rule, the patient should be transfused to a hematocrit of 30% or greater to optimize maternal and fetal oxygen consumption and to provide a reserve in the event of further heavy bleeding. Continuous reassessment as to the risk-to-benefit ratio of aggressive expectant management is required. The patient should be delivered as soon as fetal maturity is reached or maternal condition demands. Expectant management, availability of sophisticated surgical services, and blood bank facilities have lowered the maternal mortality rate from 25% to less than 1% and the total perinatal mortality rate from 60% to under 10%. Most perinatal deaths are still due to these patients being delivered before 32 weeks and to a lesser extent due to massive maternal hemorrhage.

Tocolytic Therapy

The use of tocolytic agents in the management of placenta previa is controversial. Patients with placenta previa may experience ruptured membranes, spontaneous labor, or some other complications prompting tocolysis or delivery before 37 weeks. The choice of tocolytic can influence the maternal and fetal outcome. The use of betamimetics in placenta previa results in maternal tachycardia, palpitations, and can be misdiagnosed as hypovolemia. If betamimetics are used when maternal hypovolemia exists, serious maternal hypotension results, which may be resistant to treatment with ephedrine and crystalloid administration. Administration of calcium chloride (10 mg/kg) slightly increases maternal cardiac output but does not substantially improve maternal mean arterial pressure, uterine blood flow, or fetal oxygenation.[6] Magnesium sulfate ($MgSO_4$) compared with ritodrine in terms of cardiovascular stability during hemorrhage in ewes worsens the maternal hypotensive and fetal-acid base responses to hemorrhage.[7] Hypermagnesemia attenuates maternal compensatory response to hemorrhage.

■ **KEY POINT:** Patients with complete previa who are on tocolytic therapy and undergoing regional anesthesia for cesarean section can experience significant hypotension, which requires aggressive therapy.

Surgical Considerations

The choice of uterine incision in placenta previa can influence blood loss and therefore has an impact on the anesthetic management. A transverse uterine incision is indicated in the following: a well-formed lower uterine segment, a posterior placenta (or anterior placenta that is below or just above the bladder reflection), and fetal lie that is longitudinal. In most other situations, a vertical low incision (either a low vertical or a classic) that avoids the placenta as far as possible is usually recommended.

The presence of an anterior placenta implanted in the lower segment is not an absolute contraindication to a transverse lower uterine segment incision. In this situation the surgeon has two choices: to deliver the fetus through the placenta or to make the incision above the placental edge. Both techniques can result in excessive blood loss if the surgeon is inexperienced and takes too much time in delivering the fetus.

Severe postpartum bleeding may occur after delivery of the placenta because the lower uterine segment contracts poorly. Bleeding from the placental implantation site is common and may be controlled by hemostatic sutures, manual compression, and medical therapy as described above in the section on abruptio placentae. If bleeding remains uncontrolled, surgical options such as bilateral uterine artery ligation, bilateral hypogastric artery ligation, or hysterectomy may need to be exercised. The recent development of the argon beam coagulator (Kline Medical, Houston, TX), a specialized diathermy device that carries the electrical charge to the tissue in a beam of argon gas, avoids mechanical contact with the bleeding sinuses and may help to control hemorrhage from the implantation site. There are no published data on its use in placenta previa, but this technology may offer promise.

ANESTHETIC MANAGEMENT

Anesthetic management of placenta previa should take into consideration four different scenarios:

1. Double setup for vaginal delivery/cesarean section;
2. Cesarean section in hemodynamically stable patients;
3. Cesarean section in actively bleeding and hemodynamically unstable patients;

4. Placenta accreta/percreta undergoing cesarean hysterectomy.

Double SetUp

Rarely is a definitive diagnosis of placenta previa made under "double setup." Double setup entails simultaneously preparing for immediate cesarean section and making available general anesthesia with crossmatched blood. Cervical examination causing torrential hemorrhage mandates immediate delivery. *Consequently, the examination is safer when executed in the operating room.*

Preparation includes the presence of qualified anesthesia personnel, a scrub technician, instruments, experienced operating team, and a neonatologist, in addition to the obstetrician examining the patient. Volume resuscitation preparation includes having two or more large-bore intravenous lines and two units of crossmatched blood.

Parturients who have vaginal examination under double setup conditions are prepared like cesarean section patients. Preparation for general anesthesia includes administering oral clear antacid 30 to 45 minutes before examination. During preoxygenation, an assistant is available and ready to provide cricoid pressure. With left uterine displacement, the patient is prepped and draped for cesarean section and placed in a lithotomy position. An obstetrician is ready to perform immediate cesarean section if bleeding starts, whereas another obstetrician performs the vaginal examination. Cesarean section is standard procedure if the diagnosis of placenta previa is confirmed.

Hemodynamically Stable Patients

Either regional or general anesthesia is acceptable in the placenta previa patient who bled several weeks before delivery and is hemodynamically stable and normovolemic. Adequate preparation requires the placement of two large-bore intravenous catheters. Further, at least two to four units of crossmatched blood should be present in the operating room before proceeding with surgery.

General anesthesia for patients with placenta previa undergoing cesarean section is favored by some because excessive hemorrhage can occur for the following reasons: The placenta may be located anteriorly, so the obstetrician incises through the placenta; after delivery, the distended lower uterine segment does not contract as well as the fundus; and placenta previa patients with previous cesarean sections have added risk for placenta accreta. All these factors may precipitate extensive postpartum bleeding. Regional anesthesia for cesar-

ean section in placenta previa patients offers the following advantages: decreased blood loss, lower incidence of hysterectomy, and better neonatal outcome. However, hypotension induced by epidural anesthesia in the parturient may result in decreased placental perfusion. As stated previously, patients with placenta previa on $MgSO_4$ tocolytic therapy may have exaggerated hypotension. In hypermagnesemic gravid ewes, ephedrine and phenylephrine provide similar restoration of maternal mean arterial pressure, and ephedrine was superior to phenylephrine in restoring uterine blood flow during anesthesia-induced hypotension.

Actively Bleeding/Hemodynamically Unstable Patients

Copious bleeding and hemorrhagic shock associated with placenta previa can make resuscitating the mother extremely difficult. Completely correcting blood loss before surgery is not always possible because bleeding continues until the placenta is removed. Evaluation of the patient, surgical preparation, aspiration prophylaxis, monitoring, and volume resuscitation should proceed simultaneously.

Induction of general anesthesia must be preceded by left uterine displacement and preoxygenation (denitrogenation). Using a rapid sequence induction and utilizing cricoid pressure, anesthesia is induced either with 0.5 to 1.0 mg/kg ketamine or 0.3 mg/kg etomidate. Ketamine produces sympathetic nervous system stimulation and blood pressure maintenance. Etomidate is associated with stable hemodynamics and is safe in obstetrics. Sodium pentothal or propofol are not the induction agents of choice in a hypovolemic patient. Some patients on arrival to the operating room are hypotensive and moribund. In such cases, establishing an airway precedes anesthesia induction.

Maintenance agent selection depends on the degree of cardiovascular compromise. Halogenated agents administered during balanced general anesthesia cause uterine relaxation and increase blood loss during cesarean section. In a bleeding patient, it is prudent to eliminate halogenated agents and uterine relaxants. Anesthesia maintenance is achieved with oxygen, small doses of short-acting narcotics, and nitrous oxide as tolerated. Benzodiazepines will decrease the risk of intraoperative awareness.

Delivery of the fetus and removal of the placenta minimize the threat to the mother. If bleeding continues from the atonic lower uterine segment, oxytocin, methergine 15-methyl prostaglandin $F_{2\alpha}$, may be necessary to establish uterine tone. As assessed by blood pressure, CVP measurements, and urine output, adequate resuscitation normalizes the blood volume.

The neonate may also require intensive resuscitation at birth if asphyxiated, acidotic, and/or hypovolemic.

Placenta Accreta/Percreta/Increta

A patient with placenta previa or otherwise identified as high risk for placenta accreta, percreta, or increta is often scheduled for elective cesarean hysterectomy to avoid complications after vaginal delivery (Fig. 10–6). If undetected before delivery, placenta accreta is usually diagnosed if there is unusual adherence and difficulty in placental delivery. Placenta accreta removal results in catastrophic hemorrhage, particularly as the raw myometrium is exposed. The reported blood loss varies from 3.5 to 5 L, resulting in significant maternal morbidity and mortality.

Uterine atony and bleeding may be treated with pharmacologic agents listed in Table 10–5. Ultimately, one may have to perform a bilateral hypogastric artery ligation or, if that is unsuccessful, an abdominal hysterectomy. Maternal mortality ranges from 67% with conservative management to 2% with prompt hysterectomy, antibiotics, and adequate blood transfusions.

Placenta percreta is a subtype of placenta accreta. Placenta percreta causes intraperitoneal or intravesical bleeding. These patients are at high risk for hemorrhage, sepsis, and DIC. This is a life-threatening event and characteristically mimics a concealed placental abruption or uterine rupture. Placenta percreta is commonly diagnosed after delivery, because any

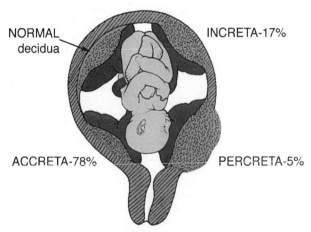

Figure 10–6 ■ Incidence of placenta accreta, increta, and percreta. (Drawn by Carl Clingman, Baylor College of Medicine.)

attempt is impossible for manual removal. It is associated with severe bleeding, shock, or acute inversion of the uterus. Hysterectomy is the treatment of choice because it causes the least morbidity and mortality.

■ **KEY POINT:** Temporizing measures of bleeding that might become absolutely necessary to save the mother include manually cross-clamping the abdominal aorta or compressing the aorta against the vertebral column, thereby reducing the pulse pressure and heavy bleeding at the surgical site.

Anesthetic Management

Cesarean Hysterectomy in Unsuspected Placenta Accreta/Percreta. The anesthesiologist with a bleeding, hypovolemic, and unstable patient undergoing cesarean hysterectomy with unsuspected placenta accreta/percreta has two priorities: evaluating the airway/oxygen administration and establishing vascular access with large-bore intravenous catheters for volume resuscitation. Blood is typed and crossmatched. Transfusion of type O negative or crossmatched blood must be initiated immediately, and the patient is transferred to the operating room. General anesthesia is as outlined in a previous section.

In a patient with functioning epidural anesthetic in situ when unsuspected placenta accreta/percreta is encountered, resulting in cesarean hysterectomy, the anesthetic can be continued provided hemodynamic stability remains, whereas a patient with development of sudden hemodynamic instability and no anesthetic on board should receive a general anesthesia, as described previously.

The development of intraoperative bleeding diathesis can worsen complications markedly. There are no published recommendations for dealing with an epidural catheter in obstetric patients who develop coagulopathy. The anesthesiologist is faced with a dilemma whether to remove an epidural catheter in a parturient with DIC. Sprung et al.[8] made the following recommendations. If there is no evidence of intraspinal bleeding, the catheter must be removed as early as possible because of the potential for intravascular catheter migration and initiation of bleeding. If bleeding is present around the catheter insertion site and possibly in the epidural/subarachnoid space, the catheter must be left in place. Frequent assessment of neurologic status is important until the underlying cause of the coagulopathy is treated and the bleeding is resolved. In case of intraspinal hematoma, leading to neurologic deficit, *immediate neurologic consult and decompression surgery is needed.*

Elective Cesarean-Hysterectomy in Suspected Placenta Accreta. Adequate preparation for massive volume resuscitation, appropriate invasive hemodynamic monitoring, warming devices, and a minimum of four units of cross-matched blood in the operating room are required. In addition, the blood bank should be notified that more blood may be required. The choice of anesthetic technique for elective cesarean hysterectomy is controversial. Patients undergoing cesarean hysterectomy under a regional anesthetic may require conversion to general anesthesia due to patient discomfort and/or inadequate operating conditions. Regional anesthesia may be inadequate for the following reasons. First, operative time for cesarean hysterectomy is twice that required for routine cesarean section. This predisposes the patient to fatigue and restlessness. Second, intraperitoneal manipulation, dissection, and traction can be excessive for cesarean hysterectomy resulting in pain, nausea, and vomiting. Third, the engorged edematous vasculature requires careful dissection facilitated by a quiet operative field, without the patient straining. However, a prospective multiinstitutional study of cesarean hysterectomy suggested that the epidural anesthesia provided optimum anesthesia and that none of the cesarean hysterectomy patients required general anesthesia if they remained hemodynamically stable.[9]

Anesthetic determination for cesarean hysterectomy depends on the evaluation of the patient's airway, preferences of the patient and the anesthesiologist, skills and experience of the obstetrician, and availability of staff. One can proceed with either general or regional anesthesia in a patient who seems to have an easily intubatable airway. Failed intubation and pulmonary aspiration of gastric contents continue to be leading causes of maternal morbidity from anesthesia. The American College of Obstetricians and Gynecologists (ACOG) Committee Opinion states that the risk of these complications can be reduced by careful antepartum assessment and greater use of regional anesthesia when possible. Committee opinion is valuable and applicable in most situations; however, this sort of reasoning in a patient with difficult airway applied to a patient who is at risk for major hemorrhage may be dangerous. Further, massive fluid resuscitation produces airway edema, making an airway that was easily intubatable into a difficult airway. Further, if the airway is questionable or difficult, the airway needs to be secured awake using a fiberscope. An airway established before surgery is sometimes preferred in patients at risk for potentially serious hemorrhage. Once the airway is secured, managing other problems, hemorrhage, and massive volume resuscitation can be dealt with.

Postoperative management after cesarean hysterectomy involves close intensive care unit-type monitoring initially postpartum. Monitoring includes assessment of serial hematocrit assessment, coagulation profile, hemodynamics, volume status, urine output, ventilatory status, and core temperature.

■ **KEY POINT:** Interventional radiologic techniques are being used more frequently in the patient with suspected placenta accreta. Angiographic placement of a balloon occlusion device may be performed preoperatively and used in the event of massive hemorrhage.

UTERINE RUPTURE

Spontaneous rupture of the gravid uterus still carries significant maternal and fetal mortality. The incidence is approximately 1 in 2000 deliveries, with a 9.7% maternal mortality rate and a rate of fetal wastage of 56%. Uterine rupture may be spontaneous, secondary to trauma, or result from rupture of a previous uterine scar. Dehiscence of a previous ceasarean section scar, with extension, is probably the most frequent etiology of uterine rupture in modern obstetrics. See Chapter 16 for a discussion of maternal mortality caused by uterine rupture.

The most common clinical presentation is vaginal bleeding, shock, and lower abdominal pain. In some instances, the area to which the fetal heart tone was initially localized is noted to have shifted. Usually acute fetal bradycardia or sudden profound "fetal distress" is noted. In cases of catastrophic rupture and fetal demise, inability to detect fetal heart tones may occur concomitantly with acute abdominal pain, hypotension, vaginal bleeding, appearance of frank blood in the urinary catheter (indicative of anterior rupture into the bladder), and retraction of the fetal presenting part (indicative of fetal expulsion into the abdomen).

If the fetus is still undelivered or if uterine bleeding is believed to be secondary to a uterine or cervical defect, immediate laparotomy is indicated. If a defect is found at the time of postpartum examination after a vaginal birth after cesarean section (VBAC) but no bleeding is noted and the patient is hemodynamically stable, close observation is warranted, with resort to laparotomy if the patient shows signs of decompensation.

> **■ KEY POINT:** A sudden increase in baseline uterine tone or sudden absence of uterine pressure coupled with evidence of acute fetal bradycardia, indicates uterine rupture and mandates an immediate abdominal delivery.

ANESTHETIC MANAGEMENT IN SITUATIONS REQUIRING UTERINE RELAXATION

Uterine relaxation may be required emergently to allow obstetric maneuvers in complicated situations such as retained placenta and inverted uterus (Fig. 10-7). Although not always life threatening, the aforementioned situations can lead to significant maternal morbidity secondary to hemorrhage. These situations can constitute emergencies, thus demanding immediate intervention of the anesthesia care team, in providing uterine relaxation and extensive volume resuscitation.

Classically, amylnitrate, diethylether, and halogenated inhalation anesthetics have been used. Usually, uterine muscle relaxation is accomplished with a potent inhalation agent. Equipotent doses of halothane, enflurane, and isoflurane depress uterine contractility. *Rapid sequence induction with cricoid pressure and endotracheal intubation is mandatory.* General anesthesia administration procedure is time consuming and exposes the parturient to an otherwise unnecessary

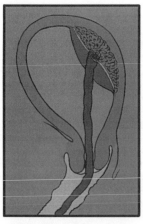 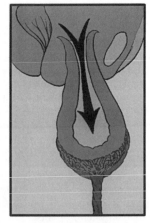

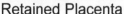

Retained Placenta   Inverted Uterus

Figure 10–7 ■ Situations that cause hemorrhage yet require uterine relaxation emergently.

general anesthetic with the attendant risks of regurgitation and aspiration.

Smooth muscle is present in the cervix, uterus, and vagina. Nitroglycerine (NTG) has been shown to be a powerful relaxant of the rat uterus myometrium strips in vitro. Intravenous NTG is also an effective smooth muscle relaxant with rapid onset of action in 30 to 80 seconds, a short plasma half-life (2 minutes), and a brief duration of action. It can be titrated to effect to produce controlled smooth muscle relaxation. A number of reports indicate that a NTG dose range of 50 to 500 μg administered intravenously has been successful in providing uterine relaxation. The higher dose of NTG (500 μg) provides effective uterine relaxation; however, it is associated with systolic hypotension requiring crystalloid or vasopressor therapy. The use of NTG doses of 200 μg or less for retained placenta appears efficacious and safe. Sublingual administration of glyceryl trinitrate by aerosol is also effective in providing uterine relaxation in various situations. Glyceryl trinitrate by aerosol in two boluses of 400 μg each relaxes the uterus in 30 to 60 seconds. The use of NTG, intravenous or aerosol, should be considered as the first line of therapy in selected patients requiring uterine relaxation. NTG use avoids the need for general anesthesia and its attendant risks. Although glyceryl trinitrate sublingual spray or intravenous NTG are not approved for marketing for obstetric applications, its use for obstetric emergencies deserves further evaluation.

CONCLUSION

Hemorrhage in the obstetric patient occurs unexpectedly and has potential for serious maternal and fetal morbidity and mortality. Different aspects of obstetric hemorrhage along with management guidelines have been reviewed. A well-equipped labor and delivery and operative suite along with expert obstetric, anesthesia, neonatal, and nursing teams lend to the successful outcome for both mother and baby. Finally, NTG provides adequate uterine relaxation in conditions like retained placenta and inverted uterus and should be considered the first line of management, thus avoiding general anesthesia and its inherent risks. Hemodynamic resuscitation is equally important in these conditions. Further, postoperative morbidity after obstetric hemorrhage is minimized by excellent postoperative/critical care management.

REFERENCES

1. Baker RN: Hemorrhage in obstetrics. Obstet Gynecol Annu 6:295, 1997.
2. Gonik B: Intensive care monitoring of the critically ill pregnant patient. In:

Creasky RK, Resnik P, eds. Maternal-Fetal Medicine, 2nd ed. Philadelphia: W.B. Saunders, 1989.

3. Suresh MS, Solanki DR, Andrews JJ, et al: Comparison of etomidate with thiopental for induction of anesthesia at cesarean section. Anesthesiology 65:A400, 1986.

4. Clark SL, Koonings P, Phelan JP, et al: Placenta previa/accreta and prior cesarean section. Obstet Gynecol 66:89–92, 1985.

5. Cotton DB, Read JA, Paul RH, et al: The conservative aggressive management of placenta previa. Am J Obstet Gynecol 137:687–695, 1980.

6. Vincent RD, Chestnut DH, Sipes SL, et al: Does calcium chloride help restore maternal blood pressure and uterine blood flow during hemorrhagic hypotension in hypermagnesium gravid ewes? Anesth Analg 74:670–676, 1992.

7. Chestnut DH, Thompson CS, McLaughlin GL, et al: Does the intravenous infusion of ritodrine or magnesium sulfate alter the hemodynamic response to hemorrhage in gravid ewes? Am J Obstet Gynecol 159:1467–1473, 1988.

8. Sprung J, Cheng EY, Patel S: When to remove an epidural catheter in a parturient with disseminated intravascular coagulation. Reg Anesth 17:351–354, 1992.

9. Chestnut DH, Dewan DM, Redick LF, et al: Anesthetic management for obstetric hysterectomy: a multiinstitutional study. Anesthesiology 70:607–610, 1989.

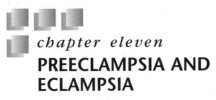

chapter eleven

PREECLAMPSIA AND ECLAMPSIA

Stephen P. Gatt, MD

INCIDENCE AND MORTALITY

Preeclampsia occurs in 2.5 to 7.0% of all pregnancies, but eclampsia is becoming progressively less frequent in developed countries. Hypertension in pregnancy accounts for close to 13% of maternal deaths in the United States (Table 11-1). Most deaths in preeclampsia occur as a result of convulsions (eclampsia) or secondary to an intracerebral insult[1] (Table 11-2).

> ■ **KEY POINT:** Preeclampsia is a multisystem disorder that remains a leading cause of maternal morbidity and mortality.

DEFINITIONS

The Australasian Society for the Study of Hypertension in Pregnancy (ASSHP) defines hypertension in pregnancy as systolic arterial systemic pressure (SAP) ≥140 mm Hg and/or diastolic arterial pressure (DAP) ≥90 mm Hg *or* a rise in SAP ≥25 mm

■ Table 11-1
MATERNAL MORTALITY IN PREGNANCY IN THE UNITED STATES BETWEEN 1980 AND 1985

Causes	Percent
Embolism	17.0
Indirect causes	15.6
Hypertension in pregnancy	12.3
Ectopic pregnancy complications	10.0
Hemorrhage	9.1
Stroke	8.4
Anesthesia	7.0
Complications of termination	5.2
Cardiomyopathy	4.2
Infection	3.5
Other	7.7

Adapted from the U.S. Maternal Mortality Surveillance, 1980-85. MMWR CDC Surveillance Summary, 1988.

■ Table 11–2
CAUSES OF DEATH IN PREECLAMPSIA IN DESCENDING ORDER OF FREQUENCY

Eclampsia
Hypertensive encephalopathy
Intracranial hemorrhage
Pulmonary edema
Abruptio placentae
Cardiac dysrhythmias
Hepatic rupture
Upper airway edema

Hg and/or a rise in DAP ≥15 mm Hg from systemic arterial pressure before conception or in the first trimester. Preeclampsia is defined by the American College of Obstetricians and Gynecologists (ACOG) as hypertension (systolic ≥140 mm Hg or ≥30 mm Hg above baseline; diastolic ≥90 mm Hg or ≥15 mm Hg above baseline) with proteinuria (≥300 mg/L/24 h or ≥1+ on dipstick), edema or both occurring after 20 weeks' gestation or in the early postpartum period. ASSHP believes the term "HELLP syndrome" (hemolysis, elevated liver enzymes, low platelets) should be abolished so that abnormal liver function, thrombocytopenia, and hemolysis are not viewed as anything but manifestations of severe preeclampsia.

Preeclampsia is said to be severe when evidence of severe end-organ damage or failure is apparent (Table 11–3).

Most severe preeclamptics present for surgery having received aggressive treatment beforehand. In this situation, a definition of *severe treated* preeclampsia is a diastolic arterial pressure of more than 100 mm Hg (as opposed to 110 mm Hg in the standard "untreated" definition) and proteinuria > 2+ *or* significant oliguria *or* neurologic or abdominal signs. The degree of proteinuria is a good yardstick whereby the anesthetist can assess grade of severity in the treated parturient.

■ Table 11–3
FEATURES THAT DIFFERENTIATE SEVERE PREECLAMPSIA FROM MILD PREECLAMPSIA

SAP ≥ 160 mm Hg
DAP ≥ 110 mm Hg
Proteinuria ≥ 5 g/24 h or dipstick ≥ 3+ to 4+
Oliguria ≤ 500 mL/24 h
Headache or visual disturbances
Epigastric or right upper quadrant abdominal pain
Pulmonary edema or cyanosis
HELLP syndrome

■ Table 11-4
ACOG CLASSIFICATION OF HYPERTENSION IN PREGNANCY

Pregnancy-induced hypertension (PIH)
    Mild
    Severe
    Eclampsia
    HELLP syndrome
Chronic hypertensive disease
    Essential hypertension
    Secondary hypertension
Chronic hypertension with superimposed PIH
Nonproteinuric gestational hypertension

CLASSIFICATION

ACOG classifies hypertension in pregnancy as shown in Table 11-4.[2] ASSHP have, in their consensus statement (which was ratified and adopted by a number of colleges and professional bodies), simplified this classification even further. ASSHP classifies hypertension in pregnancy as preeclampsia, mild and severe; chronic hypertension, essential and secondary; and preeclampsia superimposed on chronic hypertension.[3]

RISK FACTORS

In 1996, ACOG listed the risk factors for developing pre-eclampsia as chronic renal disease (20:1), angiotensin T-235 homozygous (20:1), chronic hypertension (10:1), antiphospholipid syndrome (10:1), family history of preeclampsia (5:1), twin gestation (4:1), angiotensin T-235 heterozygous (4:1), >40 years of age (3:1), nulliparity (3:1), diabetes (2:1), and African-American race (1.5:1). Low socioeconomic group and young maternal age are (probably) not risk factors for developing preeclampsia/eclampsia.[2]

ANTIHYPERTENSIVE AGENTS FOR ESTABLISHED HYPERTENSION IN PREECLAMPSIA/ECLAMPSIA

The antihypertensive agents used to manage preeclampsia can be divided into two groups: those used to control hypertension in late pregnancy and those used in acute hypertensive emergencies before delivery (Table 11-5).[4]

Although labetalol and hydralazine remain the mainstays of treatment of preeclampsia, other beta-blockers (e.g., metoprolol, atenolol) and calcium channel blockers (see below) are being used with ever-increasing frequency to control hypertension in preeclampsia.[5]

The calcium channel blockers given either orally (amlodi-

■ Table 11–5
ANTIHYPERTENSIVE AGENTS USED IN PREGNANCY TO MANAGE HYPERTENSION AND TO TREAT ACUTE HYPERTENSIVE EMERGENCIES AND CRISES

Antihypertensive Agents	Drug	Management of	
		Hypertension in Pregnancy	Acute Hypertensive Emergency
Diuretic	Thiazide	O	O
	Frusemide	O	+ + +
Beta-blocker	Atenolol, metoprolol	+ +	+ +
	Esmolol	O	+ + +
Beta/alpha-blocker	Labetalol	+ + +	+ +
Adrenergic blocker	Methyldopa	+ + + +	+ +
	Clonidine	+ /O	O
Alpha-blocker	Phenoxybenzamine	O	O
Postsynaptic alpha-blocker	Prazosin	+ +	O
Sympathetic postganglionic transmission blocker	Reserpine	+	O
Ganglion blocker	Trimetaphan	O	+ +
Vasodilator	Hydralazine	+	+ + + +
	Diazoxide	+ /O	+ + +
	Nitroprusside	O	+ + + +
	Minoxidil	O	O
	Magnesium	O/ +	O/ +
	Nitroglycerin	O	+ + +
Serotonin II antagonist	Ketanserin	+ /O	O
Sedative	Barbiturate	+	O
Calcium channel blocker	Nifedipine	+ +	+ +
Angiotensin-converting enzyme inhibitor	Captopril	+ /O	O

O, not used for this indication; +, used rarely for this indication; + + + +, drug very commonly used for this indication.

pine, nifedipine, felodipine, verapamil, diltiazem) or sublingually (nifedipine) have proven to be efficacious for control of hypertension in pregnant patients, but hypotension and respiratory embarrassment have been reported when they are used in combination with magnesium sulfate.[6]

Angiotensin-converting enzyme inhibitors (captopril, perindopril, trandolapril, ramipril, quinapril, enalapril, fosinopril, cilazapril, lisinopril) are best avoided in pregnancy because of adverse fetal and neonatal effects.[6]

PREVENTION OF PREECLAMPSIA

Though the use of aspirin to prevent preeclampsia initially seemed to show much promise, many of the original claims were not subsequently supported by a large multicenter study. Supplementation with calcium may be able to reduce the incidence of preeclampsia.

ANESTHETIC RISK ASSESSMENT

Significant proteinuria (+ +), hypoproteinemia, platelet count of <75,000, elevated serum uric acid, elevated antiphospholipid (anticardiolipin) antibody, hemoconcentration, and neurologic or hepatic symptoms suggest poor anesthetic risk. If preeclampsia is superimposed on chronic hypertension or associated with insulin-dependent diabetes, the risk is compounded.[7]

■ **K E Y P O I N T :** Preeclampsia may be associated with hematologic changes that may have an impact on the choice of anesthesia technique.

LABORATORY INVESTIGATION OF PREECLAMPSIA

Investigations that may be useful to the anesthesiologist in deciding whether a regional technique is appropriate in preeclampsia include platelet count and thromboelastography. Depressed urinary calcium and elevated cellular plasma fibronectin are laboratory tests that allow discrimination between preeclampsia and chronic hypertension. The severity of preeclampsia is reflected by the degree of hyperuricemia and proteinuria, by the serum iron and β-thromboglobulin concentration increase, and by the rise in hematocrit and hemoglobin. Severity of the HELLP syndrome is assessable with platelet count and total serum lactate dehydrogenase.

PREPARATION FOR ANESTHESIA AND SURGERY

A few hours spent in rehydration, blood pressure control, intrauterine fetal resuscitation, eclampsia prophylaxis, and stabilizing the mother's condition is time well spent. Although unnecessary delay in delivery of the infant is not desirable when evidence of diminished uteroplacental blood flow or intrauterine growth retardation exists, if there is no absolute

■ Table 11–6
ABSOLUTE AND RELATIVE MATERNAL AND FETAL INDICATIONS FOR DELIVERY OF THE FETUS IN SEVERE PREECLAMPSIA

Absolute	Relative
Maternal	Maternal
Convulsion	Severe hypertension
Cerebral irritability	Right upper quadrant
Heart failure	abdominal pain
Oliguria (to <20 mL/hr)	Heavy proteinuria
Uncontrollable hypertension	
Rising serum creatinine (>50%)	
Thrombocytopenia	
Microangiopathic blood film	
Clinical placental abruption	
Fetal	Fetal
Fetal distress	Intrauterine growth retardation

Modified from Gallery EDM: Hypertension in pregnancy. Practical management recommendations. Drugs 49:561, 1995.

indication for immediate delivery (significant fetal jeopardy, abruption of the placenta), resuscitation before anesthesia is the best course (Tables 11-6 and 11-7). Preeclamptic patients have an exaggerated hypertensive response to pain and should receive analgesia.

■ **K E Y   P O I N T :**   Neuraxial analgesia is the preferred method in the preeclamptic patient because it is the most effective technique and produces a reduction in catecholamines, which helps to normalize blood pressure.

■ Table 11–7
PREOPERATIVE RESUSCITATION OF THE WOMAN WITH SEVERE PREECLAMPSIA

Control hypertension
Gradually rehydrate
Reestablish adequate urine output
Secure seizure prophylaxis
Decide which attenuator of pressor responses to intubation and
    laryngoscopy to use
Institute hemodynamic monitoring
Look for evidence of laryngeal or upper airway edema
Assess degree of recent bleeding (if any)
Assess fetal condition
Choose the best anesthetic
    Decide whether neuraxial block is safe (remember thrombocytopenia,
        disseminated intravascular coagulation, renal or liver damage)
    Decide whether general anesthesia is safe

PRE- AND INTRAOPERATIVE MONITORING

A number of hemodynamic parameters are altered in normal pregnancy. For example, although the cardiac output (CO) is increased by about 43%, the systemic arterial vascular resistance (SVR) is decreased by 21% so that the mean arterial pressure in normal pregnancy is not altered to any appreciable extent.[8]

Severe "classic" preeclampsia superimposes upon pregnancy a set of changes. Left ventricular function is increased and the CO is increased even further than in normal pregnancy (Fig. 11-1). The SVR is increased in severe preeclampsia, often markedly such that the SVR index (SVRI) is often more than 2200 dyne-sec·cm^{-5}·m^{-2}. Mean arterial pressure rises not only to but above prepregnant levels. The picture of

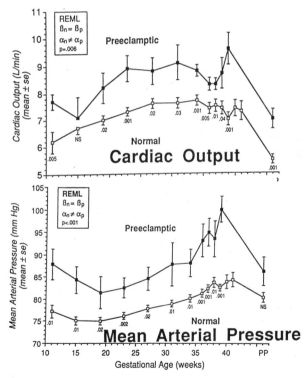

Figure 11-1 ■ The cardiac output (top) and mean systemic arterial pressure (bottom). In normal (□) and preeclamptic (■) pregnancies at different stages of pregnancy and in the postpartum period. (From Easterling TR, Benedetti TJ, Schmucker BC, Millard SP: Maternal hemodynamics in normal and preeclamptic pregnancies: a longitudinal study. Obstet Gynecol 76:1061-1069, 1990.)

■ Table 11–8
CLINICAL PICTURE OF CLASSIC, SEVERE, UNTREATED PREECLAMPSIA

Hemodynamic Parameter	Change from Normal Pregnancy Level
Left ventricular function	Marked elevation
CO	Moderate elevation
SVR	Marked elevation
Colloid osmotic pressure	Usually decreased
Mean arterial pressure	Marked elevation
Central venous pressure	Modest decrease
Plasma volume	Modest decrease
Blood viscosity	Small elevation
Red blood cell deformability	Mild increase
Pulmonary vascular resistance	Unaffected
Urine output	Moderate decrease

a hemoconcentrated, hypertensive, oliguric patient emerges (Table 11-8).

The clinical picture is made more complex because, in some patients, the picture is not "classic" even when the condition is untreated. For example, whereas the SVRI is elevated (>2200) in most patients, it is normal (1500 to 2200) in many and low (<1500) in a few. Likewise, although the cardiac index is normal (>3 L/min/m^2) or high (>5) in most severe preeclamptic patients, in some it is low (<3). To add insult to injury, large hemodynamic alterations occur intra- and immediately postpartum. Noninvasive measurement of CO has considerably simplified intraoperative assessment.[9]

There is poor correlation between central venous pressure and pulmonary capillary wedge pressure in those with severe preeclampsia at term. Indications for pulmonary artery catheter insertion at term include

- Patients who remain anuric or severely oliguric despite fluid loading,
- Patients who develop pulmonary edema resistant to standard cardiac failure therapy,
- Patients who have diastolic DAP >110 mm Hg unresponsive to aggressive antihypertensive therapy.[10]

SEIZURE TREATMENT AND PROPHYLAXIS

Seizures are initially treated by maintenance of a patent airway, rolling the patient into the left lateral position, or administration of oxygen by face mask, or they are controlled with a small dose of a barbiturate (e.g., thiopentone), a benzodiazepine (e.g., IV diazepam), or, if seizures continue or the airway

■ Table 11–9
STRATAGEM FOR THE PREVENTION OF CONVULSIONS IN THOSE WHO HAVE EITHER DEVELOPED SEVERE PREECLAMPSIA OR EXPERIENCED A PRIOR CONVULSIVE (ECLAMPTIC) EPISODE

Rigid control of blood pressure, including epidural sympathetic blockade
Magnesium sulfate
   Less commonly, phenytoin sodium
   Rarely, both phenytoin and magnesium

is compromised, by a modified rapid sequence induction followed by endotracheal intubation.

Prophylaxis against recurrence of convulsions is shown in Table 11-9. Table 11-10 reviews methods of hypertension control.

The International Multicentre Collaborative Eclampsia Trial ($n = 1680$) showed that women receiving magnesium had a 52% lower risk of recurrence of convulsions than those receiving diazepam and a 67% lower risk than those given phenytoin. Magnesium was also found to be superior to diazepam or phenytoin for the treatment of eclampsia.[11]

SPINAL, EPIDURAL, OR GENERAL ANESTHESIA?

Epidural, spinal, and general anesthesia techniques have all been used successfully to manage severe preeclamptic pa-

■ Table 11–10
A REGIMEN OF ANTIHYPERTENSIVE MEDICATION FOR SEVERE ACUTE AND MILD PREECLAMPSIA

Acute (indicated in cases of severe hypertension: blood pressure $\geq$ 170 mm Hg systolic and/or $\geq$ 110 mm Hg diastolic)
   Hydralazine, intravenously or intramuscularly
   Nifedipine, orally or sublingually
   Labetalol, intravenously
   Diazoxide, repeated minibolus intravenously
Chronic (indicated in cases of mild hypertension: blood pressure $\geq$ 160 mm Hg systolic and/or $\geq$ 90 mm Hg diastolic)
   Initial agents: methyldopa, oxprenolol, labetalol, clonidine
   Second-line agents: hydralazine, nifedipine
Avoid:
   Angiotensin-converting enzyme inhibitors
   Diuretics
   Nonsteroidal antiinflammatory agents, excluding low-dose aspirin

Modified from Brown MA, Gallery EDM, Gatt SP, et al: Management of Hypertension in Pregnancy. Consensus Statement of the Australasian Society for the Study of Hypertension in Pregnancy, Executive Summary. Med J Aust 158:700–702, 1993.

tients, but each technique carries hazards that can be minimized but not completely eliminated. Risks due to major continuous conduction anesthesia are hypotension and hemodynamic instability with potential reduction in uteroplacental and renal blood flow in those with hypovolemia and spinal bleeding with the risk of cord compression in those with clinically significant thrombocytopenia and coagulopathy. Risks due to general anesthesia are marked elevations in blood pressure and hemodynamic upheaval at laryngoscopy and endotracheal intubation and extubation and intracerebral bleeding and raised intracranial pressure.

■ **KEY POINT:** Regardless of anesthetic planned, a thorough airway examination is essential owing to the risk of airway edema and difficult intubation.

REGIONAL ANESTHESIA

Because in most institutions a "bloody" tap occurs in about 5% of epidural punctures, many anesthetists are concerned that severe preeclamptic patients could develop epidural and subdural hematomas. Platelet counts of less than 150×10^9/L occur in 11 to 50% of preeclamptic pregnancies. The risk of clinically significant hematoma increases as the number of available effective platelets drops progressively.

It seems prudent to have a cutoff point below which epidural needling and catheter placement becomes undesirable. This minimum point must be different for each patient, depending on clinical scenario. A decision to proceed with or refuse epidural analgesia is determined based on the institution's policy and patient condition. A full coagulation profile is often of little additional assistance in making such a decision. Although there is no single number below which epidural analgesia should not be performed, many practitioners use 50,000 or 75,000/mm^3 as their cutoff. Physical examination, assumed difficulty of intubation, and rate at which platelet count declined must all be considered.

■ **KEY POINT:** Epidural anesthesia and spinal anesthesia have been safely administered to women with mild preeclampsia. For women with severe preeclampsia, the use of spinal anesthesia remains controversial.

GENERAL ANESTHESIA

Preoperative Preparation

In the immediate preoperative period, attention should be paid to preoxygenation, aspiration prophylaxis, left uterine displacement, and crossmatching of blood.

Induction

A thiopental-succinylcholine rapid sequence induction with cricoid pressure is recommended. Episodes of hypertension and hypotension should be treated aggressively.

Laryngoscopy and Endotracheal Intubation

The pressor response of laryngoscopy and endotracheal intubation needs to be controlled to avoid elevation of intracranial pressure or poorly controlled hypertension. Magnesium sulfate, supplementary doses of induction agents, local anesthetics (e.g., lidocaine), short-acting opioids (e.g., remifentanil), vasodilators (e.g., α-adrenoreceptor blockers), and β-adrenoreceptor antagonists (e.g., esmolol) have all been used successfully, but no method guarantees complete ablation of pressor responses at doses free of side effects.

Maintenance

Inhalational agents, opioids, hypnotics, and nondepolarizing muscle relaxants can all be used in the preeclamptic patient.

Postoperative Analgesia

An intravenous patient-controlled analgesia, intravenous opiate infusion, or intermittent intramuscular opioid injection regimen can be used for postoperative analgesia.

Differential Diagnosis

Acute cocaine intoxication can present with signs and symptoms very similar to preeclampsia, that is, convulsions, hypertension, proteinuria, and thrombocytopenia. The differential diagnosis of preeclampsia also includes essential hypertension, renal disease, idiopathic thrombocytopenic purpura, gallbladder disease, systemic lupus, acute fatty liver of pregnancy, pheochromocytoma, cardiomyopathy, dissecting aortic aneurysm, glomerulonephritis, and ruptured bile duct. It would seem that severe preeclampsia, hemolytic uremic syndrome in pregnancy, thrombotic thrombocytopenic purpura, HELLP syndrome, and postpartum acute renal failure are often part of the spectrum of the same illness.[12]

CONCLUSION

The management of preeclamptic patients is usually straightforward, but in some patients it can be both challenging and surprisingly difficult. Fastidiousness of approach ensures a positive outcome for both mother and infant in most cases. The secret to successful management lies in simultaneous treatment of several aspects of this multifaceted disease. For example, volume replacement without pari passu vasodilatation will almost certainly tip some women into pulmonary (or worse, cerebral) edema even though these women are usually hypovolemic and oliguric. Likewise, if the vasospasm and hypertension are treated too aggressively with antihypertensives or high epidural sympathetic blockade, there will sometimes be a massive, perhaps even life threatening, fall in blood pressure.

Treatment should be seen as an exercise in timing and balance. Small parallel adjustments should be made to relieve the vasospasm, oliguria, hypertension, and hypovolemia. Most errors and pitfalls in preeclampsia management are related to the timing and degree of aggressiveness in adjustment of the continuously changing hemodynamic balance.

REFERENCES

1. Bernheim J: Hypertension in pregnancy. Nephron 76:254–263, 1997.
2. American College of Obstetricians & Gynecologists: Technical bulletin. Int J Gynecol Obstet 53:175–183, 1996.
3. Brown MA, Gallery EDM, Gatt S, et al: Consensus Statement. Management of Hypertension in Pregnancy. Australasian Society for the Study of Hypertension in Pregnancy. Sydney: New Era Printing 1993:15–46.
4. Malinow AM: Preeclampsia and eclampsia: anesthetic management *In:* American Society of Anesthesiologists 1996 Annual Refresher Course Lecture. Philadelphia: Lippincott-Raven, 1996:1–7.
5. Sibai BM: Treatment of hypertension in pregnant women. N Engl J Med 335:257–265, 1996.
6. Gallery ED: Hypertension in pregnancy. Practical management recommendations. Drugs 49:555–562, 1995.
7. Gatt SP: Gestational proteinuric hypertension. Curr Opin Anesthesiol 5:354–359, 1992.
8. Easterling TR, Benedetti TJ, Schmucker BC, Millard SP: Maternal hemodynamics in normal and preeclamptic pregnancies: a longitudinal study. Obstet Gynecol 76:1061–1069, 1990.
9. Wasserstrum N, Cotton DB: Hemodynamic monitoring in severe pregnancy-induced hypertension. Clin Perinatol 13:781–799, 1986.
10. Clark SL, Cotton DB: Clinical indications for pulmonary artery catheterization in the patient with severe preeclampsia. Am J Obstet Gynecol 158:453–458, 1988.
11. Eclampsia Trial Collaborative Group: Which anticonvulsant for women with eclampsia? Evidence from the Collaborative Eclampsia Trial. Lancet 345:1455–1463, 1995.
12. Redman CW, Roberts JM: Management of pre-eclampsia. Lancet 341:1451–1454, 1993.

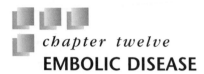

chapter twelve
EMBOLIC DISEASE
Andrew M. Malinow, MD

Pregnant women are afflicted by three types of emboli: amniotic fluid embolism, pulmonary thromboembolism (PTE), and venous air embolism. All have been reported to occur at any time in pregnancy, although most are associated with parturition. In the extreme, all three are associated with sudden dramatic alteration in cardiorespiratory function, leading to cardiac arrest and death. Together, these disorders make up the most common cause of direct maternal mortality.[1] The anesthesiologist is often involved in resuscitation of patients. Early recognition, diagnosis, and treatment are necessary to reduce the morbidity and mortality.

■ **KEY POINT:** Embolism in the pregnant patient is a common cause of maternal morbidity and mortality.

AMNIOTIC FLUID EMBOLISM

Amniotic fluid embolism was first reported in 1926,[2] but it was not until 1941 that Steiner and Lushbaugh[3] reviewed a series of autopsies and described the syndrome of sudden peripartum shock characterized by pulmonary edema.

Incidence

In the United States, the incidence of amniotic fluid embolism is approximately 3 per 100,000 live births.[4] Amniotic fluid embolism accounts for as many as 12% of maternal deaths.[1] The overall mortality for afflicted parturients is as high as 60 to 80%, and 63% succumb within the first 5 hours.[5, 6] In a recent review by Clark et al.[6] of 46 patients collected from a national registry for amniotic fluid embolism, only 8% of patients who survived a cardiac arrest were judged neurologically intact.

Pathophysiology

The etiology of the amniotic fluid embolism syndrome is unclear. The amount of particulate matter found in the lungs does not correlate with the severity of the clinical presentation. However, the presence of meconium at clinical presentation is associated with a uniformly dismal prognosis.[6] It is suggested that this is due to the presence of a heat-stable pressor agent in meconium, which enhances the cardiopulmonary response to the infusion of autologous amniotic fluid in goats.[7] However, in only 30% of cases was meconium-stained amniotic fluid demonstrated.[6] Others have suggested that arachidonic acid metabolites, especially leukotrienes, are responsible for the clinical and pathophysiologic features of amniotic fluid embolism.[5]

There have been two cases of successful pregnancy outcomes in women who survived amniotic fluid embolism in earlier pregnancies, suggesting the role of a qualitatively abnormal amniotic fluid, which may be different in a subsequent pregnancy, as opposed to any unusual maternal sensitivity to amniotic fluid per se in the genesis of this condition.[6]

A *biphasic* response to amniotic fluid embolism has been described.[7] The *early phase* consists of transient (but perhaps intense) pulmonary vasospasm, which probably results from the release of vasoactive substances. This may account for the right heart dysfunction that is often fatal.[7] Low cardiac output leads to increased ventilation–perfusion mismatch, hypoxemia, and hypotension. This phase probably has a duration of less than 30 minutes.[7] Of interest, right heart function and pulmonary artery pressures are usually close to "normal" by the time hemodynamic monitoring is begun in humans resuscitated from amniotic fluid embolism.[5, 8] A *second phase* of left ventricular failure and pulmonary edema occurs in those women who survive the initial insult.[5, 8, 9] Case reports that include invasive hemodynamic monitoring have consistently noted the occurrence of left ventricular dysfunction in women afflicted with amniotic fluid embolism.[5, 8, 9] The etiology of the left ventricular dysfunction is unclear.

Disruption of the normal clotting cascade occurs in as many as 80% of women with amniotic fluid embolism.[5, 6] Uterine atony (perhaps a result of a circulating myometrial depressant factor or uterine hypoperfusion) occurs in some women.[5, 6] Massive hemorrhage may also contribute to a consumptive coagulopathy.[5, 6]

Clinical Presentation

Amniotic fluid embolism has also occurred during first-trimester abortion, in the second trimester, at delivery, after abdominal trauma, and even in the postpartum period.[5] In the review of the National Registry for Amniotic Fluid Embolism, only 70% of amniotic fluid embolisms were diagnosed before delivery but less than 10% occurred more than 5 minutes after delivery.[6] Overall, labor was not tumultuous. Only 50% of patients had received oxytocin and none demonstrated uterine hyperstimulation.[6] Thirty-eight of 46 patients had already undergone spontaneous or artificial rupture of membranes at the time of diagnosis.[6] In six of these patients, artificial rupture of membranes and placement of an intrauterine pressure

▪ Table 12–1

SIGNS AND SYMPTOMS NOTED IN 46 PATIENTS DIAGNOSED WITH AMNIOTIC FLUID EMBOLISM

Sign/Symptom	Incidence (%)
Hypotension	100
Fetal distress	100
Pulmonary edema/ARDS	87
Cardiopulmonary arrest	83
Cyanosis	83
Coagulopathy	83
Dyspnea	49
Seizure	48
Uterine atony	23
Bronchospasm	15
Transient hypotension	11
Cough	7
Headache	7
Chest pain	7

ARDS, acute respiratory distress syndrome.
From Clark SL, Hankins GDV, Dudley DA, et al: Amniotic fluid embolism: analysis of the national registry. Am J Obstet Gynecol 172:1156–1169; 1995.

catheter was followed within 3 minutes by signs and symptoms of amniotic fluid embolism.[6]

The diagnosis of amniotic fluid embolism is one of exclusion (Table 12–1). The clinical presentation is often compatible with other malignant obstetric (e.g., abruptio placentae, eclampsia), nonobstetric (e.g., other embolic events, sepsis, myocardial infarction, anaphylaxis), and anesthetic (e.g., total spinal anesthesia, local anesthetic toxicity) events.

In the past, physicians thought that detection of fetal squamous cells in the pulmonary circulation was pathognomonic of amniotic fluid embolism.[5] However, in those patients diagnosed with amniotic fluid embolism, cells of fetal origin were found in the pulmonary circulation in only 73% of those patients who expired and underwent autopsy.[5] Overall, cells of fetal origin were found in only 50% of patients diagnosed with amniotic fluid embolism who had aspirates of pulmonary arterial blood.[5] Indeed, obstetricians have detected fetal squames in the pulmonary circulation of both antepartum and postpartum patients with no clinical evidence of amniotic fluid embolism.[5]

▪ **KEY POINT:** Amniotic fluid embolism should be considered if a parturient experiences sudden dyspnea or cardiovascular collapse. Amniotic fluid embolism can occur at any time during labor and delivery and remains unpredictable, unpreventable, and often untreatable.

Management

Prompt recognition and institution of resuscitative measures may influence maternal and fetal outcome (Table 12–2). Several cases have been published of patients who survived amniotic fluid embolism.[5, 6] Resuscitative measures should be aggressive. The heroic (and successful) use of cardiopulmonary bypass for treatment of postpartum shock caused by amniotic fluid embolism has been reported.[10] A decision must be made almost immediately during resuscitation as to delivering the fetus. Greater than a 15-minute delay in delivery after maternal cardiac arrest significantly decreases the chance for delivery of a neurologically intact neonate.[6] Resuscitation efforts, including ensuring venous return and closed chest compressions, may be made easier with delivery of the fetus.

If the patient received regional anesthesia before the onset of amniotic fluid embolism, subsequent coagulopathy should alert physicians and nurses to the potential for epidural hematoma. Neurologic function should be assessed frequently. An indwelling epidural catheter should be removed as soon as possible, preferably after the transfusion of blood and replacement of coagulation factors has temporarily created a state of normal coagulation.

■ Table 12–2
RESUSCITATION OF THE PATIENT WITH AMNIOTIC FLUID EMBOLISM

Initiate CPR/ACLS as indicated
  Establish and maintain airway (e.g., tracheal intubation)
    Establish adequate ventilation with 100% oxygen initially
    Support maternal circulation
      Volume resuscitation
      Intravenous access (several large-gauge catheters)
      Inotropic support if needed (e.g., dopamine, norepinephrine)
Monitoring
  Maternal
    Insert intraarterial catheter
    Insert pulmonary artery catheter
  Fetal
    Make a decision regarding delivery (either before impending
      maternal demise or to improve chances of maternal resuscitation)
Treat the coagulopathy
  Component therapy vs. fresh whole blood (if available)
  Consultation with hemopathologist to inform blood bank of situation
  Prepare for laparotomy (i.e., hysterectomy, hypogastric artery ligation)
Manage sequelae of shock (e.g., cardiac, renal, and hepatic failure;
    neurologic sequelae; respiratory failure—pulmonary edema, ARDS)
  Establish the location for appropriate intensive care

CPR, cardiopulmonary resuscitation; ACLS, advanced cardiac life support; ARDS, acute respiratory distress syndrome.

PULMONARY THROMBOEMBOLISM

Incidence

PTE occurs in approximately 0.05% of all pregnancies.[11] It most often occurs secondary to deep vein thrombosis, but it can also occur after superficial vein, puerperal septic pelvic vein, and puerperal ovarian vein thrombosis.

Approximately 33% of patients with untreated septic pelvic vein thrombosis experience a pulmonary embolus. However, most cases of PTE during pregnancy occur as a result of deep vein thrombosis.[11] Interestingly, given that most deep vein thromboses occur in the antepartum period, almost two thirds of all pulmonary embolisms associated with pregnancy occur in the postpartum period. Approximately 13 to 24% of pregnant patients with untreated deep vein thrombosis experience a pulmonary embolus. Treatment of deep vein thrombosis reduces the incidence of PTE to 0.7 to 4.5%[12, 13] and the mortality rate to 0.7%.[14] Although the incidence of maternal mortality from PTE has declined by over 50% during the last two decades, PTE still accounts for approximately 12 to 25% of direct maternal mortality.[1, 15]

Etiology

One half the cases of thromboembolism in women of childbearing years occur during pregnancy or the puerperium.[16] In fact, pregnancy results in a five- to sixfold increase in the relative risk of thromboembolism when compared with nonpregnant women.[15] The increased frequency of thromboembolic disease in pregnancy is a result of at least three factors: an increase in pelvic and lower extremity venous stasis (due to caval compression), the hypercoagulable state of pregnancy (and the decreased fibrinolytic activity immediately postpartum), and the vascular injury associated with vaginal or cesarean delivery.

A history of previous thromboembolism increases the risk of PTE during pregnancy.[17] In addition, coincidental diseases, which further increase the risk of thromboembolism in obstetric patients, include obesity, lupus anticoagulant, protein S and C deficiencies, antithrombin III deficiency, and dysfibrinogenemia.[14]

Pathophysiology

The manifestations and prognosis of PTE depend on the size and number of emboli, concurrent cardiopulmonary function, the rate of clot fragmentation and lysis, and the presence or absence of a source for recurrent emboli.[18] After a pulmonary embolus occurs, respiratory failure results from either extensive occlusion of the pulmonary vasculature (which results in cardiorespiratory decompensation) or pulmonary edema.[18]

Pulmonary hypertension may result from direct vascular obstruction by a large embolus (e.g., a saddle embolus). However, a small embolus may also be associated with severe pulmonary hypertension, especially if there is underlying cardiac or pulmonary disease or recurrent pulmonary embolization.[18] In any case, right ventricular overload can occur. In addition, disruption of normal capillary integrity may occur.[18] Simultaneous cardiorespiratory compromise may prompt aggressive intravenous volume replacement. The increase in hydrostatic forces and the disruption of normal capillary integrity predispose to pulmonary edema.[18]

Diagnosis

Clinical

The diagnosis of a pulmonary embolus requires a high index of suspicion and prompt evaluation. The patient may complain of dyspnea, palpitations, anxiety, and chest pain, which is sometimes pleuritic. The patient may appear cyanic and diaphoretic. The patient may have a cough, with or without hemoptysis. Findings on physical examination are listed in Table 12-3.

Embolism leads to a redistribution in pulmonary blood flow, possibly leading to "hyperfusion" of otherwise low ventilation–perfusion zones in unaffected areas of the lung. In cases of right ventricular failure, a decrease in cardiac output will lead to decreased mixed-venous oxygen content, which enhances the effects of ventilation–perfusion mismatch. Arterial hypoxemia often results. However, 5 to 14% of all patients with a pulmonary embolus have a Pao_2 greater than 85 mm Hg.

Diagnostic Imaging

Chest x-ray findings may show atelectasis, pleural effusion, elevated hemidiaphragm, and a peripheral segmental or sub-

■ Table 12–3
**PHYSICAL FINDINGS OF
PULMONARY EMBOLISM**

Finding	Percent of Patients
Tachypnea	85
Tachycardia	40
Fever	45
Accentuated second heart sound	50
Localized rales	60
Thrombophlebitis	40
Supraventricular dysrhythmia	15

From Spence TH: Pulmonary embolization syndrome. In: Civetta JM, Taylor RW, Kirby RR, eds. Critical Care. Philadelphia: J.B. Lippincott, 1988:1091–1102.

segmental infiltrate. However, the chest radiograph is neither specific nor sensitive in the diagnosis of PTE. In fact, 25 to 40% of patients with a pulmonary embolus have a normal chest x-ray study. The chest x-ray examination facilitates the interpretation of the nuclear scan because not all perfusion defects on lung scan are a result of PTE. In addition, it aids in the diagnosis of other conditions (e.g., pleurisy, pneumothorax, and fractured rib) that may mimic PTE.

If the perfusion scan is normal, the diagnosis of PTE can be excluded. Multiple perfusion defects and ventilation–perfusion mismatch on lung scan suggest a high probability of a pulmonary embolus.[19] A high clinical suspicion of PTE and a high-probability lung scan (e.g., segmental perfusion defect with normal ventilation) indicate initiation of heparin therapy. If the lung scan reveals subsegmental defects with normal ventilation or matched perfusion and ventilation defects, the probability of PTE is between 10 and 40%. Pulmonary angiography (preferably performed via the brachial route) should be considered if clinical suspicion is high.

Although the physician should limit unnecessary fetal radiation exposure, small amounts of radiation exposure probably increase fetal risk to a very limited degree. Most studies suggest that fetal radiation exposure to less than 5 rads does not result in an increased incidence of teratogenesis.[19]

It is possible to use a chest x-ray study, ventilation-perfusion scan, and pulmonary angiography to make the diagnosis of PTE, with a total fetal radiation exposure of less than 60 mrads. Even when pulmonary angiography must be done via the femoral route, the total fetal radiation exposure is less than 400 mrads.

Although not as sensitive as pulmonary angiography in the detection of a pulmonary artery embolus, echocardiographic confirmation of a clot may obviate the need for the more invasive procedure (especially if there is a delay in beginning the angiography procedure) and may hasten the time to anticoagulation.[20]

Therapy

Approximately 10% of all afflicted patients die within the first hour after a pulmonary embolus.[21] Of those who survive this acute phase, long-term survival depends on rapid diagnosis and institution of therapy. Therapy focuses on providing adequate maternal and fetal oxygenation; support of maternal circulation, including uteroplacental perfusion; and immediate anticoagulation or venous interruption to prevent recurrence of a (perhaps lethal) pulmonary embolus. Acute decompensation from a pulmonary embolus warrants fibrinolytic therapy and in severe cases, surgical embolectomy.

Heparin is the anticoagulant of choice. Heparin therapy should be started immediately. A bolus intravenous dose of

150 U/kg is followed by a continuous infusion of 15 to 20 U/ kg/h to maintain the partial thromboplastin time (PTT) at twice-normal values.

Inferior vena caval interruption should be considered in any patient who cannot be anticoagulated or who suffers from recurrent emboli while on anticoagulant therapy. In nonpregnant patients, insertion of an inferior vena caval filter has a mortality rate of less than 1% and a recurrence rate of lethal emboli of less than 1%. Transvenous placement of a Greenfield filter has a long-term patency rate of 97%.

Thrombolytic therapy should be considered in patients with a massive pulmonary embolus. A suggested dose of urokinase therapy is an initial dose of 4400 U/kg followed by 4400 U/kg/h. Although an increase in the PTT and fibrin degradation products can be used to follow thrombolytic therapy, the most sensitive measure is the thrombin time. The thrombin time should be no greater than five times normal. Nonetheless, the risk of bleeding is always present. Antepartum and intrapartum complications include maternal hemorrhage and abruptio placentae.

Recombinant tissue plasminogen factor has been used successfully in pregnant women suffering massive pulmonary embolism.[22] Minimal bleeding complications have been reported.

Surgical embolectomy is an extreme measure reserved for the rapidly deteriorating patient.[23] It is associated with a high mortality rate.

■ **KEY POINT:** Therapy for PTE focuses on providing adequate maternal and fetal oxygenation. Approximately 10% of all afflicted patients die within 1 hour of the embolus.

Anesthetic Management

Cardiopulmonary sequelae of PTE often dictate the anesthetic management for labor and vaginal or cesarean delivery. More often, asymptomatic women with a history of deep vein thrombosis present for labor and vaginal or cesarean delivery. The anesthesiologist must then consider the risks (essentially epidural hematoma) versus the benefits of regional anesthesia. The risk of epidural hematoma associated with each specific therapy is unquantifiable. Obviously, both the anesthesiologist and the patient would like reassurance of little or no increase in risk when compared with that for the patient who is not receiving anticoagulation therapy. Suggested guidelines for induction of regional anesthesia are proposed in Table 12–4.

If needed, incremental doses of protamine can be given up

■ Table 12–4
SUGGESTED GUIDELINES FOR REGIONAL ANESTHESIA IN THE ANTICOAGULATED PARTURIENT

1. Heparin is discontinued with the onset of active labor.
2. Regional anesthesia is induced when the PTT is normal or the blood heparin concentration is near zero.
3. If these conditions are not met, the patient is offered intravenous opioid analgesia for labor until the PTT or blood heparin concentration levels are near normal.
4. Protamine (incremental doses up to a calculated dose of 1 mg protamine/100 U of heparin and titrated to surgical hemostasis) may be administered in selected patients who require emergency cesarean delivery. Regional anesthesia is administered only if a coagulation profile is normal. We do not routinely reverse heparin therapy with protamine to allow administration of regional anesthesia.
5. If cesarean delivery is needed in a patient with abnormal coagulation, general anesthesia is administered.
6. The anesthesiologist and obstetrician should discuss the reinstitution of anticoagulation therapy after delivery. Removal of the epidural catheter may cause venous disruption and bleeding into the epidural space. It therefore seems optimal to remove the epidural catheter before the reinstitution of heparin therapy or as soon as possible.

to a calculated dose of 1 mg protamine/100 U of heparin. The dose should be titrated to surgical hemostasis.

Fibrinolytic agents are associated with a significant risk of abruptio placentae and maternal hemorrhage. Therefore, labor and delivery represent relative contraindications to the use of fibrinolytic therapy, and the question regarding epidural anesthesia is moot.

Peripartum anticoagulation or fibrinolytic therapy (administered before, during, or after administration of regional anesthesia) requires that the anesthesiologist, obstetrician, and nursing staff remain vigilant for any of the signs and symptoms that herald epidural hematoma, including severe unremitting backache; neurologic deficit, including bowel or bladder dysfunction or radiculopathy; tenderness over the spinous or paraspinous area; and unexplained fever. Suspicion of epidural hematoma should lead to immediate diagnostic imaging of the spinal cord and neurosurgical consultation for possible spinal cord decompression.

> ■ **KEY POINT:** If a parturient has had anticoagulation with heparin or warfarin, prothrombin time, activated PTT, activated clotting time, and thromboelastogram can be used to assess the degree of reversal before initiation of a neuraxial block.

VENOUS AIR EMBOLISM

Numerous case reports of venous air embolism in obstetric patients have appeared in the medical literature since the early 19th century.[24]

Incidence

Venous air embolism (as determined by precordial Doppler, echocardiography, and analysis of end-tidal nitrogen) occurs in essentially all parturients undergoing cesarean delivery[25] and has been reported at vaginal delivery.[26]

■ **KEY POINT:** The vascular structure of the gravid uterus allows air entrance during cesarean section, and air embolism is a frequent subclinical finding, especially on exteriorization of the uterus.

Pathophysiology

A gradient as small as -5 cm H_2O between the surgical field and the heart allows a significant amount of air to be entrained into the venous circulation. Routine left uterine displacement and use of the Trendelenburg position (which is often requested during cesarean delivery) increase this gradient. In theory, any cause of decreased central venous pressure (e.g., hemorrhage) may also increase the chance for venous air embolism. Deep Trendelenburg is probably best avoided. Placement of the table in an exaggerated reverse Trendelenburg probably does not significantly decrease the incidence of venous air embolism. However, uterine exteriorization is associated with an increased incidence of Doppler changes suggestive of venous air embolism during cesarean section.[27]

Morbidity and mortality from venous air embolism are related to the volume and rate of infusion of air into the central circulation and the site of embolization. Large volumes (more than 3 mL/kg) of air may lead to fatal right ventricular outflow tract obstruction (i.e., "air lock"). Smaller amounts of air can result in ventilation–perfusion mismatch, hypoxemia, right heart failure, arrhythmia, and hypotension, and paradoxical air embolus into the arterial circulation (via a patent foramen ovale) can lead to cardiovascular and neurologic sequelae and morbidity.

Clinical Presentation

Massive venous air embolism can present as a sudden, dramatic, and devastating event with hypotension, hypoxemia, and even cardiac arrest. However, venous air embolism causes significant hemodynamic compromise (i.e., a more than 20% decrease in blood pressure) in only 0.7 to 2% of parturients at delivery. Usually, the clinical picture is much less dramatic. Venous air embolism has been associated with chest pain (less than 50% of cases), decreased SaO_2 (25% of cases), and dyspnea (20 to 50% of cases). It is unclear whether venous air embolism is responsible for these electrocardiographic changes (e.g., ST-segment depression) seen in 25 to 50% of all patients undergoing cesarean delivery.[28] The clinical significance of these electrocardiographic changes is also unclear.

Recommendations

Although there is evidence that venous air embolism is a common occurrence during cesarean section, maternal morbidity and mortality are rare. I do not recommend the routine use of precordial Doppler monitoring during cesarean section. However, high-risk patients (those who are hypovolemic or those with known intracardiac shunts) may benefit from the use of precordial Doppler monitoring. A high index of suspicion should accompany any complaints of chest pain or dyspnea, decreased SaO_2, hypotension, or arrhythmia. Early recognition of these signs and symptoms associated with venous air embolism should prompt the appropriate response (Table 12-5).

SUMMARY

Embolic disease in the gravida may manifest as an acute dramatic event. Anesthesiologists must be ever vigilant for the signs and symptoms of embolic phenomena in the obstetric

■ Table 12–5
RESUSCITATION OF THE PATIENT WITH MASSIVE VENOUS AIR EMBOLISM

- Prevent further air entrainment (e.g., flood surgical field, change position).
- Discontinue nitrous oxide and give 100% oxygen.
- Support ventilation as needed.
- Support circulation.
- If hemodynamic instability persists, consider placement of a multiorifice central venous catheter to attempt aspiration of air.
- Expedite delivery.
- If there is delayed emergence from general anesthesia, consider neurodiagnostic imaging to rule out intracerebral air. Patients with evidence of paradoxical cerebral arterial gas embolism may benefit from hyperbaric oxygen therapy.

patient. Often, it has been early diagnosis and aggressive intervention that has led to a successful outcome.

REFERENCES

1. Berg CJ, Atrash K, Koonin LM, et al: Pregnancy-related maternal mortality in the United States, 1987-1990. Obstet Gynecol 88:161-167, 1996.
2. Meyer JR: Embolia pulmonar amnio-caseo. Bras Med 2:301-303, 1926.
3. Steiner PE, Lushbaugh CC: Maternal pulmonary embolism by amniotic fluid. JAMA 117:1245-1254, 1941.
4. Price TH, Baker VV, Cefalo RC: Amniotic fluid embolism: three cases with a review of the literature. Obstet Gynecol Surv 40:462-475, 1985.
5. Clark SL: New concepts of amniotic fluid embolism: a review. Obstet Gynecol Surv 45:360-368, 1990.
6. Clark SL, Hankins GDV, Dudley DA, et al: Amniotic fluid embolism: analysis of the national registry. Am J Obstet Gynecol 172:1156-1169, 1995.
7. Hankins GDV, Snyder RR, Clark SL, et al: Acute hemodynamic and respiratory effects of amniotic fluid embolism in the pregnant goat model. Am J Obstet Gynecol 68:1113-1130, 1993.
8. Clark SC, Cotton DB, Gonik B, et al: Central hemodynamic alterations in amniotic fluid embolism. Am J Obstet Gynecol 158:1124-1126, 1988.
9. Clark SL, Montz FJ, Phelan JP: Hemodynamic alterations associated with amniotic fluid embolism: a reappraisal. Am J Obstet Gynecol 151:617-621, 1985.
10. Esposito RA, Grossi EA, Coppia G, et al: Successful treatment of postpartum shock caused by amniotic fluid embolism with cardiopulmonary bypass and pulmonary artery thromboembolectomy. Am J Obstet Gynecol 163:571-574, 1990.
11. Weiner CP: Diagnosis and management of thromboembolic disease during pregnancy. Clin Obstet Gynecol 28:107-118, 1985.
12. Bolan JC: Thromboembolic complications of pregnancy. Clin Obstet Gynecol 26:913-922, 1981.
13. Villasanta U: Thromboembolic disease in pregnancy. Am J Obstet Gynecol 93:142-160, 1965.
14. Sipes SL, Weiner CP: Venous thromboembolic disease in pregnancy. Semin Perinatol 14:103-118, 1990.
15. Franks AL, Atrash HK, Lawson HW, et al: Obstetrical pulmonary embolism mortality: United States 1970-1985. Am J Public Health 80:720-721, 1990.
16. Bonnar J: Venous thromboembolism and pregnancy. Clin Obstet Gynecol 8:455-473, 1981.
17. Bremme K, Lind H, Blomback M: The effect of prophylactic heparin treatment in enhanced thrombin generation in pregnancy. Obstet Gynecol 78:78-83, 1993.
18. Spence TH: Pulmonary embolization syndrome. In: Civetta JM, Taylor RM, Kirby RR, eds. Critical Care. Philadelphia: J.B. Lippincott, 1988:1091-1102.
19. Barron WM: The pregnant surgical patient: medical evaluation and management. Ann Intern Med 101:683-691, 1984.
20. Rosenberg JM, Lefor AT, Kenien G, et al: Echocardiographic diagnosis and surgical treatment of postpartum pulmonary embolism. Ann Thorac Surg 49:667-669, 1990.
21. Dalen JE, Alpert JS: Natural history of pulmonary embolism. Prog Cardiovasc Dis 17:259-270, 1975.
22. Baudo F, Caimi TM, Redaelli R, et al: Emergency treatment with recombinant tissue plasminogen activator of pulmonary embolism in a pregnant woman with antithrombin III deficiency. Am J Obstet Gynecol 163:1274-1275, 1990.
23. Splinter WM, Dwane PD, Wigle RD, et al: Anaesthetic management of emergency cesarean section followed by pulmonary embolectomy. Can J Anaesth 36:689-692, 1989.

24. Amussat JZ: Recherces sur l'Introduction Accidentelle de l'Air Dans les Veins. Paris: Germer Bailliere, 1839:255.
25. Malinow AM, Naulty JS, Hunt CO, et al: Precordial ultrasonic Doppler monitoring during cesarean delivery. Anesthesiology 66:816–819, 1987.
26. Flanagan J, Slimack J, Black D, et al: The incidence of venous air embolism in the parturient [abstract]. Reg Anesth 15:A10, 1990.
27. Bromage PR, Hohman WA: Uterine posture and incidence of venous air embolism (VAE) during cesarean section (CS) [abstract]. Reg Anesth 15:S29, 1991.
28. McLintic AJ, Pringle SD, Lilley S, et al: Electrocardiographic changes during cesarean section under regional anesthesia. Anesth Analg 74:51–56, 1992.

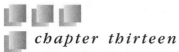

chapter thirteen

ANESTHETIC MANAGEMENT OF THE PREGNANT SURGICAL PATIENT

Corey A. Burchman, MD

Nonobstetric surgery in the pregnant patient is a serious matter. It is almost always urgent in nature. About 4 million infants are born annually in the United States. Up to 2% of pregnant women undergo a surgical procedure each year. Thus, the potential exists for nearly 80,000 pregnant patients requiring some form of anesthesia each year.

■ **KEY POINT:** A large number of women undergo nonobstetric surgery during pregnancy. Most of these women will need anesthesia for these surgical procedures. Many different anesthetic agents have been safely used for these patients.

The anesthetic management of the pregnant surgical patient requires an in-depth knowledge of the physiologic alterations seen during pregnancy and the anesthetic implications of these alterations. With this must come an intimate knowledge of fetal development and physiology, particularly as it pertains to how drugs influence and alter the homeostasis of the unborn child.

Anesthetic issues of major concern include

- Avoiding teratogenic agents;
- Avoiding and treating premature labor;
- Maintaining normal uteroplacental perfusion;
- Avoiding fetal asphyxia;
- Ensuring maternal safety.

There are risks and benefits associated with all anesthetic techniques. Considerations now must take into account both the mother and the child. Furthermore, obstetric complications can complicate the conduct of the anesthetic. Although no single "correct" management exists, this chapter may serve as a guide.

■ **KEY POINT:** If elective surgery can be delayed, it should not be performed in the pregnant patient. If it must be performed but is nonemergent, surgery should be avoided in the first trimester because of the risks associated with surgery and anesthesia during organogenesis.

FETAL CONSIDERATIONS

The pregnant surgical patient will have major concern for the well-being of her infant. What reassurance can *you*, the anesthesiologist, offer her regarding the risks to the fetus for birth defects? Teratogenicity is influenced by several factors:

- Genetic factors of the fetus (you cannot control for this);
- Fetal stage of development (you cannot control for this);
- Nature of the anesthetic agent;
- Dosage and access of the drug to fetal circulation.

The period of greatest susceptibility to teratogenic agents is from days 15 to 30 postconception, the period of organogenesis. The rate of organogenesis continues but declines from days 30 to 90. From the 13th week of gestation, the fetus enters the stage of growth and development.

Insofar as the most vulnerable period for a developing fetus is from days 15 to 90, all females of childbearing age must be questioned about their menstrual history. If there are any lingering doubts about such a history, a pregnancy test should be obtained.

Almost all anesthetic agents exhibit *some* teratogenic effects in *some* animals. Before nidation, the embedding of the early embryo into uterine mucosa, teratogenicity will lead to spontaneous abortion. Large retrospective studies in the United States and Great Britain looked at chronic exposure of trace amounts of anesthetic gases in female anesthetists and wives of male anesthetists. There was a statistically significant increased incidence of congenital anomalies and spontaneous abortion. The validity of the results of these studies, however, has been called into question because of methodologic problems.

No anesthetic agent used in pregnancy, with the exception of cocaine, has been specifically linked to human teratogenicity. One cannot, however, categorically state that anesthetics are not teratogenic. Populations in published studies are just too small to make any study valid.

Interpretation of human teratogenicity data from animal studies is problematic. Many drugs known to be teratogenic in small animals demonstrate no such effect in humans. Conversely, thalidomide produces no defect in rodents, whereas offspring of pregnant humans who took thalidomide during pregnancy had multiple developmental lesions. Furthermore, it may be difficult to control hemodynamic, ventilatory, and metabolic parameters in animals while exposure to potential agents occurs, as would be the case in a well-conducted anesthetic. Perhaps the perturbation in physiologic homeostasis contributes to adverse developmental effects. Hypoxia, hypotension, and hypercarbia will always contribute to the creation of malformation and to death.

Animal studies[1] have demonstrated a large safety margin with the following agents. Additionally, these drugs have been "time tested" and are generally regarded as safe in humans:

- Morphine sulfate
- Alfentanil
- Sufentanil
- Meperidine
- Sodium thiopental
- Ketamine
- Etomidate
- Methohexital
- Succinylcholine
- Curare

A probable link has been found between the following drugs and human birth defects:

- Warfarins—bone anomalies
- Benzodiazepines—facial abnormalities, including cleft lip

Teratogenicity of Inhaled Agents

Animal studies have failed to show that the inhalational agents halothane, enflurane, isoflurane, desflurane, and sevoflurane are associated with birth defects. Although extensive studies are available for the latter two newer inhalational agents, they have not stood the rigors of time like the other three.

The potential teratogenicity of nitrous oxide deserves some discussion. There is a large degree of controversy surrounding this issue. Some animal studies have shown that nitrous oxide inhibits methionine synthetase activity, which can in turn inhibit DNA synthesis in a developing fetus.[2] Human studies do not fully support this finding. Retrospective epidemiologic investigations show no correlation between the use of nitrous oxide in anesthetics in early pregnancy and the incidence of congenital malformations or abortions. Still, because of the animal data, many centers in the United States routinely advocate against its use during pregnancy.

■ KEY POINT: It has been suggested that nitrous oxide is a teratogen in animals; however, recent human studies have failed to show an association between nitrous oxide exposure and reproductive risk.

Outcome studies of females who have received anesthesia during pregnancy have failed to demonstrate any anesthetic agent (again with the exception of cocaine) as being teratogenic.[3] There is a statistically significant increase in fetal loss, however, from preterm labor in these patients. Given the relatively small number of episodes of preterm labors when compared with the total number of pregnant women and the inability to conduct a randomized controlled study on the population and to control for the surgical procedure or presurgical condition, it is not possible to determine the cause of the loss of the pregnancy.

A major Canadian study compared over 2500 pregnant women who had surgery with age-matched pregnant females who did not have surgery.[4] Although no statistically significant difference in birth defects was apparent, the risk of spontaneous abortion was more common among patients in whom general anesthesia was used. That was not the case for patients who received central neuraxial anesthetics or no anesthesia at all. Unfortunately, as in many similar studies, it is difficult to differentiate the effects of anesthesia from those of the surgical procedure.

Gestational Viability

The increased incidence of preterm labor in the pregnant surgical patient appears to correlate with the site and nature of surgery. Spontaneous abortion was more highly associated with pelvic and intrabdominal procedures. As previously mentioned, patients who underwent general anesthesia also had a higher incidence of spontaneous abortion than age-matched control subjects who did not have general anesthesia. Reasons for this are not clear. Regardless of the cause of spontaneous abortion, meticulous attention to uterine activity should be made both intraoperatively and in the postoperative period, particularly in the second and third trimester when electronic fetal monitoring can often be effectively used.

If uterine contractions develop, tocolysis should be used aggressively, and a few obstetricians recommend the use of prophylactic tocolysis in all pregnant patients undergoing surgery. The anesthesiologist, however, does need to appreciate that both β-adrenergic agonists (ritodrine, terbutaline) and magnesium sulfate have anesthetic implications. The β agonist can cause tachycardia and a myriad of tachyarrhythmias. As such, β-sympathomimetic agents such as ephedrine and ketamine must be administered judiciously. Drugs that can result in tachycardia, such as atropine, glycopyrrolate, and pancuronium, must also be used with a degree of caution. Magnesium sulfate, the other major tocolytic agent, has muscle relaxant properties. As such, it can act synergistically with both depolarizing and nondepolarizing muscle relaxants. Even a "defasciculating" dose of a nondepolarizer before the injection of succinylcholine may result in major motor paralysis in a patient with high magnesium levels. The actions of magnesium on the neuromuscular junction can be antagonized by the careful administration of calcium.

> ■ **KEY POINT:** Monitoring for uterine contractions should be performed intraoperatively when possible and postoperatively as well, so that if preterm labor occurs, tocolytic therapy can be quickly instituted. The use of prophylactic tocolytic therapy is controversial.

MATERNAL CONSIDERATIONS

The physiologic changes that occur during pregnancy have major effects on the maternal organ systems. These changes have anesthetic implications. This subject is covered in Chapter 1.

Cardiovascular System

The pregnant mother's circulatory system is hyperdynamic. Increases in cardiac output begin as early as 8 weeks. Increases in cardiac output and circulatory volume exceed 40% of the prepregnant values by week 28. Then, they slowly decline to about 20% of the normal nonpregnant state. Because of these increases in circulatory dynamics, pregnant patients may present with both heart murmurs and electrocardiographic changes not seen in the nonpregnant state. At the bedside, these frequently cannot be distinguished from pathologic states.

By about week 20, the gravid uterus can cause aortocaval compression when the patient assumes the supine position. The pregnant patient should be tilted by a wedge under her right hip. This will displace the uterus laterally to the left, favoring less of a chance of compressing the vena cava or partially occluding the descending thoracic aorta. As a general rule, uterine displacement should be carried out both pre-, intra-, and postoperatively. This includes during transport of the patient.

Respiratory System

There is a 70% increase in alveolar ventilation as pregnancy approaches term. Both the increase in baseline respiratory rate and the increase in tidal volume contribute to a more rapid uptake of inhalational agents, corresponding to a more rapid induction and emergence from anesthesia. There is a significant risk of the rapid development of hypoxia and acidosis, due to a combination of a 20% decrease in functional residual capacity and increases in basal metabolic rate and oxygen consumption. Before the induction of general anesthesia, denitrogenation with 100% oxygen is essential. The respiratory mucosa and glottic aperture may be edematous or engorged. They are quite prone to bleeding with any form of instrumentation. A 6.0- to 7.0-mm endotracheal tube is recommended. Enlarged breasts may further hamper attempts at intubation.

Gastrointestinal System

The parturient is particularly susceptible to aspiration because of the character, quantity, and "environment" of her gastric contents. High circulating levels of progesterone during pregnancy result in increased basal rates of gastrin secretion. As a result, there is more gastric acid secreted. The pregnant patient may have a delayed gastric emptying time and also a humoral effect, which is worsened by the adminstration of opioids. The gravid uterus presses upward, against the stomach, and can actually pose a mechanical obstruction to the duodenum. The expanding uterus actually displaces the esophageal barrier to reflux superiorly. Progesterone further decreases lower esophageal sphincter tone. The pregnant surgical patient is an aspiration waiting to happen.

The most significant treatment measure is prophylaxis. General anesthesia is to be avoided if possible. When general anesthesia is indicated, classic full-stomach precautions must be taken. Premedicants such as 30 mL of nonparticulate antacid, such as sodium citrate (Bicitra), should be administered. Some recommend the addition of an H_2 blocker and metoclopramide as well.

Central Nervous System

The minimum alveolar concentration (MAC) for inhalational agents decreases by up to 40% in pregnancy. Even in major central neuraxial regional anesthetics, pregnant patients experience a more rapid onset and higher level block than those of age-matched cohorts. This is probably a humoral effect. For these reasons, pregnant patients must be administered neuroactive drugs prudently, and drugs must be titrated to effect.

Renal System

Renal hemodynamics undergo major changes during pregnancy. Renal plasma flow increases by up to 80% and glomerular filtration rate by 50% by week 16. The clinical implications of this are great. The pharmacokinetics of drugs primarily excreted by the kidney are altered. Laboratory values such as blood urea nitrogen and creatinine are decreased, and one must be careful in assigning "normal" values to pregnant women.

■ Table 13–1
SUMMARY OF ANESTHETIC CONSIDERATIONS

	First Trimester	Second and Third Trimesters
Agents to avoid	Nitrous oxide, benzodiazepines, α_1 agonists (can cause uterine vasoconstriction)	NSAIDs (can cause closure of ductus arteriosus)
Probably safe to use	Narcotics, barbiturates, local anesthetic (except cocaine), inhalational agents, muscle relaxants	Narcotics, barbiturates, local anesthetics (except cocaine), inhalational agents, muscle relaxants
Major concerns	Avoiding teratogenic drugs	Avoiding maternal hypoxemia and hypotension. Maintain uteroplacental blood flow, use left uterine displacement after 18 weeks, monitor fetal heart rate and tocodynamics after 18 weeks, and intraoperatively, if possible

NSAIDs, nonsteroidal anti-inflammatory drugs.

Hematologic System

The physiologic "anemia" associated with pregnancy is secondary to the 20% increase in red blood cell mass and concomitant 40% increase in plasma volume. This does not result in an attenuation of oxygen delivery because the increase in cardiac output actually *increases* oxygen delivery at the tissue level. Serum proteins are diluted, however. Therefore, the pharmacokinetics of highly protein-bound agents are altered.

The platelet count of the parturient is usually increased, as are coagulation factors I, VII, X, and XII. These values can result in a hypercoagulable state, increasing the risk of thromboembolic complications. For these reasons, antithrombotic pumps should be used in the pregnant surgical patient. If patients must be confined to bed for a prolonged recovery, minidose heparin has been used in the perioperative period without ill effects. Anesthetic considerations are summarized in Table 13–1.

INTRAOPERATIVE MANAGEMENT

Regional anesthesia is preferable if surgically feasible. Anesthetic management should be altered to conform to the physiologic changes of pregnancy and all drugs should be titrated to effect. With general anesthesia, denitrogenation with 100% oxygen should be carried out for up to 3 to 4 minutes if possible. Alternatively, four maximally deep inspirations of 100% oxygen over 30 seconds will result in end-tidal nitrogen concentrations of less than 4%. Rapid sequence induction with cricoid pressure is mandatory, and endotracheal intubation is used to decrease the risk of aspiration. Ketamine, thiopental, etomidate, and propofol are all acceptable agents for induction of general anesthesia.[5] Ketamine can increase uterine tone in the first trimester if doses of greater than 2 mg/kg are used.

Maintenance of general anesthesia with inhalational agents (to levels less than two times MAC) is most common and actually preferred to decrease uterine tone and inhibit contractions. If hypotension ensues during the course of an anesthetic, which is refractory to pharmacologic therapy, consider surgical packs and retractors to be a cause, which in combination with the gravid uterus can cause aortocaval compression.

■ **KEY POINT:** Laparoscopic surgery can be performed in the pregnant patient when indicated. However, several recommendations should be followed, including monitoring the fetal and uterine status, the maternal end-tidal CO_2, and watching arterial blood-gas measurements. An open technique should be used to enter the abdomen, and pneumoperitoneum pressures should be maintained below 15 mm Hg.

Muscle relaxants are highly ionized and not found to cross the placenta to any appreciable extent when used in the normal dose range. Reversal agents such as endrophonium, pyridostigmine, and neostigmine are all quaternary molecules and also will not readily cross the placental barrier. Anticholinergic agents such as atropine and glycopyrrolate should be used in conjunction with an anticholinesterase drug. A "defasciculating" dose of a nondepolarizing muscle relaxant is unnecessary before the administration of succinylcholine, because the pregnant patient usually does not fasciculate and therefore does not get the resultant muscle pain.

With regional anesthesia, the cardinal principle of ensuring maternal hemodynamic stability is the best measure to ensure fetal safety. Adequate preloading of crystalloid is necessary before the induction of spinal or epidural anesthesia. Again, the simple yet effective technique of left uterine displacement is a ready means to avoid maternal hypotension. Ephedrine is the pressor of choice if low blood pressure ensues; however, phenylephrine may be used safely in situations where hypotension is refractory to treatment with ephedrine.

No one technique is the correct technique. Although it may seem simplistic and somewhat redundant, if you avoid the "classic four H's" (maternal *hypotension*, *hypoxia*, *hypercarbia*, and *hypovolemia*), as an anesthesiologist you are doing most of what you can do to maintain the integrity of the pregnancy.

■ **KEY POINT:** Maternal events that cause severe hypotension, hypoxia, or acidosis present a greater risk to the fetus than the anesthetic itself. Transient mild decreases in maternal Po_2 are well tolerated by the fetus. Severe maternal hypoxia, however, will quickly lead to fetal hypoxia and ultimately to fetal morbidity and mortality.

POSTOPERATIVE AGENDA

In addition to the usual monitors of electrocardiogram, oxygen saturation, capnography, and blood pressure measurements, a tocodynamometer should be used, if at all possible, to detect premature labor. A fetal heart rate monitor can also be used to gauge fetal well-being in a viable fetus. It is useful to have a labor nurse with the patient in the postanesthesia care unit (PACU) who has familiarity with these types of monitors. Electronic fetal monitoring should be maintained in the postoperative period.

FETAL SURGERY

First described in 1963, fetal surgery is performed for a variety of reasons. From exchange transfusions to the antenatal placement of urinary diversion catheters, under ultrasonic or fluoroscopic guidance, fetal surgery is being performed with increasing frequency.

As previously mentioned, maintaining maternal hemodynamic and respiratory integrity still apply. Local, general, and regional anesthesia and monitored anesthetic care have been applied to the mother undergoing fetal surgery. Adequate uterine relaxation can be reliably obtained with general anesthesia, which is the anesthetic technique usually chosen.

It has been shown that preterm infants who undergo surgery experience multiple hormonal responses indicative of stress. Direct IM or IV administration of nondepolarizing neuromuscular blockers such as pancuronium, atracurium, and *d*-tubocurarine have been used successfully to arrest fetal movement. Atracurium in the dose range of 0.4 mg/kg, injected directly into the umbilical vein, will result in complete cessation of movement for 30 to 60 minutes.

> **■ KEY POINT:** Fetal surgery has been used in situations in which anomalies are present that can cause harm to the fetus during a period in which fetal lung maturity has not developed. Examples include bilateral hydronephrosis, cystic adenomatoid malformations, and congenital diaphragmatic hernia.

POSTPARTUM SURGERY

Many physiologic changes accompanying pregnancy do not correct themselves in the immediate postpartum period. With vaginal delivery, an autotransfusion of 500 to 700 mL of blood occurs. Cardiac output increases sharply after delivery and gradually returns to normal 2 to 4 weeks postpartum. The immediate postpartum period is considered one of high risk for patients with stenotic valvular disease and pulmonary hypertension. Elevated levels of progesterone still exist for 2 to 3 weeks. This may delay gastric emptying. Consequently, full stomach conditions still apply.

The only elective postpartum procedure performed with regularity is sterilization (tubal ligation). This can be performed either with a general endotracheal or regional anesthetic, although most anesthesiologists prefer regional anesthesia and many actually refuse to electively administer general anesthesia for these cases. Frequently, if a patient received epidural analgesia for labor and delivery, the epidural catheter can be used for a postoperative tubal ligation, although these epidurals, if dormant for a period, may fail to provide adequate anesthesia. The fundus of the uterus remains at the level of the umbilicus for about 2 days postpartum. Thus, timely performance of this surgery in the postdelivery period is essential.

> **■ KEY POINT:** Because of the risk of gastroesophageal reflux, regional anesthesia is preferred for postpartum tubal ligation. If an epidural is already in situ, it can be used. However, if surgery is delayed more than 10 hours following use of the epidural, there is an increased likelihood of catheter failure. In cases in which postpartum tubal ligation is delayed, spinal anesthesia is the preferred anesthetic technique.

The most common reason for emergency surgery in the postpartum period is obstetric hemorrhage. This is usually secondary to uterine atony, retained placental tissue, or a laceration somewhere in the birth canal. As previously mentioned, the considerations of physiologic alteration come into play. The postpartum patient for emergency surgery is usually hypovolemic. Large-bore intravenous catheters should be started. Warmed crystalloids should be infused and serial hematocrits obtained. The availability of blood products should be sought.

Ketamine 1 mg/kg is frequently the drug of choice for induction of general anesthesia in a hemorrhaging patient. A rapid sequence induction should be used. Volatile agents should be avoided because they may contribute to uterine relaxation, resulting in more brisk bleeding, stressing an already hyperdynamic cardiovascular system. Nitrous oxide, narcotics, and muscle relaxants work well for anesthesia maintenance. Coagulopathy and thrombocytopenia are not uncommon. Provisions should be made for blood product availability should the need for transfusion arise.

CONCLUSION

There are risks and benefits associated with all anesthetic techniques. In the case of the pregnant patient who is preordained to visit the operating room, factors must now be weighed for both the mother and the infant. Further, obstetric complications can entangle the conduct of anesthetics. No one anesthetic technique is the right technique, and the anesthesiologist must always have backup plans.

REFERENCES

1. David TJ: Drug and environmental agents in the pathogenesis of congenital malformations. In: Eskes T, Finster M, eds. Drug Therapy During Pregnancy. Boston: Butterworths, 1985:259–268.
2. Crawford JS, Lewis M: Nitrous oxide in early human pregnancy. Anaesthesia 41:900–905, 1986.
3. Mazze RI, Kallen B: Reproductive outcome after anesthesia and operation during pregnancy: a registry study of 5405 cases. Am J Obstet Gynecol 161: 1178–1185, 1989.
4. Duncan PG, Pope WDB, Cohen MM, et al. Fetal risk of anesthesia and surgery during pregnancy. Anesthesiology 64:790–794, 1986.
5. Gin T: Propofol during pregnancy. Acta Anaesthesiol Sin 32:127–132, 1994.

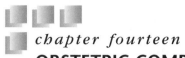

chapter fourteen

OBSTETRIC COMPLICATIONS

Regina Fragneto, MD

The anesthesiologist providing care in the labor and delivery suite will be confronted on a regular basis with patients presenting with some common obstetric complications, including premature labor, vaginal birth after cesarean (VBAC), fetal malpresentation, multiple gestation, and multiparity. It is important for the anesthesiologist to have a clear understanding of the obstetric and anesthetic implications of these clinical situations so an appropriate anesthetic plan can be formulated for each parturient.

PREMATURE LABOR

Premature labor and delivery is a serious obstetric complication whose incidence is increasing. Approximately 10% of all births in the United States are preterm, and such a high incidence has certainly contributed to the United States' high infant mortality rate.[1] The morbidity associated with preterm labor and birth also results in significant burdens to the infant, the family, and to society. Although the etiology of premature labor remains unclear in most cases, multiple risk factors have been associated with its development. Common risk factors are listed in Table 14-1. In caring for these patients, it is essential that the anesthesiologist has a clear understanding of the obstetric plan.

First, the diagnosis of premature labor must be confirmed. Gestational age less than 37 weeks and regular contractions of at least four in 20 minutes must be present. However, to distinguish premature labor from false labor, documented change in cervical dilation or effacement, cervical dilation of

■ Table 14–1
RISK FACTORS FOR PREMATURE LABOR

- Previous preterm birth
- Previous second trimester loss
- Young teenager
- Low socioeconomic class
- Drug use (especially tobacco and cocaine)
- Physically demanding work
- Infection (genital and urinary tract)
- Overdistended uterus (multiple gestation, polyhydramnios)
- Uterine abnormalities
- Cervical incompetence
- Antepartum hemorrhage (placenta previa, abruptio placentae)
- Premature rupture of membranes

■ Table 14–2
MgSO₄ THERAPY: DOSING AND SIDE EFFECTS

Dosing:	4-g load over 20–30 min; continuous infusion of 1–4 g/h to maintain Mg level 5–7 mg/100 mL
Common side effects:	chest pain/tightness; flushing; headache; nausea; sedation; transient hypotension; pulmonary edema

2 cm, or effacement of 80% must also be present. Once the diagnosis has been established, initial treatment frequently consists of bedrest and intravenous hydration. If unsuccessful, the obstetrician will then decide whether to institute tocolytic therapy. Generally, tocolysis is reserved for pregnancies less than 34 weeks' gestation. Contraindications to tocolysis include the presence of chorioamnionitis, severe antepartum hemorrage, evidence of in utero fetal compromise, and advanced cervical dilation. Many obstetricians also consider rupture of membranes a contraindication. Even in cases where long-term tocolysis is not indicated, the obstetrician may decide to administer a tocolytic agent for a short period (24 to 48 hours) to allow time for the maternal administration of a glucocorticoid to accelerate fetal lung maturity. Many of the physiologic effects of tocolytic agents will produce significant interactions with anesthetic agents and techniques. Commonly used tocolytics include magnesium sulfate, β-adrenergic agents, prostaglandin synthetase inhibitors, and calcium channel blocking agents.

Magnesium sulfate is often the first-line tocolytic therapy. Table 14–2 includes the dosing regimen and common side effects of this agent. Magnesium acts by preventing an increase in the free intracellular calcium concentration. As a result, the interaction of actin and myosin necessary for uterine contraction is decreased. The hypermagnesemia resulting from tocolytic therapy also produces abnormal neuromuscular function and potentiates the action of both depolarizing and nondepolarizing muscle relaxants. Magnesium toxicity is a serious complication of tocolytic therapy that can be prevented by carefully monitoring patients for continued presence of deep tendon reflexes. The clinical signs of toxicity with corresponding systemic Mg levels are listed in Table 14–3. If toxicity occurs, intravenous calcium gluconate is an effective treatment.

■ **KEY POINT:** Magnesium sulfate treatment can increase the likelihood of hypotension and alters the maternal hemodynamic response to vasopressors. Magnesium sulfate also causes abnormal neuromuscular function, potentiating the action of both depolorizing and nondepolarizing muscle relaxants.

■ Table 14–3
SIGNS OF MAGNESIUM TOXICITY

Clinical Sign	Mg Level
Loss of deep tendon reflexes	10 mEq/L
Respiratory depression	12–15 mEq/L
Respiratory arrest	15 mEq/L
Cardiac arrest	20–25 mEq/L

β-Adrenergic drugs are also commonly used as tocolytic agents. Although ritodrine is the only β-adrenergic agent approved by the U.S. Food and Drug Administration for use as a tocolytic, terbutaline is the agent most frequently used. Table 14-4 lists the dosing regimen and common side effects of terbutaline. These agents produce tocolysis via stimulation of the β_2 receptors in the myometrium, resulting in uterine muscle relaxation. Prolonged administration of these agents is limited by the relatively greater cardiovascular side effects (compared with $MgSO_4$) and decreased effectiveness secondary to downregulation of the β_2 receptors. The etiology of pulmonary edema in patients receiving tocolytic agents remains unclear. Most clinicians, however, believe it is noncardiogenic and in some patients may include a component of volume overload.

Indomethacin, a prostaglandin synthetase inhibitor, has been used for tocolysis of premature labor. Its use has been limited, however, because it may cause premature closure of the patent ductus arteriosus in utero, resulting in persistent fetal circulation if delivery occurs. Generally, it is administered for only 24 to 48 hours to patients with gestational ages less than 32 weeks. If a high likelihood of delivery within 24 hours exists, indomethacin should not be used. Some anesthesiologists have expressed concern about the effects of indomethacin on platelet function and the safety of performing regional anesthesia on parturients who have recently received the drug. The effects on platelet function, however, are only transient, and there are no published cases of epidural hematoma in pregnant women who have recently received indomethacin. Therefore, I will perform regional anesthesia on these

■ Table 14–4
TERBUTALINE: DOSING AND SIDE EFFECTS

Dosing:	initial infusion 2.5 mcg/min and increasing 2.5 mcg/min every 20 min as needed to maximum of 20 mcg/min or 0.25 mg subcutaneously over 3 hours
Common side effects:	tachycardia, cardiac arrhythmias, supraventricular tachycardia (SVT), hypotension, pulmonary edema, hyperglycemia, hypokalemia

parturients without obtaining a test of platelet function, such as thromboelastography.

Calcium channel blocking agents, especially nifedipine, have become increasingly popular as a second-line treatment for premature labor. These agents act by decreasing the amount of available intracellular calcium. Actin–myosin interactions are therefore decreased, resulting in relaxation of the myometrial smooth muscle. The dosing regimen and side effects are listed in Table 14-5. Caution is necessary because neuromuscular weakness may develop in patients who are receiving combination therapy of nifedipine and $MgSO_4$.

Various factors must be considered in the anesthetic management of premature labor and delivery. These include the special obstetric considerations associated with preterm delivery, interactions between anesthetic and tocolytic drugs, and effects of anesthetic agents on the preterm fetus.

Epidural analgesia is an ideal technique for premature labor and delivery. Because the premature fetus does not tolerate labor as well as a term fetus, the incidence of fetal jeopardy requiring an emergency cesarean delivery is greater. The presence of an epidural in such a situation will decrease the likelihood that general anesthesia with all its associated risks will be required. When a vaginal delivery is planned, epidural analgesia can also contribute to the obstetrician's ability to perform an optimal delivery. Because the preterm infant is more susceptible to intracranial hemorrhage from traumatic delivery, the obstetrician's goal is to avoid precipitous delivery and to perform a controlled atraumatic delivery of the neonate's head. Epidural analgesia can provide a relaxed pelvic floor and perineum to facilitate such a delivery. In addition, the parturient who is receiving adequate analgesia during the second stage of labor may be better able to cooperate with the obstetrician's instructions during delivery.

■ **KEY POINT:** Previous administration of tocolytics (including magnesium and adrenergic agents) is not a contraindication of neuraxial anesthesia.

Usually, administration of epidural analgesia to women in premature labor occurs only after tocolysis has failed. These patients may therefore be in advanced labor. In such a situa-

■ Table 14–5
NIFEDIPINE: DOSING AND SIDE EFFECTS

Initial dosing:	10 mg orally repeated q 20 min (if contractions persist) to maximum 30 mg
Maintenance dosing:	10–20 mg orally q 6 hr
Common side effects:	headache, nausea, flushing, postpartum uterine atony

tion, a combined spinal–epidural technique could be an excellent alternative to epidural analgesia. Epidural analgesia is usually delayed until the obstetrician has determined that labor cannot be arrested. However, there are some special situations where one must consider placing an epidural catheter while a tocolytic agent is still being administered. These would include cases where success of tocolysis is unlikely or where, due to an obstetric consideration (such as a breech presentation), an urgent cesarean delivery would be required once tocolysis has failed. The anesthesiologist should also consider early epidural placement when confronted with a patient in whom the administration of general anesthesia in an emergency situation would be problematic (such as the patient with a difficult airway).

When choosing analgesic and anesthetic drugs for use in the parturient experiencing premature labor, the effects of these drugs on a premature fetus should be considered. Various physiologic differences between the preterm and term fetus suggest that the preterm fetus may be more susceptible to any depressant effects of maternally administered drugs. These differences include less protein binding capacity, resulting in increased free drug concentrations; incomplete blood–brain barrier, allowing greater drug access to the central nervous system; and less efficient metabolism and excretion of drugs. Therefore, when providing epidural analgesia for labor or epidural anesthesia for cesarean section, use the smallest doses and concentrations of local anesthetic and opioid drugs that will provide adequate analgesia or anesthesia to the mother.

Tocolytic agents may also have an impact on the administration of epidural anesthesia. Because patients who have received terbutaline or $MgSO_4$ are at risk for developing pulmonary edema, the fluid preload given before induction of epidural anesthesia should be limited. Epidural anesthesia should be induced slowly, and additional crystalloid should be administered as needed to maintain a normal blood pressure during induction and maintenance of epidural anesthesia. If maternal hypotension occurs, ephedrine remains the pharmacologic treatment of choice in parturients who have received $MgSO_4$ or a β-adrenergic agent.[2, 3] However, if a patient has significant tachycardia due to terbutaline therapy, the administration of small doses of phenylephrine for treatment of hypotension is recommended.

Premature labor patients are more likely than term parturients to require cesarean delivery due to fetal malpresentation or failure to tolerate labor. Due to the depressant effects of general anesthetic agents on the preterm fetus and the established risks of general anesthesia in all parturients, regional anesthesia is the anesthetic of choice whenever possible. If tocolysis has produced tachycardia or other cardiovascular instability, slow induction of epidural anesthesia is often preferable to single-shot spinal anesthesia. If fetal jeopardy occurs in a parturient who has a functioning epidural catheter, epidural medications should be administered via the catheter to achieve surgical anesthesia. The drug of choice in this situation would be 2-chloroprocaine because of its rapid onset and lack of "ion trapping" in the acidotic fetus.

In cases of profound fetal distress (agonal tracing, profound bradycardia), general anesthesia may be required if an epidural catheter is not in place already. Administration of general anesthesia in this situation will be similar to that in the term patient, but with two additional considerations taken into account. Because the premature fetus may be more susceptible than the term fetus to the depressant effects of anesthestic agents, particular attention should be paid to administering the smallest doses of these agents that will provide adequate anesthesia to the mother. In patients who have received MgSO$_4$, the effects of both depolarizing and nondepolarizing neuromuscular blocking agents will be potentiated. The intubating dose of succinylcholine (100 mg) should not be decreased. However, recovery from this initial dose should be confirmed with a nerve stimulator before administering any additional muscle relaxants. Subsequent doses of neuromuscular blocking agents should be reduced and the patient's response meticulously monitored.

Premature neonates are likely to experience several problems at birth. Therefore, a pediatrician or healthcare professional other than the anesthesiologist responsible for care of the mother who is trained in neonatal resuscitation should be present at all deliveries of premature infants.

VBAC AND UTERINE RUPTURE

From 1970 to the late 1980s there was a steady rise in the cesarean section rate in the United States (5.7% in 1970 to 24.7% in 1988).[4] The practice of routinely performing a repeat cesarean section in women with a prior cesarean delivery contributed significantly to this rise. In response to this marked rise in cesarean section rates, the federal government and the American College of Obstetricians and Gynecologists (ACOG) began a campaign to educate the public and physicians about the option of VBAC. Most importantly, maternal morbidity and possibly perinatal morbidity and mortality are lower with VBAC. In addition, vaginal delivery is significantly less expensive than cesarean delivery. As a result of this patient and physician education, VBAC has become common obstetric practice in the 1990s.

Because the feared complication of VBAC is uterine rupture, the type of uterine scar from a prior cesarean delivery determines whether a woman is a candidate for VBAC. The incidence of uterine rupture is quite high (10 to 12%) in women with a prior classical incision (vertical incision in upper portion of uterus) so these patients are generally not allowed to labor. Most patients, however, have undergone a low transverse uterine incision. The incidence and severity of uterine rupture is low (0.8 to 2%) in these patients,[5, 6] and ACOG recommends that patients with one low transverse incision are encouraged to undergo a trial of labor. Although there are limited data, it also appears safe for women with more than one previous cesarean delivery through low transverse incisions to undergo VBAC. Most obstetricians will recommend a trial of labor to patients with a previous low vertical incision only if there is documentation that the incision was confined to the lower uterine segment. Because uterine rupture is an obstetric emergency that can result in both fetal and maternal distress, VBAC should only be attempted at hospitals capable of responding in a timely manner to such an emergency, including the ability to perform a cesarean delivery. Generally, the indication for a previous cesarean section is not a factor in determining whether a woman is an appropriate candidate for a trial of labor. VBAC is successful in approximately 75% of patients. Even when the indication for previous cesarean delivery was dystocia or cephalopelvic disproportion, the success rate for a subsequent trial of labor remains high.

The anesthesiologist caring for patients attempting VBAC should be aware of the signs and symptoms of uterine rupture and its management. It is important to distinguish between uterine dehiscence and uterine rupture. Uterine dehiscence is a defect or separation of the uterine wall without expulsion of fetal parts or placenta into the abdominal cavity and does not result in fetal distress or severe hemorrhage. Frequently, the dehiscence is asymptomatic, and the diagnosis is made incidentally when cesarean section is performed for another obstetric indication. Uterine rupture involves complete separation of the uterine wall with communication of the uterine cavity with the abdominal cavity, resulting in fetal distress or significant maternal hemorrhage. Although most uterine wall separations in patients with a classic incision scar result in a frank rupture, a significant number of the uterine wall defects that occur in patients with a low transverse scar are asymptomatic dehiscences. The incidence of catastrophic rupture in these patients is 0.8%.[5] Table 14–6 lists signs and symptoms of uterine rupture.

Fetal distress is the most common sign of rupture. Patients with a catastrophic rupture will require emergency laparotomy and cesarean section. Once delivery of the fetus has been accomplished, either uterine repair or cesarean hysterectomy will be necessary.

■ **KEY POINT:** Neuraxial analgesia is not contraindicated in women undergoing a trial of labor. Continuous electronic fetal heart rate monitoring is the best method to detect uterine rupture.

■ Table 14–6
SIGNS AND SYMPTOMS OF UTERINE RUPTURE

- Abrupt change in fetal heart rate pattern (bradycardia and prolonged decelerations)
- Sudden onset constant suprapubic or abdominal pain
- Vaginal bleeding
- Uterine tenderness
- Maternal tachycardia
- Recession of presenting fetal part
- Abrupt change in uterine activity or pressure

Obstetric care for the parturient attempting VBAC is similar to that for any parturient. Because fetal distress is the most reliable sign of uterine rupture, most obstetricians consider continuous electronic fetal heart rate monitoring mandatory in these patients. When VBAC was gaining popularity, some obstetricians considered the administration of oxytocin contraindicated in these patients because they believed it increased the risk of uterine rupture. However, studies have not found a greater incidence of uterine rupture or dehiscence in patients receiving oxytocin augmentation,[6] and ACOG has stated that the risk of oxytocin administration is no greater in women attempting VBAC than in the general obstetric population.[7]

Preparation for a possible uterine rupture and concerns about the safety of epidural analgesia are the major issues in the anesthetic management of women undergoing a trial of labor. Although the incidence of uterine rupture is low, patients attempting VBAC should have intravenous access established early in labor with at least an 18-gauge catheter. These patients should also have a valid type and screen in the hospital's blood bank.

When VBAC first became a standard obstetric practice, many obstetricians withheld epidural analgesia from these patients because of a concern that abdominal pain associated with uterine rupture or dehiscence would be masked by the analgesia and diagnosis would therefore be delayed. There was also a concern that the sympathectomy produced by epidural analgesia would attentuate the compensatory responses to maternal hemorrhage caused by uterine rupture. Not only could this loss of compensatory responses such as maternal tachycardia and vasoconstriction jeopardize the mother's hemodynamic status, it could also delay diagnosis by preventing the development of one of the signs of rupture, maternal tachycardia. Experience in the management of women attempting VBAC, however, has not borne out these concerns. In fact, abdominal pain and maternal tachycardia are not always reliable signs of uterine rupture. In addition, epidural analgesia with the dilute local anesthetic solutions currently used in obstetric anesthesia practice has not masked the abdominal pain that some women have developed with uterine rupture.

Based on significant experience with VBAC, most obstetricians and anesthesiologists now believe that epidural analgesia is an ideal technique of pain relief for parturients undergoing a trial of labor. Many studies have reported the successful use of epidural analgesia in VBAC patients. In women who have been receiving satisfactory epidural labor analgesia, the sudden development of "breakthrough" abdominal pain may be an early sign of uterine rupture or dehiscence. Therefore, the administration of epidural analgesia in patients attempting VBAC could actually aid in the diagnosis of uterine rupture. In addition, if anesthesia is ultimately required for an operative delivery, epidural analgesia can quickly be converted to a safe surgical anesthetic. Even in cases of laparotomy for repair of a uterine dehiscence or rupture, epidural anesthesia can be administered, avoiding the risks of general anesthesia, provided the patient is hemodynamically stable without severe hemorrhage. Finally, many women are more likely to choose VBAC rather than elective repeat cesarean section if they know the superior labor pain relief of epidural analgesia is available to them.

Generally, dosing an epidural for labor analgesia in patients attempting VBAC should not be different from dosing strategies used in the general obstetric population. Attention should be paid to using the smallest doses and concentrations of drugs that provide satisfactory analgesia. Large doses and concentrations that could produce anesthesia rather than analgesia should not be administered, to avoid the possiblity of masking abdominal pain resulting from rupture or dehiscence. If a patient receiving satisfactory labor analgesia experiences a sudden loss of analgesia, this should be a warning to the anesthesiologist that uterine rupture may be occurring and the obstetrician should be advised immediately.

Because combined spinal–epidural analgesia is a new technique, its use in parturients undergoing a trial of labor is not yet well established. However, it seems unlikely that abdominal pain associated with uterine rupture would be masked by the spinal analgesia provided for labor. Some anesthesiologists might argue that patients attempting VBAC are at increased risk for requiring an emergency cesarean section, and therefore one should determine immediately upon insertion that the epidural catheter is functioning. However, because the incidence of catastrophic uterine rupture is exceedingly rare, combined spinal–epidural analgesia should be considered a viable option for VBAC patients.

MALPRESENTATION

Patients with fetal malpresentation, including breech and transverse lie, have an increased incidence of obstetric complications. Optimal management of these patients requires coordination and cooperation between the obstetrician and anesthesiologist. Obstetric and anesthetic plans should be established early in labor. Breech presentation is the most common malpresentation, with an incidence of approximately 3 to 4% of term pregnancies. The incidence among preterm fetuses can be as high as 40%, depending on gestational age. Three types of breech presentation exist, as depicted in Figure 14–1. Frank breech, in which the hips are flexed and the knees are extended, is the most common breech presentation. Incomplete, or footling, breech is common among preterm fetuses. The least common form of breech presentation is complete breech, where both the hips and knees are flexed.

The obstetrician must make several clinical decisions when a parturient with a breech fetus presents to the labor and delivery suite, and the anesthesiologist, as in all patients, must be aware of the obstetric plan. If the patient is in early labor, an attempt may be made at external cephalic version. In fact, some patients at 36 to 39 weeks' gestation are admitted to labor and delivery specifically for a version attempt. If version to the vertex presentation is successful, vaginal delivery will be accomplished at essentially the same rate as the general obstetric population. Risks of external cephalic version include abruptio placentae and umbilical cord compression, which could result in acute fetal distress. Therefore, whenever this procedure is attempted, a preanesthetic evaluation should be performed and an anesthesiologist should be readily available in case an emergency cesarean delivery is required.

The preferences and practice of the obstetrician and anesthesiologist will determine whether additional anesthetic involvement occurs during an external cephalic version attempt. Because epidural analgesia will decrease patient discomfort and may improve the success rate for the procedure,[8] some obstetricians will request that epidural or spinal anesthe-

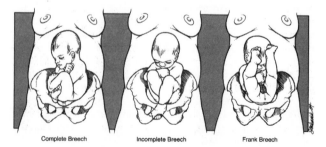

Complete Breech   Incomplete Breech   Frank Breech

Figure 14–1 ■ Three possible breech presentations. The complete breech demonstrates flexion of the hips and flexion of the knees. The incomplete breech demonstrates intermediate reflexion of one hip and knee. The frank breech demonstrates flexion of the hips and extension of both knees. (From Seeds JW: Malpresentations. In: Gabbe SG, Niebyl JR, Simpson JL, eds.: Obstetrics: Normal and Problem Pregnancies, 3rd ed. New York: Churchill Livingstone, 1996:479.)

sia is initiated before proceeding with version. If fetal distress occurs, extension of the epidural block could provide anesthesia for cesarean section. Some obstetricians, however, believe that excessive force, which could increase the risk of placental separation, is more likely to be applied if epidural analgesia is provided and do not advocate its use.

■ **KEY POINT:** Neuraxial analgesia offers several potential advantages for external cephalic version. The patient is more comfortable and the process rate may be improved.

If external cephalic version is unsuccessful or not attempted, the obstetrician and patient must then decide on the mode of delivery. A preterm fetus in the breech presentation will usually be delivered via cesarean section because vaginal breech delivery of a fetus less than 1500 g may increase the risk of birth trauma and cerebral hemorrhage. The preferable mode of delivery for a term fetus in the breech presentation is more controversial. In current obstetric practice, most of these patients will undergo cesarean delivery. However, many obstetricians will offer vaginal delivery to women who meet certain criteria, including frank breech presentation, adequate pelvimetry, estimated fetal weight of 2500 to 3800 g, and flexed fetal head. If a breech vaginal delivery is planned, it is essential that anesthesia coverage be immediately available.

There are three types of breech vaginal delivery: spontaneous breech delivery in which no traction is applied, assisted breech delivery in which the obstetrician assists delivery of the chest and head with forceps after the neonate has spontaneously delivered to the umbilicus, and total breech extraction in which traction is applied on the feet and ankles to deliver the entire body. The latter is used only to deliver a second twin.

Increased perinatal morbidity and mortality associated with breech deliveries is accounted for in part by significant complications that may occur during delivery. These include umbilical cord prolapse, which is increased 5- to 20-fold, and entrapped fetal head, which occurs in 8.8% of breech deliveries.[9] Both are true obstetric emergencies, and the anesthesiologist must be prepared to respond to them emergently.

Epidural analgesia is an ideal anesthetic technique for labor and vaginal breech delivery. In fact, many obstetricians will not attempt such a delivery unless the patient accepts an epidural. The advantages of this technique include superior labor analgesia, inhibition of early pushing before the cervix has become fully dilated, provision of a relaxed pelvic wall and perineum at delivery, and the ability to extend the block if an emergency cesarean section is necessary. However, it can be quite a challenge to meet all of these goals when providing epidural analgesia to a patient attempting vaginal breech delivery. During the first stage of labor, the epidural block must be dense enough to prevent early pushing. However, once the second stage of labor is reached, the epidural block must not inhibit the patient's ability to push effectively because it is essential that the infant deliver spontaneously to the umbilicus. The anesthesiologist must also be able to quickly provide dense perineal anesthesia if the obstetrician decides to assist delivery with forceps.

If the aftercoming head becomes entrapped, the obstetrician will request cervical relaxation to facilitate delivery. Intravenous nitroglycerin 50 to 100 μg may provide adequate uterine relaxation. At the same time that this is administered, however, preparation for rapid sequence induction of general anesthesia should also be made. If the nitroglycerin does not provide the desired effect, the definitive treatment is the administration of a high concentration of a volatile agent, such as isoflurane 2 to 3 MAC, once the airway has been secured.

Most women presenting with breech presentation will undergo elective cesarean section. Regional anesthesia is the technique of choice unless contraindications exist. Even with an abdominal delivery, uterine relaxation may be required to facilitate delivery of the breech infant. Diluted nitroglycerin should therefore be immediately available. The neonate delivered in the breech presentation is more likely to be depressed at delivery and has a higher incidence of morbidity and mortality. Therefore, it is essential that trained personnel, preferably a neonatologist, are available at all breech deliveries, both vaginal and abdominal.

■ **KEY POINT:** Intravenous or sublingual nitroglycerin is the first-line treatment for uterine relaxation to treat fetal entrapment during vaginal breech delivery.

Transverse lie, or shoulder presentation, is another malpresentation that may occur, especially in preterm fetuses. Unless an external cephalic version is successful, cesarean delivery is required with this presentation. If the fetus is positioned with the back down, a classical uterine incision may be required. The risk of umbilical cord prolapse is especially high with this presentation.

Other malpresentations that may occur include face, brow, and compound presentations. These are much rarer than breech or transverse lie presentations. Although vaginal delivery may be attempted, these patients are more likely than patients with a vertex presentation to require cesarean delivery.

PROLAPSED CORD

Prolapse of the umbilical cord, requiring emergency cesarean delivery, can occur at any time during labor. When this problem is identified, a member of the obstetric team must elevate the fetal head off the cord to prevent prolonged compression until cesarean delivery can be accomplished. If an epidural catheter is in place, the anesthesiologist should quickly extend anesthesia with 3% 2-chloroprocaine. However, the anesthesiologist should also be prepared to induce general anesthesia in case an adequate block is not present when the obstetrician is ready to begin surgery. If epidural analgesia is not already established, general anesthesia is usually required due to the time factor and the inability to position the patient for regional anesthesia while the fetal head is being elevated. Occasionally, the parturient can be placed in the lateral position while the obstetrician elevates the fetal head, so that a spinal anesthetic can be performed. If this is attempted, fetal heart rate must be closely monitored during attempted spinal anesthetic placement.

MULTIPLE GESTATION

With the increasing use of assisted reproductive technologies, the frequency of multiple gestation has increased. Between 1973 and 1990, twin births increased at twice the rate of singleton births. The resulting frequencies of occurrence changed from one in 55 to one in 43 births for twins and from one in 3323 to one in 1341 for triplet+ births.[9] The frequency of higher order multiple gestation has also increased significantly. Both perinatal and maternal morbidity and mortality are increased with multiple gestation. Maternal complications that occur more frequently with multiple gestation include premature labor, preeclampsia, uterine atony, and postpartum hemorrhage. Preterm delivery, intrauterine growth restriction, malpresentation, cord entanglement, and umbilical cord prolapse are fetal complications that occur with greater frequency in multiple gestation.

The implications of multiple gestation in the obstetric and anesthetic management of these parturients is significant and presents challenges to obstetricians and anesthesiologists. Some maternal physiologic changes of pregnancy are exaggerated by multiple gestation. The larger uterine size of women with multiple gestation results in a greater decrease in functional residual capacity. Hypoxemia, therefore, will develop more rapidly if a situation of apnea or hypoventilation occurs. Aortocaval compression and the supine hypotensive syndrome are also likely to be more severe in these patients due to the greater uterine size and weight. Uterine atony and postpartum hemorrhage are more likely to occur in these patients and may cause hemodynamic instability, the need for transfusion, and, rarely, hysterectomy.

In planning the obstetric management for a patient with multiple gestation, the route of delivery must first be decided. The presentation of the first twin usually determines whether a vaginal delivery will be attempted, with most obstetricians requiring vertex presentation of the presenting twin. Once twin A is delivered vaginally, a decision must be made concerning the route of delivery for twin B. First, presentation must be confirmed by ultrasound because presentation of twin B can change after delivery of the first twin. Fetal heart tones must also be evaluated because fetal bradycardia in the second twin can develop after delivery of twin A. If the second twin is also in the vertex presentation and the fetal heart rate pattern is reassuring, the obstetrician will generally proceed with vaginal delivery. If twin B has a nonvertex presentation, the obstetrician must decide among external cephalic version, internal podalic version, total breech extraction, or cesarean delivery. Communication regarding the planned delivery method for twin B must occur between obstetrician and anesthesiologist, so that appropriate anesthesia and uterine relaxation can be provided, if necessary. Generally, triplets and higher order multiple gestation are delivered via cesarean section.

■ **KEY POINT:** Epidural analgesia is not contraindicated in the healthy woman with twin gestations; rather, it is the method of choice. It provides effective pain relief, optimal delivery conditions, and the route for a rapid induction of anesthesia should an emergency cesarean section be required for twin B.

The anesthetic management for labor and vaginal delivery of twins is similar to that for a breech vaginal delivery. There is an increased incidence of prolapse of the umbilical cord of the second twin after delivery of twin A that would necessitate emergency cesarean delivery. If a breech delivery of the second twin is attempted, one must be prepared to respond to an entrapped fetal head.

■ **KEY POINT:** Cord prolapse is an obstetric emergency that often results in profound fetal bradycardia. If this occurs, the fetal head must be elevated until cesarean delivery occurs. If an epidural catheter is in place, it can be used to provide surgical anesthesia if the fetus is stable.

Because of a likelihood that some form of manipulation will be required for delivery of twin B, augmenting the depth and height of the sensory block during delivery of twin A should be considered. Denser anesthesia is required for a total breech extraction and may also contribute to the success of an external cephalic version. The anesthesiologist may also need to provide uterine relaxation for either of these procedures. Usually, intravenous nitroglycerin 50 to 100 μg will provide the necessary relaxation, but one also must be prepared to provide rapid sequence induction of general endotracheal anesthesia followed by the administration of a high-dose volatile agent.

Because the incidence of postpartum hemorrhage is increased in these patients, large-bore venous access should be established early in labor, and a current type and screen must be present in the blood bank. These patients are also more prone to supine hypotensive syndrome, and particular attention must be paid to maintaining left uterine displacement.

MULTIPARITY

Some clinical scenarios more frequently associated with multiparous patients present management challenges to the anesthesiologist and obstetrician. These women frequently present to the labor and delivery suite in advanced labor and may experience a precipitous delivery. Fulfilling the patient's request for labor analgesia in such a situation can truly be a challenge. This is the ideal scenario for combined spinal–epidural analgesia (see Chapter 5 for dosing options).

Patients with high parity are also more likely to develop uterine atony, which may lead to postpartum hemorrhage. The initial treatment of this postpartum hemorrhage includes uterine massage, but frequently pharmacologic treatment of the atony is also required. Table 14–7 summarizes the pharmacologic options for management of uterine atony and postpartum hemorrhage. The anesthesiologist will frequently become involved in providing fluid resuscitation for these patients and anesthesia for uterine exploration. If atony persists after pharmacologic treatment and uterine exploration, a gravid hysterectomy may be required. This procedure typically involves large blood loss requiring aggressive fluid resuscitation

■ Table 14–7
PHARMACOLOGIC TREATMENT OF UTERINE ATONY

Oxytocin
  First-line drug
  Dosing: 20 units in 1000 mL NS or LR; administer as rapid IV infusion
  Side effects: vasodilatation and hypotension when administered as IV bolus
15-Methyl prostaglandin $F_{2\alpha}$
  Second-line drug
  Dosing: 250 μg intramyometrial or IM; may repeat q 15 min to maximum dose 2 mg
  Side effects: bronchospasm (especially in asthmatics), vasoconstriction with resulting hypertension (especially in patients with preexisting hypertension), diarrhea
Methergine
  Third-line drug
  Dosing: 0.2 mg IM (should not be administered IV)
  Side effects: hypertension, vasoconstriction including coronary artery, cerebral vascular accident in patients with preexisting hypertension, bronchospasm, nausea and vomiting

NS, normal saline; LR, lactated Ringer's solution.

and blood replacement. Occasionally, this surgery can be performed under epidural anesthesia if a block had already been established before hemorrhage. In many cases, however, general anesthesia is required.

Acute uterine inversion is a rare but very serious obstetric complication that may occur more frequently in women with high parity due to their predisposition to uterine atony. Immediately after inversion, neurogenic shock develops as a result of traction on the round ligaments and ovaries, and the patient will experience bradycardia and hypotension. Hemorrhage and hypovolemic shock will quickly follow. Obstetric management includes replacing the inverted uterus as soon as possible. Although this can be done without anesthesia, it is easier to perform in the patient who has existing epidural analgesia. A cervical ring quickly develops that makes replacement very difficult. If the obstetrician's initial attempt is unsuccessful, a tocolytic agent should be administered in an attempt to relax the cervical ring. Incremental doses of nitroglycerin 50 to 100 μg provide rapid relaxation; this is considered the drug of choice by most obstetricians and anesthesiologists. If replacement still fails after nitroglycerin administration, manual replacement under general anesthesia with a high concentration of volatile agent should be attempted. If all attempts at manual replacement of the uterus are unsuccessful, surgical replacement or hysterectomy is necessary. Once the inversion is corrected, an oxytocic drug should be administered to keep the uterus contracted and prevent a recurrent inversion. In addition to providing anesthesia and uterine relaxation, the anesthesiologist also must provide aggressive fluid resuscitation during this obstetric emergency.

REFERENCES

1. National Center for Health Statistics: Health, United States, 1991. Hyattsville, MD: US Department of Health and Human Services Public Health Service, 1991.
2. Chestnut DH, Weiner CP, Wang JP, et al: The effect of ephedrine upon uterine artery blood flow velocity in the pregnant guinea pig subjected to terbutaline infusion and acute hemorrhage. Anesthesiology 66:508-512, 1987.
3. Sipes SL, Chestnut DH, Vincent RD, et al: Which vasopressor should be used to treat hypotension during magnesium sulfate infusion and epidural anesthesia? Anesthesiology 77:101-108, 1992.
4. Stafford RS: The impact of nonclinical factors on repeat cesarean section. JAMA 265:59-63, 1991.
5. Farmer RM, Kirschbaum T, Potter D, et al: Uterine rupture during trial of labor after previous cesarean section. Am J Obstet Gynecol 165:996-1001, 1991.
6. Rosen MG, Dickinson JC, Westhoff CL: Vaginal birth after cesarean: a meta-analysis of morbidity and mortality. Obstet Gynecol 77:465-470, 1991.
7. American College of Obstetricians and Gynecologists Committee on Obstetrics: Maternal and Fetal Medicine. Guidelines for Vaginal Delivery After a Previous Cesarean Birth. ACOG Committee Opinion no. 64. Washington, DC, 1988, American College of Obstetricians and Gynecologists.
8. Carlan SJ, Dent JM, Huckaby T, et al: The effect of epidural anesthesia on safety and success of external cephalic version at term. Anesth Analg 79:525-528, 1994.
9. Luke B: The changing pattern of multiple births in the United States: Maternal and infant characteristics, 1973 and 1990. Obstet Gynecol 84:101-106, 1994.

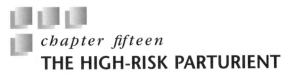

chapter fifteen
THE HIGH-RISK PARTURIENT
Ronald Hurley, MD

The parturient is classified as "high risk" when the presence of systemic disorders increase the maternal and/or neonatal morbidity and mortality. Obstetric and anesthetic management of these patients requires a thorough understanding of the physiology of pregnancy and the pathophysiology of the disease states. Early consultation and constant communication between the obstetric and anesthesia teams are essential.

DIABETES MELLITUS

The diagnosis of diabetes mellitus in a parturient before the isolation of insulin in 1921 was a death sentence. Most diabetics were too ill to conceive. Modern management has reduced the maternal and perinatal mortality to a rate near that of the normal population. However, significant morbidity still occurs, and complacency can lead to disaster. There is no disease entity that requires more cooperation and communication between the obstetrician, internist, anesthesiologist, and pediatrician.

■ **KEY POINT:** Pregnancy is associated with a progressive increase in insulin resistance.

Pathophysiology

Pregnancy results in two major opposing forces that affect glucose metabolism: accelerated starvation and insulin resistance. Overnight fasting glucose levels in pregnant patients are 15 to 20 mg/dL lower than in nonpregnant women. After fasting for 12 hours, plasma glucose levels may fall to 40 mg/dL, whereas hydroxybutyrate and acetoacetate rise to levels two to four times that of nonpregnant patients. Thus, ketoacidosis can occur despite the lack of a dramatic hyperglycemia. However, pregnancy is also characterized by a relative insulin resistance that is probably secondary to a rise in the pregnancy-related hormones estrogen, progesterone, prolactin, and human placental lactogen.

Classification

The National Diabetes Data Group classifies diabetes into the primary form, where no other systemic illness is responsible, and the secondary form, where the altered glucose homeostasis results from a second systemic disease such as pancreatitis or pheochromocytoma. The primary form is subdivided into two types. Though type 1 is often synonymous with insulin-dependent diabetes mellitus and type 2 synonymous with non–insulin-dependent diabetes mellitus, the type designation actually refers to the pathogenetic mechanism of immune mediated (type 1) and non-immune mediated (type 2). The subtypes also designate the patients that are prone to ketoacidosis (type 1) and those that are ketoacidosis resistant (type 2).

Classification During Pregnancy

Diabetes complicating pregnancy can be either a preexisting condition or gestational. The White classification was devised to attempt to correlate increasing severity of disease with infant survival. The classification was modified by the American College of Obstetricians and Gynecologists in 1986 and is summarized in Table 15–1.

Problems Complicating the Diabetic Pregnancy

The pathophysiology of diabetes mellitus affects every organ system, and the medical, obstetric, and anesthetic management can be extremely challenging.

Diabetic Ketoacidosis

Diabetic ketoacidosis (DKA) is a threat to the lives of mother and fetus and results from the absolute or relative deficiency in insulin and a relative or absolute increase in the counterregulatory hormone, glucagon. Typical inciting events include the failure to take insulin, infection, and the treatment

■ Table 15–1
MODIFIED WHITE CLASSIFICATION OF DIABETES IN PREGNANCY

Class	Age of Onset (y)		Duration (y)	Vascular Disease?	Insulin?
A-1	Any		Gestational	No	Diet only
A-2	Any		Gestational	No	Yes
B	>20		<10	No	Yes
C	10–19	or	10–19	No	Yes
D	<10	or	>20	Benign retinopathy	Yes
F	Any		Any	Nephropathy	Yes
R	Any		Any	Proliferative retinopathy	Yes
H	Any		Any	Heart disease	Yes

of premature labor with β agonists and glucocorticoids. Decreased peripheral glucose uptake and increased gluconeogenesis cause a hyperglycemia that leads to an osmotic diuresis and the dehydration typical of DKA. The hypoinsulinemia and β stimulation increase the production of hydroxybutyrate and acetoacetate, fixed acids that depress bicarbonate with a resultant anion gap and metabolic acidosis.

Treatment of DKA consists of

1. Volume replacement. Parturients in DKA are significantly volume depleted secondary to the osmotic diuresis. A separate venous access for noninsulin, nonglucose-containing crystalloid is essential. Remember to place a urinary catheter and consider a central line.
2. Electrolytes. Initial serum Na^+ and K^+ may be normal, although this masks a significant total body depletion. Insulin therapy will move K^+ into cells so K^+ must be added. Some authorities recommend the initial potassium is administered as the phosphate. Phosphate is also depressed in DKA, which may lead to a decrease in 2,3-diphosphoglycerate (DPG) and a leftward shift of the oxygen dissociation curve. Check the electrolytes frequently and consider an electrocardiogram during K^+ replenishment.
3. Insulin. Avoid subcutaneous insulin. Administer regular insulin as an intravenous infusion.
4. Blood gases. Consider an arterial line as periodic pH determinations and frequent electrolyte levels will need to be drawn.
5. Fetal monitoring. The metabolic acidosis may lead to fetal distress and premature labor may be present. β Agonist therapy is relatively contraindicated and magnesium sulfate is considered to be the tocolytic of choice.

Placental Insufficiency

Placental abnormalities may be present even with tight glucose and insulin therapy. Uteroplacental flow may be decreased by 35 to 40%.

Oxygen Transport Deficiency

Poor glucose control will lead to higher levels of glycosylated hemoglobin. Glycosylated hemoglobin and lower levels of 2,3-DPG may impair oxygen release in the placenta.

Hypertension and Preeclampsia

Patients with preexisting insulin-dependent diabetes mellitus have higher systolic and diastolic blood pressures and are three times more likely to develop pregnancy-induced hypertension.

Fetal Effects

Maternal hyperglycemia leads to fetal hyperglycemia and postdelivery hypoglycemia. It is important to have tight control of the maternal glucose level (80 to 100 mg/dL) at the time of delivery. Alert the pediatricians in the event of poorly controlled maternal glucose levels so they can be prepared for fetal hypoglycemia.

Fetal macrosomia is common in diabetic parturients. The need for cesarean delivery is increased and the possibility of a shoulder dystocia during a vaginal delivery may be present. Congenital anomalies are a leading cause of perinatal mortality in diabetic parturients.

Respiratory distress syndrome may be more common in the neonate. Assessment of the fetal lung maturity with appropriate validated tests (saturated phosphatidylcholine) is indicated.

Insulin Requirements

Insulin requirements drop dramatically after delivery. Frequent glucose determinations will guide therapy.

■ **KEY POINT:** Insulin requirements usually decrease during the first stage of labor and increase during the second stage. Insulin requirements decrease again after delivery.

Stiff Joint Syndrome

Stiff joint syndrome with limited mobility of the atlantoaxial joints may make endotracheal intubation difficult. The "prayer sign" or inability to approximate the palmar surfaces of the phalangeal surfaces may be a clue to the presence of the syndrome.

Autonomic Neuropathy

The presence of an autonomic neuropathy may make the parturient more susceptible to hypotension after major neural blockade. Gastroparesis may aggravate the already poor gastric emptying present in pregnant patients.

Retinopathy

Eye complications of diabetes are the leading cause of blindness in the United States. Proliferative retinopathy is very common in patients with long-standing insulin–dependent diabetes mellitus.

Nephropathy

Renal disease from diabetes causes 30% of end-stage renal disease in the United States. Proteinuria present in patients with nephropathy may complicate the diagnosis of preeclampsia.

Atherosclerosis

The development of atherosclerosis is accelerated in the diabetic, and the possibility of significant coronary artery disease should not be overlooked.

Anesthetic Management of the Diabetic Parturient

Vaginal Delivery

Moderate doses of parenteral narcotics, either pure agonists (morphine and meperidine) or mixed agonist–antagonist agents (nalbuphine), may be administered in early labor, but the potential for respiratory depression in a compromised neonate limits their use. Paracervical block is usually contraindicated because fetal hypoxia has been reported secondary to umbilical and uterine artery vasoconstriction. Lumbar epidural analgesia, with or without the utilization of the combined spinal epidural technique, offers numerous advantages. The excellent pain relief afforded will reduce maternal catecholamine levels that will then reduce maternal lactate production. The epidural catheter may be supplemented later with 2% lidocaine with epinephrine or 3% 2-chloroprocaine for cesarean or forceps delivery. If no epidural catheter is present, spinal anesthesia for forceps delivery can be provided with 1.5% lidocaine with 7.5% glucose or 0.75% bupivacaine in 8.25% glucose. At the Brigham and Women's Hospital, the epidural is initiated with 12 mL of 0.25% bupivacaine in divided doses followed by an infusion of 0.125% bupivacaine with 2 μg/mL of fentanyl at 10 mL/h. The combined technique consists of an initial dose of either 25 μg of fentanyl or 5 μg of sufentanil with 2.5 mg of plain bupivacaine in the subarachnoid space followed by immediate activation of the epidural with 0.125% bupivacaine plus 2 μg of fentanyl per mL at 10 mL/h.

Cesarean Delivery

The diabetic patient presenting for cesarean delivery requires careful attention to detail. Despite recent studies that have called into question the value of fluid loading, most practitioners still rapidly infuse 1.0 to 1.5 L of *glucose-free* crystalloid before major regional anesthesia. Sodium citrate oral antacid 30 mL plus 10 mg of intravenous metoclopramide to aid gastric emptying should be administered. The advantages of spinal versus epidural anesthesia continue to be debated. Epidural anesthesia with 2% lidocaine with epinephrine, 3% 2-chloroprocaine, or 0.5% bupivacaine offer the advantage of slow onset and perhaps a lower risk of hypotension in a patient especially at risk for this complication. Bupivacaine 0.5% has the slowest onset of this trio. 2-Chloroprocaine has the advantage of a rapid metabolic breakdown that minimizes the risk of local anesthetic accumulation in an acidotic fetus. Fentanyl (50 to 100 μg) may be added, though the advantage may be minimal with chloroprocaine. Preservative-free morphine sulfate, 3 mg via the epidural catheter, provides excellent postoperative analgesia. Perispinal morphine has proven safe provided a carefully considered nursing protocol is in place to guard against the possibility of delayed respiratory depression. Epidural anesthesia may be most appropriate for the severe diabetic (class FR, superimposed pre-eclampsia, proven atherosclerosis, and the transplant patient).

Spinal anesthesia is appropriate for the diabetic cesarean delivery if special attention is given to the avoidance of hypotension. Small (5 to 10 mg) doses of ephedrine given intravenously just after the spinal is placed and a rapid infusion of crystalloid may be helpful. The spinal is done in the right lateral decubitus or sitting position. The usual mixture at the Brigham and Women's Hospital consists of 1.6 mL of 0.75% hyperbaric bupivacaine with 10 μg of fentanyl and 0.2 mg of preservative-free morphine sulfate.

General anesthesia has become increasingly rare for the pregnant patient, even the pregnant diabetic patient. When it becomes necessary, however, it can be performed safely. It is usually reserved for the truly emergent cesarean section and for the usual contraindications to regional anesthesia (patient refusal, coagulopathy, infection at the spinal/epidural site, significant hypovolemia). Care must be taken to closely evaluate the airway and check for the possibility of stiff joint syndrome.

■ **KEY POINT:** Inability to approximate the palmar surfaces of the phalangeal joints despite maximal effort is a sign of the diabetic stiff joint syndrome, which may be a cause of failed intubation.

Left uterine displacement and tight maternal glucose control at the time of delivery are important no matter what form of anesthesia is chosen for the diabetic parturient.

ASTHMA

Bronchial asthma, estimated to affect 1 to 4% of pregnant women, is one of the most common medical disorders of pregnancy. The National Asthma Education Program has noted a trend of increasing morbidity and mortality from asthma during pregnancy. Studies have shown no consistent pattern on the effect of pregnancy on asthma, with as many improving as there are experiencing a worsening of their respiratory symptoms.

■ **KEY POINT:** The course of asthma may improve, worsen, or remain the same during pregnancy. When asthma is carefully managed, it generally does not adversely affect perinatal outcome.

Objective Evaluation

Wheezing and dyspnea are the classic symptoms of bronchospasm, but unfortunately they do not always correlate well with the severity of the attack. Peak flow meters, pulmonary function testing, arterial blood gas analysis, and pulse oximetry are the mainstays of objective evaluation.

Peak expiratory flow rate is normally 380 to 550 L/min with normally no change due to pregnancy. A reduction of 20% from baseline would be considered significant. A reduction below 100 L/min would indicate severe obstruction and impending respiratory distress.

In pregnancy there is normally an increase in tidal volume and minute ventilation, with decreases in forced vital capacity, residual volume, and functional residual capacity. A forced expiratory volume in 1 second-to-forced vital capacity ratio of less than 0.75 is typical of obstructive disease. A forced expiratory volume in 1 second of less than 1 L may correlate with significant hypoxemia.

Normal arterial blood gas values are affected by pregnancy (Table 15-2). Note that the "normal" P_{CO_2} of 40 in the nonpregnant patient may indicate severe obstruction and impending respiratory failure in the parturient. Pulse oximetry is a late indicator of respiratory insufficiency but is useful for following trends in oxygenation during treatment.

Treatment Regimens

β_2 Agonists remain the mainstay of acute treatment of exacerbations, as reviewed in Table 15-3. Inhaled corticosteroids, although important for chronic maintenance have no place in acute attacks. Atropine derivatives such as ipratropium have seen limited use in pregnancy and have the disadvantage of a fairly slow onset. Aminophylline and its salt derivative, theoph-

■ Table 15–2
ASTHMATIC EXACERBATION

Respiratory Pattern	pH	P_{O_2}	P_{CO_2}
Normal	7.4–7.45	95–106	28–32
Mild obstruction	Increased	Normal	Decreased
Severe obstruction	Normal	Decreased	Normal
Respiratory failure	Decreased	Decreased	Increased

■ Table 15–3
TREATMENT OF ACUTE ASTHMATIC OBSTRUCTION

Medication Class	Dose and Route of Delivery
Parenteral β agonist	Epinephrine: 0.2–0.5 mg SC (1/1000); repeat q 15–20 min × 2
	Terbutaline: 0.25 mg SC; repeat × 1 in 20 min
Inhaled β agonists	Albuterol: 0.5 mL of 0.5% solution in 2.5 mL normal saline
	Metaproterenol: 0.3 mL of 5% solution in 2.5 mL normal saline given q 20–30 min for three doses then q 1 hr prn
Corticosteroids	Methylprednisolone: 1 mg/kg IV q 6–8 hr

ylline, have fallen out of favor for use in the pregnant patient but still have advocates. These methylxanthines were purported to be phosphodiesterase inhibitors that increased the level of cyclic AMP. However, their mechanism of action is unclear because the level of enzyme inhibition seen is insufficient to cause bronchodilatation. Aminophylline levels can be significantly affected by pregnancy and the administration of other pharmaceuticals.

Anesthetic Management

Labor should be managed with lumbar epidural analgesia with or without the combined spinal epidural modification. A protocol similar to that described for the diabetic patient can be followed. Controversy arises when one considers the best form of anesthesia for the asthmatic patient scheduled for cesarean delivery. Elective cases should be delayed if significant obstructive disease is present as measured by the objective criteria delineated above. "Emergency" cases require the anesthesiologist to remember that the first responsibility is to the mother. If it is necessary to proceed, it must be remembered that major regional anesthesia has only minor effects on inspiratory effort but may have a significant effect on expiratory effort. Of the two commonly used forms of neuraxial anesthesia, epidural anesthesia produces less motor block and a more controllable level, which may be advantageous in the bronchoconstricted patient.

General anesthesia is avoided whenever possible, because the endotracheal tube may aggravate the bronchospasm. However, as the treatment for respiratory failure includes intubation, general endotracheal anesthesia may occasionally become necessary. The anesthesia circuit should be prefitted with a β agonist dispenser. After administering agents for aspiration prophylaxis (Bicitra and metoclopramide), the patient should be appropriately preoxygenated. During an acute asthma attack, general anesthesia should be induced with ketamine (≤1.5 mg/kg) and succinylcholine. General anesthesia should be maintained with a volatile agent. Halothane is not a drug of choice, however, because the concomitant use of halothane and β agonists may sensitize the myocardium and produce dysrhythmias. Uterine atony and postpartum hemorrhage may arise due to excessive uterine relaxation from the anesthetic vapor, and bronchospasm may return as the patient "lightens" at the end of the procedure. Judicious use of nonhistamine-releasing narcotics and ketamine may help when navigating this difficult course.

CARDIAC DISEASE

Cardiac disease complicates approximately 1% of pregnancies. The marked hemodynamic changes of pregnancy may have a dramatic effect on the patient with intrinsic heart disease. The physiologic changes of pregnancy are reviewed in Chapter 1 but warrant repetition here. The most important change as regards stress to the patient with underlying cardiac disease is the increase in cardiac output of 30 to 50%. This is accomplished by an increase in the heart rate and stroke volume and a decrease in total peripheral resistance. Half of the increase is in place by 8 weeks of gestation and, contrary to earlier reports, the cardiac output does not decrease after 32 weeks, although the output will decrease if aortocaval compression is allowed to occur. Labor will increase demands on the heart still further, with highest cardiac output demands during the second stage of labor and immediately after delivery.

■ **KEY POINT:** Cardiac patients often have worsening of their symptoms between 20 and 24 weeks of gestation.

Valvular Heart Disease

Mitral Stenosis

Decreasing the mitral valve area below 2.5 cm² impairs left ventricular filling and may herald the onset of symptoms. Patients with mitral stenosis tolerate tachyarrhythmias poorly. Digoxin, beta-blockers, and, if necessary, cardioversion are used to slow the heart rate. Volume control is critical, and the use of pulmonary artery catheterization may help to navigate the fine line between pulmonary edema and hypotension secondary to decreased left ventricular filling. Epidural anesthesia is certainly indicated to avoid the tachycardias associated with pain and high catecholamine secretion, if the patient is not anticoagulated.

Mitral Regurgitation

Pregnant women normally tolerate mitral regurgitation quite well. The lowering of the total peripheral resistance actually benefits this lesion. Epidural analgesia for labor gives excellent pain relief and lowers peripheral resistance further. The lower resistance unloads the left ventricle and favors forward over regurgitant flow.

Mitral Valve Prolapse

Mitral valve prolapse is the most common disorder of valvular function and occurs in 5 to 10% of the population. These patients may be more prone to tachyarrhythmias. Antibiotic prophylaxis is indicated.

Aortic Stenosis

The normal cross-sectional area of the aortic valve is 2.6 to 3.5 cm^2. Critical stenosis occurs with a reduction of the area below 1 cm^2 and represents the most dangerous of all the valvular lesions. These patients do not tolerate the lowering of peripheral resistance. An adequate diastolic pressure is required to perfuse their thickened myocardium, and hypotension may be impossible to reverse. Tachyarrhythmias must be avoided. Epidural analgesia has been used but may produce life-threatening hypotension and so must be used very carefully, if at all. For that same reason, one-shot spinal anesthesia should not be used in these patients. Phenylephrine is pressor of choice because it maintains afterload without tachycardia.

■ **KEY POINT:** Aortic stenosis and pulmonary hypertension are not absolute contraindications to regional anesthesia; however, slow induction of neuraxial block is necessary and one-shot techniques should not be attempted.

Aortic Regurgitation

Aortic regurgitation is similar to mitral regurgitation in that it is usually well tolerated by the parturient. Afterload reduction benefits the lesion; therefore, epidural analgesia is favored. With the decrease in rheumatic fever, most cases of aortic regurgitation seen today are due to connective tissue disorders such as Marfan's syndrome and bacterial endocarditis. All significant valvular lesions require antibiotic prophylaxis against bacterial endocarditis.

Congenital Heart Disease

Advanced cardiac surgical techniques and close medical supervision have allowed women that would not have survived in the past to reach the childbearing years. Shunts at the atrial or ventricular level may be partially or completely repaired. Women with repaired tetralogy of Fallot or Ebstein anomaly have become pregnant and may present at the labor floor. It is beyond the scope of this chapter to review the detail of the congenital lesions except to point out the dangers of pulmonary hypertension. The hypertension may be primary or secondary to atrial, ventricular, or aortopulmonary shunts. When the pulmonic pressures approach systemic and the shunt becomes bidirectional (Eisenmenger's syndrome), the situation can become lethal. Perinatal mortality may exceed 50%, and these lesions are not generally amenable to surgical correction.

MUSCULOSKELETAL AND NEUROLOGIC DISEASE

Pregnant women may present with a wide variety of neurologic symptoms, commonly including low back pain (with or without sciatica), a history of surgery for scoliosis, paraplegia, and multiple sclerosis (MS). It is important to carefully document the extent of the patient's deficit before anesthetic intervention so that true complications of anesthesia can be differentiated from exacerbations of the preexisting condition.

Sciatica

Low back pain with sciatica is extremely common during pregnancy and in the postpartum period. There is usually no contraindication to epidural or spinal block in these patients, although the patient should be cautioned that aggravation of her symptoms is possible.

■ **KEY POINT:** Low back pain is common during pregnancy and does not contraindicate the use of neuraxial techniques.

Spinal Surgery (Harrington Rods)

Obstetric anesthesia consultation for the patient with Harrington rods is not unusual and should be arranged well before labor. Retrieval of the operative record and relevant radiographs and a discussion with the neurosurgeon or orthopedist will aid in planning. Epidural analgesia is sometimes possible if the level of the reinforcing rods is at a distance from the usual lumbar approach used by anesthesiologists. Unfortunately, the surgery may have obliterated the epidural space, and therefore spread of epidural medications may be limited. The subarachnoid space is usually spared, however, and if a spinal can be placed below the level of the cord at L-2, analgesia for labor or anesthesia for cesarean delivery can be provided via that route.

Paraplegia

Increasingly sophisticated care has increased the survival rate of spinal cord trauma patients. Parturients with lesions below T-10 may feel the pain of contractions and request analgesia. There is no contraindication to a lumbar epidural catheter in these patients. Autonomic hyperreflexia is not usually seen with lesions below T-7 but occurs in about two thirds of the patients with lesions higher than T-7. Stimulation of the gut, bladder, or uterus may provoke the syndrome, with the patient complaining of headache, facial flushing, and diaphoresis. Autonomic hyperreflexia results from afferent impulses reaching a disinhibited spinal cord, which causes a massive secretion of catecholamines and potentially lethal hypertension. The baroreceptors are intact, so bradycardia occurs. Continuous epidural analgesia is indicated despite the patient's inability to report any sensation. Standard epidural infusion mixes are appropriate.

Multiple Sclerosis

MS is a demyelinating disease that commonly affects women of childbearing age. The effect of pregnancy may result in an amelioration of symptoms prepartum but result in a two to threefold increase in exacerbations in the months after delivery. General anesthesia has been regarded as safe for the MS parturient, but regional anesthesia is more controversial because of the demyelinating nature of the disease and the waxing and waning nature of its symptomatology. It is the practice at Brigham and Women's Hospital to administer lumbar epidural analgesia with the standard low concentrations of bupivacaine to MS patients after careful explanation that all the risks are not known and that an exacerbation of the disease is not unusual postdelivery.

■ **KEY POINT:** Regional anesthesia is not contraindicated in parturients with MS. Symptoms may worsen post partum regardless of the anesthetic used.

OBESITY

Morbid obesity is one of the most common yet difficult problems encountered on the labor floor. Morbidly obese parturients are often hypertensive, diabetic, and may have respiratory insufficiency in the supine position. They have a higher incidence of cesarean delivery, often have difficult epidural placements with a high incidence of failure and dural puncture, may have unpredictable levels after spinal anesthesia, have large volumes of gastric contents with a low pH, and laryngoscopy with endotracheal intubation may be difficult or impossible.

Principles of successful management include the following:

1. Early consultation by the obstetric anesthesia service either before or at least early in labor so that the patient can be carefully evaluated and the anesthetic options and risks discussed with the patient and obstetric providers.
2. Early epidural placement. According to some, the combined spinal–epidural technique is less attractive because it is desirable to "prove" that the catheter is properly placed if an emergent situation ensues. A continuous spinal option may be considered, especially in cases of difficult epidural placement. There is some evidence that the incidence of postdural puncture headache is reduced in the morbidly obese. Extra long spinal and epidural needles should be available.
3. In the case of a "difficult" airway, a "stat" cesarean delivery may not be possible, and this message should be clearly conveyed to the obstetric staff. The anesthesiologist's first responsibility is to the mother and the difficult airway may preclude a rapid sequence induction of general anesthesia. A difficult airway cart with fiberoptic bronchoscopy, laryngeal masks, and other airway alternatives should always be readily available.

■ **KEY POINT:** In the obese parturient with a difficult airway, every effort should be made to initiate an early regional anesthetic via a catheter technique. Should difficulty arise with placement of an epidural, a continuous spinal technique should be considered.

MALIGNANT HYPERTHERMIA

Malignant hyperthermia has been only rarely described in pregnancy. The principles of management are similar to those of the nonpregnant patient with a few caveats:

1. The malignant hyperthermia protocol should be posted at each anesthetizing location with the telephone number of the Malignant Hyperthermia Association of the United

States (800-644-9737 or 800-MH-HYPER) hotline prominently displayed.
2. The labor suite should have its own dantrolene supply if significantly distant from the main operating rooms.
3. Dantrolene crosses the placenta and reaches a level about 60% of the maternal plasma concentration.
4. Most anesthesiologists are comfortable with using either ester or amide local anesthetics for regional anesthesia.
5. Avoidance of triggering agents and treatment of hyperthermic events should proceed as with nonpregnant patients.

■ **KEY POINT:** Parturients susceptible to malignant hyperthermia should be encouraged to receive epidural analgesia, so that if a cesarean section becomes necessary, the epidural can be utilized.

ANTICOAGULATION AND REGIONAL ANESTHESIA

Heparin has been the preferred anticoagulant for use during pregnancy because it does not cross the placental barrier. Warfarin (Coumadin) is contraindicated in early pregnancy, because it crosses to the fetus and may cause fetal malformations. Usually, heparin may be withdrawn during labor and delivery and restarted after delivery. However, this decision depends on the indication for anticoagulation, and any modification of the treatment regimen should be a joint decision of the appropriate physicians. Heparin may be reversed with protamine if necessary, although it is preferable to let the heparin "wear off" and not risk an allergic reaction to protamine if time permits.

In 1993 low-molecular-weight heparins (LMWHs) were introduced to the American market. Their safety and efficacy encouraged wide use. However, as perhaps the differences between the LMWHs and standard heparin were not appreciated, complications including spinal hematomas were reported. The U.S. Food and Drug Administration took steps to notify physicians of the potential for complications after neuraxial blockade in patients receiving LMWHs in the perioperative period. A consensus conference on neuraxial block and anticoagulation was convened in May 1998.[1] A synopsis of the recommendations follows.

1. Administration of other antiplatelet or oral anticoagulant with LMWH heightens the risk of spinal hematoma.
2. A "bloody tap" with a spinal or epidural needle should delay initiation of LMWH for 24 hours.

3. Major neuraxial blocks should be delayed 12 hours after the standard dose of LMWH and 24 hours after high-dose (enoxaparin 1 mg/kg twice daily) administration.
4. LMWH may be administered postoperatively. If a continuous catheter is in place, wait 2 hours after removal before the LMWH administration.
5. LMWH + epidural = extreme vigilance. Dilute local anesthetic/opioid solutions should be used. Investigate any progressive motor block immediately.
6. Anti-Xa monitoring is not indicated because it has not been shown to correlate with bleeding.

REFERENCE

1. Horlocter TT, Wedel DJ: Neuraxial block and low-molecular weight heparin: Balancing perioperative analgesia and thromboprophylaxis. Reg Anesth Pain Med 23(suppl 2): 164–177, 1998.

Key References

Bonica JJ, McDonald JS: Principles and Practice of Obstetric Analgesia and Anesthesia, 2nd ed. Baltimore: Williams & Wilkins, 1995.

Burrow GN, Ferris TF: Medical Complications During Pregnancy, 4th ed. Philadelphia: W.B. Saunders, 1994.

Datta S: Anesthetic and Obstetric Management of High-Risk Pregnancy. St. Louis: Mosby Yearbook, 1991.

Datta S: The Obstetric Anesthesia Handbook, 2nd ed. St. Louis: Mosby, 1995.

Ferris TF: Medical disorders during pregnancy. In: Fauci AS, Braunwald E, Isselgacher KJ, et al (eds): Harrison's Principles of Internal Medicine, 14th ed. New York: McGraw-Hill, 1998, pp 24–26.

Foster DW: Diabetes mellitus. In: Fauci AS, Braunwald E, Isselgacher KJ, et al (eds): Harrison's Principles of Internal Medicine, 14th ed. New York: McGraw-Hill, 1998, pp 2060–2081.

James FM, Wheeler AS: Obstetric Anesthesia: The Complicated Patient. Philadelphia: F.A. Davis, 1982.

Malinow AM, Ostheimer GW: Anesthesia for the high-risk parturient. Obstet Gynecol 69:00–00, 1987.

McFadden ER: Diseases of the respiratory system. In: Fauci AS, Braunwald E, Isselgacher KJ, et al (eds): Harrison's Principles of Internal Medicine, 14th ed. New York: McGraw-Hill, 1998, pp 1419–1426.

Repke JT: Intrapartum Obstetrics. New York: Churchill Livingstone, 1996.

Stoelting RK, Dierdorf SF: Anesthesia and Co-Existing Disease, 3rd ed. New York: Churchill Livingstone, 1993.

Van Zundert A, Ostheimer GW: Pain Relief in Anesthesia and in Obstetrics. New York: Churchill Livingstone, 1996.

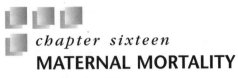

chapter sixteen
MATERNAL MORTALITY
Barry Corke, MD

Despite its dramatic decline over the years, maternal mortality remains an important subject and therefore merits inclusion in texts related to obstetric anesthesia. This chapter will deviate from most chapters related to maternal mortality by concentrating primarily on clinical issues. The chapter is not intended to be an encyclopedic review of statistics. Such information is readily available from larger obstetric anesthesia textbooks.

■ **KEY POINT:** Maternal mortality can be direct (obstetric causes); indirect (non-obstetric causes); or unrelated. Although deaths from anesthesia are usually classified as indirect, the ICD-9 (International Classification of Diseases) lists anesthesia as a distinct cause of maternal mortality.

The more important causes of maternal mortality are discussed. Emphasis is placed on procedures that are intended to reduce or, it is hoped, eliminate such danger. Where possible, there is an indication as to the prevalence of fatality and how this has changed with time.

Original estimates of maternal mortality used units of deaths per 1000 pregnancies. United Kingdom figures estimated maternal mortality in 1937 to be 4 per 1000 pregnancies. Before 1935, the United States figure was 60 deaths per 10,000 births.[1] Since that time there has been a dramatic decline in deaths, and maternal mortality is now estimated in deaths per 100,000. By the years 1985 to 1987, the United Kingdom maternal mortality rate had fallen to 7.6 per 100,000.[2] In less-developed areas, maternal mortality rates are more difficult to estimate but are likely to be higher than this figure. The United States rate is thought to be of the order of 9.1 per 100,000 but is very much influenced by socioeconomic factors and varies from area to area.

There has as yet been no consensus on the definition of maternal mortality. Death must occur during pregnancy or within a specified period after the termination of pregnancy. The American Medical Association includes all deaths during pregnancy or within 90 days of the termination of pregnancy. The International Classification of Disease includes all deaths during pregnancy or within 42 days of the termination of pregnancy. The International Federation of Gynecology and Obstetrics also includes all deaths during pregnancy or within 42 days of the termination of pregnancy. The Confidential Enquiries into Maternal Deaths in England and Wales extends the limit to 1 year after the termination of pregnancy.

It should be noted that estimates from British studies are likely to be the most accurate. A formalized reporting system has been in place for many years. Many studies from the United States have in the past been limited to reports from individual states. Maternal mortality has been shown to vary in the United States, according to the socioeconomic status of the area. In the past, reporting may have also been influenced by medicolegal concerns.

An important feature of the Confidential Enquiry is the division of cases into preventable deaths and nonpreventable deaths. Studies of the volumes of this document provide a valuable source of case presentations illustrating the dangers inherent in the management of anesthesia during pregnancy.

The more frequent complications of pregnancy are discussed with particular reference to the way in which each complication has an impact on maternal mortality. For a more detailed description of each complication, the relevant chapter should be consulted.

HEMORRHAGE

Peripartum hemorrhage continues to result in maternal mortality. The frequency of death resulting from hemorrhage has continued to fall during the 20th century. Although the total number of maternal deaths from hemorrhage has fallen significantly, the percentage of deaths related to this complication remains significant. Between 1979 and 1986, hemorrhage accounted for 18% of maternal deaths in the United States.[3] Reports from the United Kingdom indicate that 30 of 343 maternal deaths were caused by hemorrhage in the years 1970 to 1972.[4] For the years 1985 to 1987 there were 10 deaths of 139 related to hemorrhage. Between 1985 and 1987, hemorrhage was the fourth leading cause of maternal mortality in the United Kingdom.[2] Sachs et al.[5] reported that maternal deaths from hemorrhage decreased 10-fold from the mid-1950s to the mid-1980s. Hemorrhage-related deaths may be associated not only with birth but also with ectopic pregnancy and abortion.

Antepartum Hemorrhage

The most common causes of hemorrhage in the antepartum period are placental abruption and placenta previa.

Placental abruption, an emergency situation, endangers the life of both the mother and fetus. The danger is compounded by the presence of occult blood loss. A high percentage of the lost blood may be concealed behind the placenta. Placental abruption is also associated with a coagulopathy that increases the risk of massive blood loss.

The ability to diagnose placenta previa has been dramatically enhanced with the introduction of high-resolution ultrasound. The likelihood of an undiagnosed placenta previa presenting for delivery is now remote. Major hemorrhage is likely to occur from a vaginal examination if a placenta previa is not recognized. The requirement to perform a double setup before delivery is now a rarity. The double setup entailed performing a vaginal examination in an operating room and the ability to perform an immediate rapid sequence induction of general anesthesia if significant hemorrhage occurred after the examination.

Intrapartum Hemorrhage

Uterine rupture, although uncommon, remains a potentially lethal complication of delivery. Uterine rupture is most commonly associated with a multigravid patient experiencing very rapid labor. With the increased incidence of vaginal delivery after cesarean section, the incidence of uterine rupture could potentially increase.

■ **KEY POINT:** Uterine rupture is a rare but potentially catastrophic event that can cause maternal and fetal mortality. The diagnosis of uterine rupture should be considered when vaginal bleeding, cessation of labor, and fetal bradycardia occur. Unlike pain, which does not always occur, "fetal distress" is a reliable sign of uterine rupture.

Cesarean section has become a relatively safe procedure. The occurrence of significant hemorrhage is now rare. If hemorrhage does occur, the risk of maternal death is very low provided that the facility where the surgery takes place is optimally equipped. This includes the immediate availability of blood, either type specific or O negative, as well as of rapid infusion devices.

Postpartum Hemorrhage

The two principal causes of bleeding in the postpartum period are uterine atony and retained products of conception. Although bleeding may be significant, particularly if a coagulopathy exists, maternal death is now unlikely.

Reports from sources in the United States place hemorrhage as either the second or third leading cause of maternal mortality.[5] Worldwide, hemorrhage may be the leading cause of maternal mortality. Factors contributing to the very significant decrease in mortality from hemorrhage include improved nutritional states with a reduction in the incidence of severe anemia, availability of blood transfusion services, and awareness of the dangers of hemorrhage and the availability of trained personnel to deal with the emergency. This includes the ability to provide anesthesia in a safe and expeditious manner. Failure to do so is likely to contribute to maternal mortality.

HYPERTENSIVE DISEASE

In the past, the reporting of hypertensive disease during pregnancy was confused by misleading terminology. The term "pregnancy-induced hypertension" (PIH) is now the accepted term. This condition is further divided into preeclampsia and eclampsia. The primary feature of eclampsia is the occurrence of convulsions not related to a preexisting condition. Eclampsia and preeclampsia may account for up to 40% of obstetrically related deaths in reports from 1969 to 1973.[6] Conditions that accompany preeclampsia and lead to it being then defined as severe preeclampsia are the principal explanation for maternal deaths.

Respiratory Complications

Fluid retention and oncotic pressure changes are potential causes of pulmonary edema. In most cases, pulmonary edema can be managed by appropriate fluid management with or without the use of invasive monitoring. If the condition progresses to acute respiratory distress syndrome, the potential for a lethal outcome is considerably increased. In the United Kingdom from 1985 to 1987, of the 27 deaths related to hypertensive disease, 12 were from pulmonary complications.[2]

Intracerebral Hemorrhage

As with any hypertensive disease, the risk of cerebral hemorrhage is increased. If a cerebral hemorrhage occurs, mortality exceeds 80%. In the United Kingdom from 1985 to 1987, 11 of 27 deaths related to hypertension were from cerebral hemorrhage.[2]

Bleeding Disorders

Severe preeclampsia may be accompanied by a coagulopathy. Disseminated intravascular coagulopathy (DIC) may ensue and become a factor in the etiology of maternal mortality.

Renal Failure

Renal failure secondary to PIH is also a contributing factor to maternal mortality. The availability of facilities to dialyze patients has significantly reduced the likelihood of death from this complication.

Eclampsia

The occurrence of seizures heralds the onset of eclampsia and is seen most frequently in the third trimester. Eclampsia is frequently preceded by the signs of severe preeclampsia but may also occur unheralded. With aggressive management, the expected maternal mortality is less than 1%. Magnesium sulfate is the preferred preventive medication for seizures and has proved very effective.

■ **KEY POINT:** Optimal management of the eclamptic parturient decreases the risk of maternal mortality. Airway support, administration of oxygen, cricoid pressure, and left uterine displacement should all be initiated immediately. If airway protection is necessary, endotracheal intubation should be performed.

THROMBOEMBOLIC DISEASE

The risk of thromboembolic phenomena occurring is increased during pregnancy. Death from pulmonary embolism is a leading cause of maternal mortality. Although there has been a marked reduction in deaths from pulmonary embolism during pregnancy, there remains a group of women who are at greater risk of death from pulmonary embolism. African-American women have a three to four times greater risk than white women.[7] Increased age and obesity are further factors associated with an increased risk of pulmonary embolus.

The hypercoagulable state that exists during pregnancy is at its height in the immediate postpartum period. For this reason, death from thromboembolic disease is most likely to occur after delivery.

There has been an increased awareness of the dangers of thromboembolism and an increased understanding of the disease and the population at most risk. This has led to a 50% reduction in deaths from pulmonary embolus.

AMNIOTIC FLUID EMBOLISM

Amnotic fluid embolism is a potentially lethal complication of pregnancy and is not related to any other condition. The incidence of amnotic fluid embolism is approximately 3 per 100,000 pregnancies, and the mortality rate is as high as 86%.[8] Because of its lethal potential, it accounts for 10 to 12% of all maternal deaths.

Clinically, amniotic fluid embolism presents as dyspnea, hypoxia, hypotension, and coagulopathy. The diagnosis is usually made by exclusion of other complicating conditions. Because there is no definitive treatment, management of hemodynamic and respiratory complications is required in a prompt manner if survival is to occur.

CARDIAC DISEASE

Maternal mortality has been subdivided into direct and indirect causes. Deaths related to cardiac disease are classified as indirect. The preexisting cardiac disease may be aggravated by the physiologic changes that occur during pregnancy. Because congenital heart disease is now increasingly treatable, the likelihood of such patients becoming pregnant is increased. Between 1 and 2% of obstetric patients may have a significant heart lesion. Maternal mortality rates vary between 1 and 30% for obstetric patients with a significant heart lesion. The highest rates are seen in patients with life-threatening conditions, including Eisenmenger's syndrome, who become pregnant despite advice to the contrary. With the increased sophistication of management of cardiac disease during pregnancy, maternal mortality is now uncommon. Older statistics no longer apply and are not relevant to modern practice.

It should be remembered that coronary artery disease is increasing in incidence in the female population. Coronary artery disease is most likely to occur in patients with diabetes, smokers, and older parturients.

Deaths related to cardiac disease are classified together with other indirect causes of maternal mortality. Deaths from cardiac disease, both aquired and congenital, constitute the largest entity in this classification.

INFECTION

The role of infection in maternal mortality is now mainly of historical interest. The dread of puerperal sepsis existed into the 20th century. The use of antibiotics has made the condition exceedingly rare. Three conditions remain that have an impact on maternal mortality:

- Human immunodeficiency virus (HIV) is now becoming a more important consideration because most HIV-infected women are of reproductive age. There is no evidence that pregnancy hastens the onset of AIDS symptoms.
- Septic abortion—Since the legalization of abortion in many countries, the incidence of septic complications, including death, has fallen dramatically.

- Infection after cesarean section remains a cause of maternal mortality. Gram-negative sepsis with ensuing septic shock is a potentially lethal complication of surgery.

There were 30 deaths related to infection from a total of 343 maternal deaths reported in England and Wales in the years 1970 to 1972.[3] This number had fallen to 6 of 139 maternal deaths by the years 1985 to 1987.[2]

MATERNAL DEATHS RELATED TO ANESTHESIA

This section is the most relevant to the subject of this book. Anesthetic techniques have advanced, and consequently the safety of anesthesia for patients has improved. It should be noted, however, that despite the obvious improvement in outcome after anesthesia, the percentage of deaths related to anesthesia has either remained constant or risen. Although this increase in percentage of deaths related to anesthesia indicates that other causes of death have decreased at a faster rate, it has been incorrectly used to show a worsening of anesthesia outcomes. It is therefore imperative to view these statistics carefully and to look at the whole picture and not individual factors. Failure to do so may lead to an incorrect conclusion. A syndicated report appearing in several major newspapers gave such misleading information to the public. Questions were asked as to why anesthesia was causing an increased number of maternal deaths. It was, however, the percentage that had increased and not the overall number. The actual numbers had fallen.

■ **KEY POINT:** Anesthesia continues to be a cause of maternal mortality. Most recent reports indicate that these deaths are often secondary to mishaps during general anesthesia.

General Anesthesia

The two major factors that have contributed to maternal mortality associated with general anesthesia are aspiration of stomach contents and hypoxia secondary to difficulties in airway management. In some cases, these two factors are present in the same incident. This particular combination is particularly likely to result in a fatal outcome.

Mendelson[9] described the features of aspiration of stomach contents in 1946. His series of 66 cases had a mortality rate of only 3%. This is surprising in view of the lack of sophistication of critical care facilities available at that time. More recent estimates of mortality have been of the order of 30%. It is likely that the criteria used to diagnose aspiration and the volume and content of aspirate account for the large difference in the quoted mortality rates.

It has been recognized for many years that gastric emptying is significantly reduced during active labor. This reduction in gastric emptying is further enhanced by the administration of narcotic analgesics. Fortunately, this information has led to the generally held belief that oral intake during labor should be discontinued. Thus, most patients before anesthesia will have relatively empty stomachs. Despite this fact, it should always be assumed that the stomach is not empty and appropriate techniques used to guard against aspiration:

- Premedication with nonparticulate antacid;
- Rapid sequence induction if general anesthesia is used;
- Use of cricoid pressure until airway secured before intubation.

There is some merit in emptying the stomach after the airway has been secured. There is no place in current management for emptying the stomach before induction of anesthesia.

Awareness of the dangers of aspiration during general anesthesia for cesarean section has led to a very significant fall in the incidence of maternal mortality related to this complication. Knowledge of the dangers of aspiration and a better understanding of its etiology have improved the quality of anesthesia, because more experienced anesthesia personnel are now more likely to be involved in the administration of general anesthesia for pregnant patients.

■ **KEY POINT:** Aspiration of gastric contents and subsequent pneumonitis may occur following difficult or failed intubation. These risks should be explained to patients who request to eat during labor, and physicians should continue to restrict oral intake of solids during labor.

The ability to provide regional anesthesia as an alternative to general anesthesia for operative delivery has been a significant factor in the reduction of deaths from aspiration. Many patients requiring cesarean section have received epidural analgesia during labor. The epidural block can be extended to provide conditions adequate for surgery. Elective procedures may be undertaken with either epidural or spinal anesthesia.

■ **KEY POINT:** The most effective measure to decrease the risk of mortality due to aspiration is to avoid the routine use of general anesthesia in obstetrics.

The realization that gastric aspiration is a danger during general anesthesia and the adoption of the measures outlined in the previous paragraphs have resulted in the percentage and the total number of deaths related to aspiration falling. The most prevalent complication related to general anesthesia leading to maternal death is now difficulty with airway management with an episode of hypoxia as a result.

Difficulties in airway management are especially likely to occur in the pregnant patient:

■ Often an emergency situation is present—requirement for a rapid sequence induction with little or no time for assessment of the airway.
■ Obesity compounded by pregnancy may be a factor.
■ Inadequate induction dosage in an attempt to avoid neonatal depression.
■ Abnormal airway anatomy. Significant edema of laryngeal structures may occur in the presence of preeclampsia.
■ Failure to provide adequate equipment for the management of the difficult airway.
■ Inexperienced anesthesia provider.
■ Lack of a well-formulated plan to safely manage the airway when attempts at intubation are unsuccessful.

Since the introduction of reliable monitors to verify endotracheal intubation, the number of accidents related to esophageal intubation has markedly decreased. Pulse oximetry and end-tidal carbon dioxide detection are a minimum requirement for the management of anesthesia in the pregnant patient.

Training in the management of anesthesia for the pregnant patient is improving. The existence of a subspecialty organization, Society for Obstetric Anesthesia and Perinatology (SOAP), has also been of importance in disseminating information related to obstetric anesthesia and airway management of the parturient.

Sachs et al.[10] reported on 37 maternal deaths related to anesthesia occurring between 1954 and 1985. It was shown that anesthesia accounted for 4.2% of all deaths. For the years 1985 to 1987 the Confidential Enquiry[2] found six deaths related to anesthesia, which was 4.3% of the total.

Regional Anesthesia

Major regional anesthesia techniques used frequently in the pregnant patient are confined to spinal and epidural blocks. The reliance on regional anesthesia for most surgical procedures in the pregnant patient has been a factor in the reduction of maternal mortality. It should be remembered that deaths do occur from regional anesthesia and are usually preventable.

After the introduction of bupivacaine into the United

States, a number of deaths related to its use were reported.[11] In an attempt to improve the safety of this local anesthetic agent, the U.S. Food and Drug administration posted warnings regarding the use of the 0.75% for epidural anesthesia. It was also determined that the use of large boluses was a dangerous practice. The drug should be administered in small increments. After each increment, assessment is made of its effect and a further increment is not administered until the assessment is satisfactorily completed. The reported deaths associated with 0.75% bupivacaine were in general due to the administration of a large bolus of bupivacaine intravenously. Bupivacaine has a very low safety threshold when compared with lidocaine. Neurologic symptoms are rapidly followed by cardiovascular collapse. It was also found that attempts at resuscitation after cardiovascular collapse were frequently not successful in a previously healthy patient.

Spinal anesthesia uses very small drug dosages and avoids the danger of toxicity. The onset of sympathetic block may be rapid and is not always predictable. An understanding of the dangers of aortocaval compression during pregnancy and its accentuation with sympathetic blockade has led to increased safety for spinal anesthesia. It should be remembered that aspiration remains a risk in the patient who is obtunded by levels that are too high. An early decision regarding airway management is very important in ensuring patient safety.

■ **K E Y   P O I N T :**   Accidental intravascular injection of large volumes of local anesthetic that were intended for the epidural space is associated with cardiovascular collapse and maternal mortality. Although multiorifice catheters allow most intravascular catheters to be identified by aspiration, many anesthesiologists continue to use single-orifice catheters. In addition, aspiration does not detect all intravascular catheters. If boluses of local anesthetic are necessary, they should be administered in incremental (divided) doses.

CONCLUSIONS

A recent report from the World Health Organization estimated that 585,000 maternal deaths occur each year and that the vast majority occur in Sub-Saharan Africa. This information was part of a news brief on the internet (1998), which is viewed by an increasing percentage of the population. It is therefore likely that patients may have questions regarding the incidence of maternal death. It is important to have pertinent information to answer these questions.

It is also vital to be aware of the potential for serious problems during the administration of obstetric anesthesia to maintain the excellent safety record that this subspecialty has attained. Continuation of this attention to detail will ensure that the incidence of maternal mortality will continue to decrease until only the unavoidable deaths remain.

REFERENCES

1. Tu EJ: Cohort maternal mortality: New York, 1917–1972. Am J Public Health 69:1052–1055, 1979.
2. Report on Confidential Enquiries into Maternal Deaths in the United Kingdom 1985–1987. London: HMSO, 1991.
3. Koonin LM, Atrash HK, Lawson HW, et al: Maternal Mortality Surveillance—United States 1979–1986. United States Public Health Service. Atlanta, GA: Centers for Disease Control, 1991.
4. Report on Confidential Enquiries into Maternal Deaths in England and Wales 1970–1972. London: HMSO, 1976.
5. Sachs BP, Brown DA, Driscoll SG, et al: Hemorrhage, infection, toxemia, and cardiac disease, 1954–86. Causes for their declining role in maternal mortality. Am J Public Health 78:671–675, 1988.
6. Gibbs CE, Locke WE: Maternal deaths in Texas 1969–1973: a report of 501 consecutive deaths from the Texas Medical Associations Committee on Maternal Health. Am J Obstet Gynecol 126:687–692, 1976.
7. Hellgren M, Blomback M: Studies on blood coagulation and fibrinolysis in pregnancy, during delivery and in the puerperium. 1. Normal condition. Gynecol Obstet Invest 12:141–154, 1981.
8. Morgan M: Amniotic fluid embolus. Anaesthesia 34:20–32, 1979.
9. Mendelson CL: The aspiration of stomach contents into the lungs during obstetric anesthesia. Am J Obstet Gynecol 52:191–205, 1946.
10. Sachs BP, Oriol NE, Ostheimer GW, et al: Anesthesia-related maternal mortality, 1954–1985. J Clin Anesth 1:333–338, 1989.
11. Albright GA: Cardiac arrest following regional anesthesia with etidocaine and bupivacaine. Anesthesiology 51:285–287, 1979.

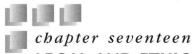

chapter seventeen

LEGAL AND ETHICAL ISSUES IN OBSTETRIC ANESTHESIA

Timothy B. McDonald, MD, JD

The purpose of this chapter is to provide basic information concerning the common and important legal and ethical issues that confront the practitioner of obstetric anesthesiology. The information contained in the first half of this chapter should help the practitioner understand and therefore prevent or successfully defend against actions in medical malpractice. The second half of the chapter concentrates on ethically complicated legal issues that confront the obstetric anesthesiologist and provides a framework to deal with those difficult issues.

LEGAL ISSUES IN OBSTETRIC ANESTHESIA

In the following excerpt from her book, Dr. Sara Charles aptly describes one of the most gut-wrenching experiences a physician can endure:

> *My first feelings after being charged with medical malpractice were of being utterly alone . . . during the five year span of my own case . . . it swallowed up my life completely, demanded constant attention and study, multiplied tension and strain, generated a pattern of broken sleep and anxiety because I felt my integrity as a person and as a physician had been damaged and might be permanently lost.*[1]

To successfully tackle or prevent the problems associated with medical malpractice, it is important to understand some basic medical–legal principles and terminology. To recover for medical malpractice, the person bringing the lawsuit (the plaintiff) must establish all of the following four elements: the existence of the physician's duty to the patient, the applicable standard of care and its violation, a causal connection between the physician's violation of the standard of care, and the resulting compensable injury to the patient.[2] Simply put, the elements needed to sustain a professional malpractice lawsuit are duty, breach, injury, and causation.

■ KEY POINT: The four essential elements that must be proved in any medical malpractice action include duty, breach, injury, and causation. *Each* one of these must be proved for the plaintiff to win.

Duty

A physician–patient relationship is normally a prerequisite to a malpractice suit filed against a physician. This relationship forms the basis for finding a duty owed by the physician to the patient. The law recognizes this duty and requires a physician to conform to a certain standard of care.

Generally, there is no legal duty to render emergency care to others. Because of this common law doctrine of no duty to aid others, most states and the District of Columbia have passed Good Samaritan statutes that encourage bystanders to render aid while immunizing them from liability against anything less than gross negligence.

Absent a Good Samaritan situation, once a physician establishes a relationship with a patient, the duty to provide reasonable care attaches. However, what constitutes a Good Samaritan situation and what constitutes a legally recognized physician–patient relationship differs widely from state to state. In some states, the Good Samaritan statute applies when three conditions are met. First, the physician encounters an emergency situation. Second, the physician has no prior relationship with the patient. Finally, the physician does not receive compensation for services rendered during the emergency.[3] Interestingly, some in-hospital physicians have successfully used the Good Samaritan statute to avoid liability in medical malpractice lawsuits. In one case, an obstetrician rendered in-hospital emergency obstetric services to a patient about whom he had no previous knowledge. He did not bill the patient for the emergency medical care. After the patient filed a lawsuit alleging medical malpractice, the physician invoked the Illinois Good Samaritan statute and successfully argued his dismissal from the lawsuit because he satisfied all three of the legislative requirements.[4] All physicians, including anesthesiologists, should review their own state's Good Samaritan statute and hospital policies to determine possible emergency situations in which they may be immunized from civil liability.

Issue: The Anesthesiologist's Duty to Provide Neonatal Resuscitation

Nowhere is the issue of legal duty more important than as it pertains to anesthesiologists and neonates in the delivery room. As with the case mentioned above, if an anesthesiologist can negate the existence of a legal duty to a neonate in the delivery room, then the anesthesiologist should be immunized from any civil liability arising from alleged negligent performance of neonatal resuscitation.

Unfortunately, a review of obstetric anesthesia medical malpractice cases from 1985 to 1993 demonstrates the legal system frequently finds anesthesiologists owe a duty to neonates in the delivery room regardless of attempts to claim otherwise. Juries have returned numerous judgments (some in excess of two million dollars) against anesthesiologists for the negligent performance of neonatal resuscitation.[5]

These adverse judgments have occurred despite the American Society of Anesthesiologists' (ASA) attempt in 1988 to more clearly define the role of anesthesiologists in the delivery room. Those ASA guidelines provide

> *Qualified personnel other than the anesthesiologist attending the mother, should be immediately available to assume responsibility for resuscitation of the newborn. The primary responsibility of the anesthesiologist is to provide care for the mother. If the anesthesiologist is also requested to provide brief assistance in the care of the newborn, the benefit to the child must be compared to the risk to the mother.[6]*

Although these ASA guidelines that tightly define the role of the anesthesiologist in the delivery room were originally approved in 1988 and amended in 1991, it is unclear whether they will have an impact on the outcome of future medical malpractice litigation as it applies to neonatal resuscitation.

For the practicing obstetric anesthesiologist, notwithstanding the ASA guidelines, it is important to ensure that hospital rules and regulations define the anesthesiologist's role in neonatal resuscitation. Hospital policies should recognize that some obstetric patients can demand all of the skill and concentration of the mother's anesthesiologist. Under those circumstances, the hospital must provide for some other healthcare provider to manage the neonate's resuscitation. Hospital rules and regulations must consider, in a manner consistent with the ASA guidelines, the anesthesiologist's primary obligation to the parturient.

Regardless of the impact of the ASA guidelines regarding delivery room care, anesthesiologists should still maintain a reasonable level of skill as it pertains to neonatal resuscitation (see Chapter 9). Courses in neonatal resuscitation or neonatal advanced life support may assist the anesthesiologist in maintaining a reasonable level of skill. In the meantime, the obstetric anesthesiologist must maintain a dialogue with obstetricians, pediatricians, and hospital administrators to clearly define the role of various healthcare personnel in providing delivery room care. This can only have a positive impact on both patient care and the outcome of litigation that involves neonatal resuscitation.

Breach

Breach is the second element necessary to sustain an action in medical malpractice. Breach is any violation or omission of a legal duty. Many states have defined a breach of the standard of medical care as a failure to exercise the required degree of care, skill, and diligence under the circumstances. It is important to note that the "required" degree of care, skill, and diligence is not the same as the "highest" degree of care, skill, and diligence.

Issue: Defining Medical "Standards of Care"

In a legal proceeding, expert medical witnesses define the applicable standard of care during either deposition testimony or at trial. If a case goes to trial, the jury ultimately chooses between the plaintiff witness's standard or the defense witness's standard for acceptable medical care and applies that standard to the facts of the case. The only situations in which expert witnesses are not necessary to define the applicable standard of care involve *res ipsa loquitor* (Latin for "the thing speaks for itself") situations where the injuries complained of do not generally occur without negligence (see below for discussion of *res ipsa loquitor*).

From the obstetric anesthesia standpoint, there are several categories of deviations from required obstetric anesthesia care (Table 17–1). One category involves the failure to provide adequate respiratory and cardiovascular homeostasis. Published reports indicate difficult tracheal intubation and pulmonary aspiration are the leading causes of maternal morbidity and mortality.[7] Other respiratory events that lead to maternal injury include esophageal intubation, bronchospasm, inadequate fraction of inspired oxygen, and premature extubation. Cardiovascular system mismanagement generally involves failure to provide adequate fluid therapy or to appropriately manage excessive blood loss.

Another category of deviations from required anesthesia care involves management of convulsions. Convulsions are much more common in obstetric anesthesia as compared with nonobstetric anesthetics. Invariably, in cases of anesthesiologist liability, obstetric patients who seize are receiving epidural anesthesia and most of these seizures are considered to be caused by toxic reactions to local anesthetics. Medical malpractice cases that allege mismanagement of maternal convulsions usually involve neurologic injury or death to the mother, the newborn, or both.

■ Table 17–1

MOST COMMON DEVIATIONS FROM ACCEPTABLE OBSTETRIC ANESTHESIA CARE

Failure to Maintain Adequate Respiratory Function
Mismanagement of the difficult tracheal intubation Pulmonary aspiration
Failure to Maintain Adequate Cardiovascular Status
Inadequate fluid therapy Mismanagement of blood loss
Failure to Properly Manage Maternal Convulsions
Toxic local anesthetic administration
Failure to Control or Prevent Maternal Pain During Delivery

A final category of damaging obstetric anesthesia events involves the failure to control or prevent maternal pain during delivery and headache, backache, or emotional distress after delivery. It has been noted that the rate of claims in this category far exceeds the rate of similar claims in the nonobstetric anesthesia population (32% vs. 4%). Some have suggested the high rate of claims in this category may reflect unrealistic expectations, general dissatisfaction with obstetric anesthesia care, or postpartum mental disturbances. Regardless of the reason, the obstetric anesthesiologist must prepare to address these potential problem areas during the postpartum visit.

■ **KEY POINT:** Anesthesiologists must be aware that there have been an increasing number of malpractice suits involving claims of inadequate control of labor pain.

Several other chapters in this book provide useful information to help the anesthesiologist maintain the required degree of care, skill, and diligence in the delivery of obstetric anesthesia care.

Injury

Unless some compensable injury to the patient accompanies the previously mentioned deviations from reasonable medical care, the plaintiff cannot sustain an action in medical malpractice. Table 17–2 lists the common obstetric anesthesia injuries triggering payments to patients.

Injuries considered unique to obstetric anesthesia obviously include the simultaneous injury to two patients—the mother and the newborn. In addition, as stated above, maternal pain during anesthesia is much more common in obstetric anesthesia- than in nonobstetric anesthesia-related cases. Furthermore, most claims for pain that occurred during anesthesia arise within the context of cesarean section performed under a regional anesthetic technique.

Issue: The Doctrine of *Res Ipsa Loquitor*

It is important to note that injury alone is usually insufficient to prove a deviation from reasonable medical care. The exception to that general rule is the well-known doctrine of

■ Table 17–2
COMMON OBSTETRIC ANESTHESIA INJURIES

Maternal death	Pain during anesthesia
Newborn brain damage	Maternal nerve damage
Headache	Emotional distress
Newborn death	Back pain

res ipsa loquitor, which eliminates the need for presenting any other evidence of negligence on the part of the physician. The doctrine of *res ipsa loquitor* has three conditions: the injury must be of a kind that ordinarily does not occur in the absence of someone's negligence, it must be caused by an agency or instrumentality within the exclusive control of the defendant, and the injury must not have been due to any voluntary action on the part of the patient.[8] When the conditions of *res ipsa loquitor* are satisfied, the patient does not need to present any other expert medical testimony bolstering the claim of unreasonable medical care.

Examples of *res ipsa loquitor* include a patient who suffers a brachial plexus nerve injury during a cesarean section, a foreign object such as the tip from an epidural catheter is left inside a patient, or a neck injury follows a patient's fall from the operating table. For the obstetric patient, many potential *res ipsa*-type injuries may not become evident until the day after surgery. The postoperative visit takes on added importance under these circumstances. The careful documentation of a normal postoperative visit can be very valuable for the anesthesiologist's defense. In the event an injury is found during the postoperative visit, the anesthesiologist can institute appropriate treatment, if necessary, and therefore mitigate any possible medical or legal consequences.

Causation

Causation is a legal term that refers to a particular action (or inaction) that produces an injury and without which the injury would not have occurred. It is one of the four elements the plaintiff must prove to sustain an action in medical malpractice. In obstetric anesthesia, the anesthesiologist's action or inaction must produce or contribute to the production of some injury. Even if an anesthesiologist owes a duty to a patient and acts negligently, the anesthesiologist's negligence must, in some way, cause or contribute to injury to the patient. Without some evidence suggesting causation of the plaintiff's injury, the anesthesiologist should prevail in an action alleging anesthesia malpractice.

In summary, to recover for negligent malpractice, the person bringing the lawsuit (the plaintiff) must establish all of the following four elements: the existence of the physician's duty to the patient, the applicable standard of care and its violation, a causal connection between the physician's violation of the standard of care, and the resulting compensable injury to the patient. Failure to establish any of these four elements should defeat the plaintiff's case.

■ **KEY POINT:** The legal trend today is to recognize patient antonomy as the most important factor.

ETHICAL ISSUES IN OBSTETRIC ANESTHESIA

Anesthesiologists, as medical professionals, have an obligation to observe rules, guidelines, principles, and moral precepts that govern their relationships with patients, colleagues, healthcare administrators, and their communities. The ASA first approved Guidelines for the Ethical Practice of Anesthesiology in 1967 and recently amended them in 1995.[9] The guidelines provide a potpourri of "do's" and "don'ts" with regard to recommended anesthesiologist behavior toward patients and colleagues. However, aside from obvious advice such as "respect your patient" and "cooperate with colleagues," the ASA guidelines offer little help to the anesthesiologist in answering the more difficult ethical questions.

Some bioethicists suggest the use of a checklist of ethical principles to apply when considering an ethical issue.[10] For the obstetric anesthesiologist, an appropriate bioethical checklist should include the principles of patient autonomy, nonmaleficence, beneficence, and truth telling. As the anesthesiologist confronts complicated legal and ethical questions, it may be helpful to consider each principle on the checklist before trying to answer those questions.

Patient Autonomy

Patient autonomy is the bioethical principle that states that the actions and choices of the patient should not be constrained by others. Under most circumstances, honoring patient autonomy allows the pregnant woman to make the final decision regarding pain control for labor, choice of anesthetic for a cesarean section, and whether she wishes to forego any medical therapy.

Nonmaleficence

This principle of *primum non nocere* (Latin for "first, do no harm") is well established within the medical community and implores physicians to avoid harming or exposing the risk of harm to their patients. Nonmaleficence requires anesthesiologists to consider the potential harm caused by obstetric anesthetics and other therapies.

Beneficence

The ethical principle of beneficence applied to obstetric anesthesia involves efforts to do what is best or most helpful for the mother and her fetus or newborn. The relationship between nonmaleficence and beneficence is sometimes referred to as the risk-to-benefit ratio.

Truth Telling

This principle requires the physician to provide all pertinent information to a patient so she can make an informed decision regarding her own health care. As applied to obstetric anesthesia, this principle implores anesthesiologists to provide all pertinent anesthetic-related information so the pregnant woman can knowledgeably decide on issues such as labor analgesia.

■ **KEY POINT:** Ethical issues in medicine are often resolved by analyzing clinical situations in the light of certain principles. Some of these principles include patient autonomy, nonmaleficence, beneficence, and truth telling.

Application of Ethical Principles to Obstetric Anesthesia

Three complicated and difficult legal/bioethical issues that confront obstetric anesthesiologists involve informed consent for labor epidurals, care for the pregnant Jehovah's Witness patient, and the role of the anesthesiologist as it relates to fetal and newborn pain. The discussion that follows attempts to apply the principles of patient autonomy, nonmaleficence, beneficence, and truth telling to these three obstetric anesthesia issues to demonstrate one approach to dealing with ethical problems.

Issue: Informed Consent for Labor Epidurals

The principles of patient autonomy and truth telling provide the foundation for the doctrine of informed consent. If a physician fails to obtain consent before performing a medical procedure, the patient may file a lawsuit alleging battery. Unlike the requirements for filing medical malpractice claims, for a battery claim the patient does not need to demonstrate any deviation from standard medical care. The patient only needs to show lack of consent.

In obstetric anesthesia, the principle of informed consent requires the anesthesiologist to honor the pregnant woman's decision regarding pain control for labor. Furthermore, it is the duty of the anesthesiologist to inform the pregnant patient in lay terms of the potential dangers of the proposed anesthetic plan. The anesthesiologist must disclose the amount of information to the pregnant woman that she needs to make an informed choice.

Courts generally recognize one of two standards for determining whether a physician has made a reasonably appropriate disclosure of potential risks of the proposed medical intervention. The traditional standard provides that the physician is required to tell the patient what any other reasonable physician under similar circumstances would tell the patient. This is known as the physician-based standard. The other standard is referred to as the patient-centered or the reasonable patient standard and provides that the physician is obliged to provide information that any reasonable patient would want to know to make an informed decision. Most anesthesiologists would agree that reasonable information relating to anesthesia, regardless of standard, includes a description of the anesthetic and its effects, a description of serious risks with an approximate probability of occurrence, and an opportunity for the patient to ask questions.[11]

With regard to serious risks and their approximate occurrence, recent concerns about labor epidurals center on whether epidural analgesia increases the frequency of forceps delivery and the frequency of cesarean section. Some studies report a substantial increase in the frequency of cesarean section in some women receiving epidural analgesia,[12] whereas other studies indicate epidural analgesia does not increase the cesarean section rate in women under slightly different circumstances.[13] For informed consent purposes, the question related to truth telling is whether the obstetric anesthesiologist is obligated to inform the parturient of the potential risks articulated in Thorp and coworkers'[12] study. For many anesthesiologists, the answer to that question may depend on whether the anesthesiologist practices in a state where there is a patient-centered standard or a physician-based standard. It could be argued that from the reasonable patient standard, the reasonable pregnant woman would want to know that a labor epidural might increase the likelihood of needing a cesarean section, whereas from the physician-based standard, the reasonable anesthesiologist does not need to discuss an issue that remains so unsettled and controversial.

To further complicate matters, as a general principle, a patient coerced or under undue influence is incapable of providing a valid consent. Some argue the pain of labor places a woman under such duress that consent is not valid under those circumstances. In addition, some have suggested that it is contrary to the best interests of the distressed laboring patient to inform her of the potential serious risks of epidural analgesia.[14] Furthermore, it is not illogical to posit that a pregnant woman who tells her obstetrician *before* she goes into labor she does not want a labor epidural is not making an informed decision because she is unable to appreciate the pain of labor she has not yet experienced.[15]

This controversy places the obstetric anesthesiologist in an awkward position. It seems unethical to withhold labor analgesia to a greatly distressed woman merely because she told her midwife "no epidural" during a period of peace and calm before going into labor. Indeed, the anesthesiologist's inaction under these circumstances appears to violate both the "do no harm" principle and the beneficence principle. Arguably, withholding analgesia from a laboring woman in excruciating pain because of concerns about a valid consent causes more harm than the amount of good labor analgesia provides. Fortunately, at least one appellate court has rejected the notion that a laboring woman is unable to give informed consent. This case suggests obtaining consent from the laboring woman should not be viewed as an impossible task.[16]

Because few "lack of informed consent" malpractice lawsuits are filed and even fewer are successfully litigated, the issues of informed consent are often more of an academic exercise than a serious practical concern. Nonetheless, all patients arguably deserve to be told information relating to anesthesia that includes a description of the anesthetic and its effects, a description of serious risks with an approximate probability of occurrence, and an opportunity for the patient to ask questions. Furthermore, the anesthesiologist should tailor the discussion of anesthetic options and risks to individual patient needs and the individual's capacity to comprehend. Obstetric anesthesiologists should not make any decisions regarding the acquisition of informed consent in a vacuum. Anesthesiologists should enlist the help of hospital risk management personnel, hospital legal counsel, and their obstetrician colleagues when they are struggling with the issues of informed consent for labor analgesia.

Issue: The Pregnant Jehovah's Witness Patient

All four ethical principles of patient autonomy, nonmaleficence, beneficence, and truth telling play a significant role in the ethical and legal controversies involving the pregnant Jehovah's Witness patient. Although the ASA guidelines recognize a primary obligation to the parturient, the anesthesiologist must always consider the impact of anesthetic interventions on the well-being of the fetus. The anesthesiologist who cares for a severely anemic laboring Jehovah's Witness is presented with an agonizing bioethical dilemma. The physician's desire to transfuse blood products into the mother to preserve the well-being of the fetus is counterbalanced by the mother's desire to maintain her own autonomy and avoid the transfusion of blood products. Patient autonomy and nonmaleficence with regard to the mother directly conflict with nonmaleficence and beneficence as they pertain to the fetus. Not surprisingly, these conflicts have forced physicians and judges to grapple with these issues over the past few several decades.

Through the 1960s many courts consistently allowed physicians to transfuse women who had already given birth because of the state's interest in preserving the life of the mother and the newborn. Many judges who ordered transfusions to Jehovah's Witnesses based their decisions on the mistaken belief that Jehovah's Witnesses were not required to refuse blood transfusions but were merely required to refuse to consent to those transfusions.[17] These judges argued that the state's interest in keeping parents alive to care for their children outweighed the Jehovah's Witness parent's autonomy interests. However, in the 1970s and early 1980s, many states reversed their decisions and began to recognize the right of competent adults to refuse blood transfusions even if their death would leave orphaned children. Presently, most courts will not approve an order to transfuse a nonpregnant Jehovah's Witness adult.

However, as stated above, the anesthesiologist who cares for a severely anemic laboring Jehovah's Witness is presented with an agonizing bioethical and legal dilemma. Because of the obvious concern for viable late-term fetuses, courts continue to struggle with approving orders to transfuse competent pregnant Jehovah's Witness adults. A recent Illinois case illustrates the conflict.

In this recent case, the court addressed the issue of a 26-year-old Jehovah's Witness beyond 34 weeks of pregnancy.[18] During the surgical removal of a urethral mass, the patient's hemoglobin dropped below 4.4 mg/dL. At that point, the physician ordered blood into the operating room. Only after the blood arrived in the room did the patient inform the operating room personnel she was a Jehovah's Witness. Awake and under regional anesthesia, the patient refused to consent to a packed red cell transfusion. After the patient's refusal, the hospital obtained a court order appointing a temporary guardian of the fetus with the right to consent to blood transfusions for the patient. After the transfusions, the patient gave birth to a healthy baby. After discharge from the hospital, the patient appealed the lower court's order.

The Appellate Court of the First District of Illinois reversed the lower court's ruling and held that the state should not order a blood transfusion to a pregnant woman against her wishes. In discussing its opinion, the appellate court recognized the right of a competent patient to refuse medical therapy, including blood transfusions. The court, however, stated that such a right to refuse therapy is not absolute. The court recognized that typically four "interests" might outweigh the patient's right to refuse: the preservation of life, the prevention of suicide, the protection of third parties, and the ethical integrity of the medical profession.

The appellate court also recognized the state's interest in preserving the viable fetus was substantial. However, the court found the state could not order invasive medical therapy in overriding the competent pregnant woman's refusal of medical therapy. In this case, the court stated a blood transfusion is invasive and therefore a court should not approve an order to give a transfusion over the pregnant patient's competent refusal. Considering the principles of patient autonomy, nonmaleficence, beneficence, and truth telling, the court concluded the interest in preserving the mother's right to make healthcare decisions (patient autonomy) and the interest in doing no harm to her (nonmaleficence) outweighed the state's interest in preserving the life of a constitutionally unprotectable fetus (beneficence).

Unfortunately for anesthesiologists in Illinois, one other appellate court has stated blood transfusions are relatively noninvasive and therefore suggested the possibility that court-approved orders allowing blood transfusions to a pregnant Jehovah's Witness might not violate a pregnant woman's constitutionally protected rights.[19] These conflicting legal opinions illustrate the need for anesthesiologists to know the law of the jurisdiction in which they practice. It is hoped that the Illinois Supreme Court, and ultimately the United States Supreme Court, will resolve the conflict between the courts on the issue of transfusions to pregnant Jehovah's Witnesses.

Until legal rules governing the care of Jehovah's Witnesses are well recognized and well established throughout the United States, individual hospital policies and procedures must accurately reflect the current status of the law that governs their hospitals and physicians. Furthermore, anesthesiologists should maintain a working knowledge of the law and hospital policies and procedures that regulate the care they provide to Jehovah's Witnesses. An anesthesiology resident trained in Boston must not be lulled into believing the same laws and regulations that governed residency will also govern an attending anesthesiology practice in Chicago.

As with policies that cover neonatal resuscitation, anesthesiologists must work closely with obstetricians, risk management committees, and hospital legal counsel to ensure the proper development of hospital policies that govern Jehovah's Witnesses health care. They must also demand appropriate widespread and thorough communication of the policies throughout the medical, nursing, and ancillary staff of their hospitals.

Some hospitals have adopted intake policies that require admitting personnel to conspicuously label the medical charts of Jehovah's Witnesses to alert all healthcare providers on the need to pay particular attention to the unique religious concerns of these patients.

Issue: The Role of the Anesthesiologist as it Relates to Fetal and Newborn Pain

Recent state and federal legislative efforts to ban a particular type of third-trimester abortion (known as "partial-birth abortion") have forced the medical community to confront the issue of fetal pain. Unfortunately, many obstetricians steadfastly refuse to acknowledge the possibility of fetal pain during third-trimester abortions. During the congressional late-term abortion debate, some obstetrician/gynecologists submitted fact sheets to Congress that claimed not only that third-trimester fetuses are incapable of experiencing pain but also that the anesthesia provided to a woman during an abortion kills the fetus.[20] These scientifically unsupported statements were quickly rebuffed by a representative of the ASA who asserted the importance of truth telling during the public discourse over such important social issues.[21]

In addition to the ASA, the American Academy of Pediatrics has promulgated a policy advocating a moral and ethical approach to fetal pain that encourages physicians to provide fetal pain relief so long as pain control interventions pose little risk to pregnant women. As professionals whose careers are dedicated to pain relief, anesthesiologists, regardless of personal convictions, should insist on modifications of potentially painful third-trimester abortion procedures so long as these modifications pose minimal risk to the pregnant women.

During a late-term abortion, the body of the fetus, sometimes as late as 38 weeks' gestation, is delivered feet first. Before the head is removed a pair of scissors is inserted into the base of the skull, an opening is made, and a large suction catheter is inserted. Through the suction catheter the intracranial contents are removed, the skull is crushed, and the remainder of the fetus is removed through the cervical opening. It has been argued that during a late-term or partial-birth abortion the obstetrician should take advantage of access to the umbilical cord to provide pain relief for the fetus before evacuating the skull contents.[22] The physician could inject substantial quantities of narcotic or barbiturate into the umbilical vessels in a manner that would not expose the woman to any additional medical or surgical risk.

However, obstetricians must first acknowledge the capacity of late-term fetuses to experience pain. Anesthesiologists familiar with recent advances in pediatric anesthesia generally accept the view that even the smallest premature infant is capable of experiencing pain. In fact, research indicates that 18- to 22-week-old fetuses are capable of withdrawing from painful stimuli and mounting a hormonal pain response similar to the response of full-term infants. Accordingly, some have advocated that those dealing with second- and third-trimester fetuses should provide adequate fetal analgesia, especially during surgical techniques that may include dismemberment.[23] Anesthesiologists should play an active role in educating the obstetric community on this issue.

Regarding another pain issue, many obstetricians refuse to acknowledge newborn circumcisions cause pain. Newborn circumcision is the only surgical procedure during which anesthesia or analgesia is routinely withheld. This practice continues despite the well-documented deleterious side effects of performing circumcision without anesthesia. These side effects, such as exaggerated physiologic and behavioral responses to subsequent noxious stimuli, may persist for more than 6 months after an unanesthetized circumcision. More importantly, the simple application of local anesthesia significantly attenuates circumcision-induced side effects. A local anesthetic cream applied to the foreskin or a local anesthetic ring block administered at the base of the penis are both adequate anesthetic techniques for newborn circumcision. Despite the widespread publication of these low-risk techniques, most newborn circumcisions are performed without analgesia. Only a disappointing 60% of all obstetric residency programs teach techniques to relieve the procedural pain of circumcision.[24]

Again, as professionals dedicated to providing pain relief, anesthesiologists have an ethical obligation to consider and communicate the principles of nonmaleficence, beneficence, and truth telling as applied to fetal and newborn pain. With a strong foundation in the physiologic, pharmacologic, and behavioral benefits of pain relief, the obstetric anesthesiologist is ideally situated to teach obstetricians, and sometimes legislators, about the existence of fetal and newborn pain (truth telling) and simple methods of providing pain relief (beneficence) without exposing the newborn or the pregnant woman, in the case of late-term abortions, to significant risk. Regardless of political, religious, or moral point of view, anesthesiologists should challenge other healthcare professionals who assert scientifically indefensible positions such as "the anesthesia provided to mothers during an abortion kills the fetus" or "circumcision without analgesia does not harm the newborn."

CONCLUSION

To successfully tackle the issues associated with the agonizing problems of medical malpractice, it is important for the anesthesiologist to understand basic medical–legal principles and terminology. To recover for medical malpractice, the person bringing the lawsuit must establish all of the following four elements: the existence of the physician's duty to the patient, the applicable standard of care and its violation, a causal connection between the physician's violation of the standard of care, and the resulting compensable injury to the patient. Failure to establish any of these four elements should defeat the plaintiff's case. Preventing or defending malpractice claims centers around these elements. Even the most careful and diligent anesthesiologist can benefit from understanding these elements and their relationship to medical malpractice.

For ethical issues, physicians may find a checklist of ethical principles helpful when they are confronted with complicated questions. For the obstetric anesthesiologist, an appropriate bioethical checklist should include the principles of patient autonomy, nonmaleficence, beneficence, and truth telling. As the anesthesiologist confronts legal and ethical questions, it may be helpful to consider each principle on the checklist before arriving at answers to those questions. Although consideration of the principles on this list does not guarantee easy answers to ethical problems, it can provide the foundation for an organized approach to understanding some of the complicated issues that confront the obstetric anesthesiologist.

REFERENCES

1. Charles SC, Kennedy E: Defendant. New York: Vintage Books, 1986.
2. Nolan JR, Nolan-Haley JM: Black's Law Dictionary. St. Paul: West Publishing Co., 1990:959.
3. Illinois Good Samaritan Statute: 745 ILCS 49/25.
4. Villamil v. Benages, 257 Ill.App.3d 81(1993).
5. Heyman HJ: Neonatal resuscitation and anesthesiologist liability. Anesthesiology 81:783, 1994.
6. Guidelines VII: guidelines for Regional Anesthesia in Obstetrics. American Society of Anesthesiologists, 1996.
7. Chadwick HS, Posner K, Caplan RA, et al: A comparison of obstetric and non-obstetric anesthesia malpractice claims. Anesthesiology 74:242-249, 1991.
8. The liability of health care professionals. In: Furrow BR, Greaney TL, Johnson SH, et al., eds. Health Law, vol 1. St. Paul: West Publishing Co., 1995:351-356.
9. Guidelines for the Ethical Practice of Anesthesiology. American Society of Anesthesiologists, 1996.
10. The study of bioethics. In: Furrow BR, Johnson SH, Jost TS, et al., eds. Bioethics: Health Care Law and Ethics. St. Paul: West Publishing Co., 1995:371.
11. Knapp RM: Legal view of informed consent for anesthesia during labor. Anesthesiology 72:211, 1990.
12. Thorp JA, Hu DH, Albin RM, et al: The effect of intrapartum epidural analgesia on nulliparous labor: a randomized, controlled, prospective trial. Am J Obstet Gynecol 169:851-858, 1993.
13. Chestnut DH, Vincent RD Jr, McGrath JM, et al: Does early administration of epidural anesthesia affect obstetric outcome in nulliparous women who are receiving intravenous oxytocin? Anesthesiology 80:1193-1200, 1994.
14. Slusarenko P, Noble WH: Epidural anaesthesia: concerns regarding informed consent. Can Anaesth Soc J 32:681-685, 1985.
15. Scott WE: Ethics in obstetric anaesthesia. Anaesthesia 51:717-718, 1996.
16. Patterson v. Van Weil, 570 P.2d 931 (1977).
17. Application of the President and Directors of Geagretown College, Inc., 331 F.2d 1000 (1964).
18. In re Fetus Brown, 689 N.E.2d 397 (1997).
19. In re Baby Boy Doe, a fetus 260 Ill. App. 3d 392 (1994).
20. H.R. Rep. 104-267, 104th Cong., 1st Sess. (1995).
21. Gianelli D: Anesthesiologists question claims in abortion debate. American Medical News, Jan. 1, 1996, p 4.
22. McDonald T: When does a fetus become a child in need of an advocate? Focusing on fetal pain. Children's Legal Rights Journal 17:12-19, 1997.
23. Giannakoulopoulos X, Sepulveda W, Kourtis P, et al: Fetal plasma cortisol and B-endorphin response to intrauterine needling. Lancet 344:77-81, 1994.
24. Howard CR, Howard FM, Garfunkel LC, et al: Neonatal circumcision and pain relief: current training practices. Pediatrics 101:423-428, 1998.

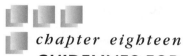

chapter eighteen

GUIDELINES FOR OBSTETRIC ANESTHESIA

Lee S. Perrin, MD

The House of Delegates of the American Society of Anesthesiologists (ASA) has over the years issued a number of documents. These documents have been variously referred to as standards, guidelines, practice guidelines, statements, positions, and protocols. The ASA's policy statement on practice parameters[1] defines some of these terms:

- *Practice parameters* include standards, guidelines, and other strategies.
- *Standards* are rules, for example, minimum requirements for sound practice. They are generally accepted principles for patient management.
- *Guidelines* are recommendations for patient management that may identify a particular management strategy or a range of management strategies.

It is important to recognize the process that created these practice parameters so that their limitations may be appreciated. Standards and guidelines were initially developed by committees of the ASA charged with their development because of a perceived need. The committees received input from the ASA membership and produced a document that was subject to review by the ASA membership and then sent to the ASA House of Delegates for review and approval. It was not unusual for a document to be sent back to the committee for further revision before being adopted. This process ensures that all interested parties are heard from and that the document is practical to implement.

The ASA has only produced four "Standards," the rest being guidelines, statements, positions, and protocols. The original document on regional anesthesia in obstetrics was a standard. Because some elements of the standard were too rigid to be "rules," the ASA House of Delegates changed this standard to its current "Guidelines for Regional Anesthesia in Obstetrics" (Appendix 18-1).

A guideline allows a significant amount of leeway to adapt to local conditions.

Members of the Society are responsible for interpreting and applying practice parameters to their own institutions and practices. The practice parameters adopted by ASA are not necessarily the only evidence of appropriate care. An individual physician should have the opportunity to show that the care rendered, even if departing from the parameters in some respects, satisfies the physician's duty to the patient under all the facts and circumstances.[1]

In addition to the guidelines for regional anesthesia in obstetrics, the ASA House of Delegates has approved the "Standards for Basic Anesthetic Monitoring" and the "Standards for Postanesthesia Care" (see Appendix 18-1). These standards have been reproduced here because they apply to all patients regardless of the setting of their anesthesia.

GUIDELINE DEVELOPMENT

Recently, the ASA developed a practice guideline in obstetric anesthesia. A practice guideline follows a slightly different path in its creation. Initially, the ASA Committee on Practice Parameters defines an area in potential need of a clinical guideline. The ASA House of Delegates then approves and funds the development of the proposed guideline.

Next, a task force of about 10 experts in the field of interest is formed to develop the guideline. These experts are representative of the different regions of the United States and of private versus academic practice. The Task Force on Obstetrical Anesthesia also includes an obstetrician. A statistician helps the committee to create a questionnaire to determine the importance, feasibility, and areas to be covered by the guideline. A total of 147 consultants, of which 115 were anesthesiologists and 32 were obstetricians, were surveyed to determine what the content of the practice guideline should be. After these data were analyzed, the task force met to determine what should be included in the proposed guideline.

A literature search, from 1940 through 1998, was performed to try to determine all areas where data might exist to support the recommendations of the guideline. Each article was classified according to the ability of the study to reach a meaningful conclusion. For example, a randomized, controlled, double-blinded study was considered to be stronger evidence than a case report. Over 4000 citations were retrieved. The final database contained 504 relevant articles from 55 journals.

The document covers the areas of perianesthetic evaluation, fasting in the obstetric patient, anesthetic choices for labor, removal of retained placenta, anesthetic choices for cesarean delivery, postpartum tubal ligation, and the management of complications.

The results are incorporated into the final document. After the task force approves the document, it is circulated at public meetings (e.g. the Society for Obstetric Anesthesia and Perinatology), so that the task force can respond to any problems, inconsistencies, or inadequacies of the proposed guideline.

Once an appropriate number of people have had an opportunity to comment on the proposed guideline, it is modified and prepared to be sent to the ASA House of Delegates. The House of Delegates has only two choices: It can recommend adoption of the guideline or reject it. The House of Delegates may not change the guideline. In the past, the House of Delegates has, in fact, rejected some proposed guidelines for a variety of reasons, including not being practical, not providing adequate scientific support, and not providing any useful guidance.

The practice guidelines for obstetric anesthesia were approved by the ASA House of Delegates on October 21, 1998. They became effective on January 1, 1999. (See Appendix 18-1.)

GUIDELINES FROM OBSTETRICS

The American College of Obstetricians and Gynecologists (ACOG) Committee on Obstetric Practice and the American Academy of Pediatrics Committee on Fetus and Newborn have together developed and published the "Guidelines for Perinatal Care."[2] This monograph defines and outlines the basic standards that an obstetric unit should strive to achieve. Its disclaimer statement says that these are not rigid rules but should provide a "firm basis on which local norms may be built."[2]

These guidelines define three types of facilities according to the types of cases and level of expertise available. In the "Basic Care Facility," "anesthesia personnel with credentials to administer obstetric anesthesia should be available on a 24-hour basis."[2] It is noteworthy that the guideline allows nonphysicians to administer the anesthetic in these institutions. In the study by Hawkins et al.,[3] in hospitals with less than 500 births per year, 55% of labor analgesia and 59% of cesarean section anesthesia was provided by a nurse anesthetist who was not being supervised by an anesthesiologist.

The "Specialty Care Facility" takes care of high-risk neonates and requires qualified maternal–fetal medicine physicians and neonatologists.

> The director of obstetric anesthesia services should be board certified in anesthesia and should have training and experience in obstetric anesthesia. Anesthesia personnel who have credentials to administer obstetric anesthesia should be readily available. Policies regarding the provision of obstetric anesthesia, including the necessary qualifications of personnel who are to administer anesthesia and their availability for both routine and emergency deliveries, should be developed.[2]

Note that the higher acuity of the cases in this type of facility requires the anesthetist to be "readily available."

The "Subspecialty Care Facility" is a referral center taking care of the most high-risk infants and mothers.

> A board-certified anesthesiologist with special training or experience in maternal-fetal anesthesia should be in charge of obstetric anesthesia services at a subspecialty care hospital. Personnel with credentials in the administration of obstetric anesthesia should be available in the hospital. Personnel with credentials in the administration of neonatal and pediatric anesthesia should be available as needed.[2]

ACOG guidelines state that "management of discomfort and pain during labor and delivery is a necessary part of good obstetric practice. Maternal request is sufficient justification for providing pain relief during labor."[2] The guidelines go on to discuss the use of childbirth preparation classes, medications, and anesthetic techniques for the relief of obstetric pain. They state

> Lumbar epidural block is the most flexible, effective, and least depressing to the central nervous system, allowing for an alert, participating mother. Lumbar epidural block has been associated with an increased incidence of operative abdominal and vaginal delivery. However, the administration of a dilute solution of local anesthetic (which results in less motor blockade) may minimize the increased incidence of operative delivery associated with epidural analgesia. Unless contraindications are present, women who request epidural anesthesia should be able to receive it.[2]
>
> The choice and availability of analgesic and anesthetic techniques depend on the experience and judgment of the obstetrician and anesthesiologist, the physical condition of the patient, the circumstances of labor and delivery, and the personal preferences of the obstetrician and patient. Because the safety of obstetric anesthesia depends primarily on the skill of the anesthesiologist, and because obstetric anesthesia must be considered emergency anesthesia, its use demands a level of competence in personnel and an availability of equipment that are similar to those required for elective surgical procedures.[2]
>
> It is the responsibility of the director of anesthesia services to make recommendations regarding the clinical privileges of all anesthesia service personnel. If obstetric anesthesia is provided by obstetricians, the director of anesthesia services should participate with a representative of the obstetric department in the formulation of procedures designed to ensure the uniform quality of anesthesia services throughout the hospital.[2]

The ACOG guidelines parallel the ASA guidelines for the supervision and monitoring of the anesthetic. The ACOG guidelines also include a list of factors that place a woman at increased risk from anesthesia and should be communicated to the anesthetist in advance of delivery. The prophylactic administration of a clear antacid is recommended before the induction of general anesthesia or a major regional block.

Regarding anesthesia for cesarean delivery, the ACOG

guidelines state that all the required personnel should be in the hospital or readily available.

> *No data correlate the timing of intervention with outcome, and there is little likelihood that any will be obtained. However, consensus has been that hospitals should have the capability of beginning a cesarean delivery within 30 minutes of the decision to operate. Not all indications for a cesarean delivery will require a 30-minute response time.*[2]

JOINT GUIDELINES

The ASA and ACOG have worked together over the years to produce a document entitled "Optimal Goals for Anesthesia Care in Obstetrics."[4] This document was created by a joint committee of the two societies and then brought to the parent societies for approval. Several modifications were proposed to the 1997 ASA House of Delegates that created some controversy in the wording of the document. The statement was referred back to the committee for more work. Subsequently, ACOG also expressed concern over parts of the joint statement. The two committees are currently working on modifications to bring back to their parent societies.

Most of the "Optimal Goals" statement contains information already available in either the ASA guidelines and standards or in the ACOG guidelines. However, there are some additional statements that are generating the controversy.

CONCLUSIONS

The development of guidelines, standards, and practice parameters is an ongoing process subject to repeated review and amendment as practices warrant. The interested reader should consult the ASA website (http://www.asahq.org) or official ASA publications for the most current guidelines.

REFERENCES

1. American Society of Anesthesiologists: Policy Statement on Practice Parameters. ASA Standards, Guidelines and Statements. Park Ridge, IL. American Society of Anesthesiologists, October, 1998.
2. Guidelines for Perinatal Care, 4th ed. Elk Grove Village, IL, and Washington, D.C. American Academy of Pediatrics and American College of Obstetricians and Gynecologists, 1997.
3. Hawkins JL, Gibbs CP, Orleans M et al: Obstetric Anesthesia Workforce Study, 1981 Versus 1992. Anesthesiology 87:135-143, 1997.
4. American Society of Anesthesiologists: Optimal Goals for Anesthesia Care in Obstetrics. ASA Standards, Guidelines and Statements. Park Ridge, IL, American Society of Anesthesiologists, October, 1998.

PRACTICE GUIDELINES FOR OBSTETRICAL ANESTHESIA*

A Report by the American Society of Anesthesiologists Task Force on Obstetrical Anesthesia

■ ■ ■

Practice guidelines are systematically developed recommendations that assist the practitioner and patient in making decisions about health care. These recommendations may be adopted, modified, or rejected according to clinical needs and constraints.

Practice guidelines are not intended as standards or absolute requirements. The use of practice guidelines cannot guarantee any special outcome. Practice guidelines are subject to periodic revision as warranted by the evolution of medical knowledge, technology, and practice. The guidelines provide basic recommendations that are supported by analysis of the current literature and by a synthesis of expert opinion, open forum commentary, and clinical feasibility data.

PURPOSES OF THE GUIDELINES FOR OBSTETRICAL ANESTHESIA

The purposes of these Guidelines are to enhance the quality of anesthesia care for obstetric patients, reduce the incidence and severity of anesthesia-related complications, and increase patient satisfaction.

FOCUS

The Guidelines focus on the anesthetic management of pregnant patients during labor, non-operative delivery, operative delivery, and selected aspects of postpartum care. The intended patient population includes, but is not limited to, intrapartum and postpartum patients with uncomplicated pregnancies or with common obstetric problems. The Guidelines do not apply to patients undergoing surgery during pregnancy, gynecological patients or parturients with chronic medical disease (e.g., severe heart, renal or neurological disease).

Reprinted from Anesthesiology 90:600-611, 1999, with permission.

Developed by the Task Force on Obstetrical Anesthesia: Joy L. Hawkins, M.D. (Chair), Denver, Colorado; James F. Arens, M.D., Galveston, Texas; Brenda A. Bucklin, M.D., Omaha, Nebraska; Robert A. Caplan, M.D., Seattle, Washington; David H. Chestnut, M.D., Birmingham, Alabama; Richard T. Connis, Ph.D., Woodinville, Washington; Patricia A. Dailey, M.D., Hillsborough, California; Larry C. Gilstrap, M.D., Houston, Texas; Stephen C. Grice, M.D., Alpharetta, Georgia; Nancy E. Oriol, M.D., Boston, Massachusetts; Kathryn J. Zuspan, M.D., Edina, Minnesota.

Submitted for publication October 29, 1998. Accepted for publication October 29, 1998. Supported by the American Society of Anesthesiologists, under the direction of James F. Arens, M.D., Chairman of the Ad Hoc Committee on Practice Parameters. Approved by the House of Delegates, October 21, 1998. Effective date January 1, 1999. A list of the articles used to develop these guidelines is available by writing to the American Society of Anesthesiologists.

Key words: Anesthesia cesarean section; analgesia labor and delivery.

APPLICATION

The Guidelines are intended for use by anesthesiologists. They also may serve as a resource for other anesthesia providers and health care professionals who advise or care for patients who will receive anesthesia care during labor, delivery and the immediate postpartum period.

TASK FORCE MEMBERS AND CONSULTANTS

The ASA appointed a Task Force of 11 members to review the published evidence and obtain consultant opinion from a representative body of anesthesiologists and obstetricians. The Task Force members consisted of anesthesiologists in both private and academic practices from various geographic areas of the United States.

The Task Force met its objective in a five-step process. First, original published research studies relevant to these issues were reviewed and analyzed. Second, Consultants from various geographic areas of the United States who practice or work in various settings (e.g., academic and private practice) were asked to participate in opinion surveys and review and comments on drafts of the Guidelines. Third, the Task Force held two open forums at major national meetings to solicit input from attendees on its draft recommendations. Fourth, all available information was used by the Task Force in developing the Guideline recommendations. Finally, the Consultants were surveyed to assess their opinions on the feasibility of implementing the Guidelines.

AVAILABILITY AND STRENGTH OF EVIDENCE

Evidence-based guidelines are developed by a rigorous analytic process. To assist the reader, the Guidelines make use of several descriptive terms that are easier to understand than the technical terms and data that are used in the actual analyses. These descriptive terms are defined below:

The following terms describe the availability of scientific evidence in the literature.

Insufficient: There are too few published studies to investigate a relationship between a clinical intervention and clinical outcome.

Inconclusive: Published studies are available, but they cannot be used to assess the relationship between a clinical intervention and a clinical outcome because the studies either do not meet predefined criteria for content as defined in the "Focus of the Guidelines," or do not meet research design or analytic standards.

Silent: There are no available studies in the literature that address a relationship of interest.

The following terms describe the strength of scientific data.

Supportive: There is sufficient quantitative information from adequately designed studies to describe a statistically significant relationship ($p < 0.01$) between a clinical intervention and a clinical outcome, using the technique of meta-analysis.

Suggestive: There is enough information from case reports and descriptive studies to provide a directional assessment of the relationship between a clinical intervention and a clinical outcome. This type of qualitative information does not permit a statistical assessment of significance.

Equivocal: Qualitative data have not provided a clear direction for clinical outcomes related to a clinical intervention and (1) there is insufficient quantitative information or (2) aggregated comparative studies have found no quantitatively significant differences among groups or conditions.

The following terms describe survey responses from Consultants for any specified issue. Responses are weighted as agree $= +1$, undecided $= 0$ or disagree $= -1$.

Agree: The average weighted responses must be equal to or greater than $+0.30$ (on a scale of -1 to 1) to indicate agreement.

Equivocal: The average weighted responses must be between -0.30 and $+0.30$ (on a scale of -1 to 1) to indicate an equivocal response.

Disagree: The average weighted responses must be equal to or less than -0.30 (on a scale of -1 to 1) to indicate disagreement.

GUIDELINES

PERIANESTHETIC EVALUATION

History and Physical Examination. The literature is silent regarding the relationship between anesthesia-related obstetric outcomes and the performance of a focused history and physical examination. However, there are suggestive data that a patient's medical history and/or findings from a physical exam may be related to anesthetic outcomes. The Consultants and Task Force agree that a focused history and physical examination may be associated with reduced maternal, fetal, and neonatal complications. The Task Force agrees that the obstetric patient benefits from communication between the anesthesiologist and the obstetrician.

RECOMMENDATIONS: The anesthesiologist should do a focused history and physical examination when consulted to deliver anesthesia care. This should include a maternal health history, an anesthesia-related obstetric history, an airway examination, and a baseline blood pressure measurement. When a regional anesthetic is planned, the back should be examined.

Recognition of significant anesthetic risk factors should encourage consultation with the obstetrician.

Intrapartum Platelet Count. A platelet count may indicate the severity of a patient's pregnancy-induced hypertension. However, the literature is insufficient to assess the predictive value of a platelet count for anesthesia-related complications in either uncomplicated parturients or those with pregnancy-induced hypertension. The Consultants and Task Force both agree that a routine platelet count in the healthy parturient is not necessary. However, in the patient with pregnancy-induced hypertension, the Consultants and Task Force both agree that the use of a platelet count may reduce the risk of anesthesia-related complications.

RECOMMENDATIONS: A specific platelet count predictive of regional anesthetic complications has not been determined. The anesthesiologist's decision to order or require a platelet count should be individualized and based upon a patient's history, physical examination, and clinical signs of a coagulopathy.

Blood Type and Screen. The literature is silent regarding whether obtaining a blood type and screen is associated with fewer maternal anesthetic complications. The Consultants and Task Force are equivocal regarding the routine use of a blood type and screen to reduce the risk of anesthesia-related complications.

RECOMMENDATIONS: The anesthesiologist's decision to order or require a blood type and screen or crossmatch should be individualized and based on anticipated hemorrhagic complications (e.g., placenta previa in a patient with previous uterine surgery).

Perianesthetic Recording of the Fetal Heart Rate. The literature suggests that analgesic/anesthetic agents may influence the fetal heart rate pattern. There is insufficient literature to demonstrate that perianesthetic recording of the fetal heart rate prevents fetal complications. However, both the Task Force and Consultants agree that perianesthetic recording of the fetal heart rate reduces fetal and neonatal complications.

RECOMMENDATIONS: The fetal heart rate should be monitored by a qualified individual before and after administration of regional analgesia for labor. The Task Force recognizes that *continuous* electronic recording of the fetal heart rate may not be possible during placement of a regional anesthetic.

FASTING IN THE OBSTETRIC PATIENT

Clear Liquids. Published evidence is insufficient regarding the relationship between fasting times for clear liquids and the risk of emesis/reflux or pulmonary aspiration during labor. The Task Force and Consultants agree that oral intake of clear liquids during labor improves maternal comfort and satisfaction. The Task Force and Consultants are equivocal whether oral intake of clear liquids increases maternal risk of pulmonary aspiration.

RECOMMENDATIONS: The oral intake of modest amounts of clear liquids may be allowed for uncomplicated laboring patients. Examples of clear liquids include, but are not limited to, water, fruit juices without pulp, carbonated beverages, clear tea, and black coffee. The volume of liquid ingested is less important than the type of liquid ingested. However, patients with additional risk factors of aspiration (e.g., morbid obesity, diabetes, difficult airway), or patients at increased risk for operative delivery (e.g., nonreassuring fetal heart rate pattern) may have further restrictions of oral intake, determined on a case-by-case basis.

Solids. A specific fasting time for solids that is predictive of maternal anesthetic complications has not been determined. There is insufficient published evidence to address the safety of *any* particular fasting period for solids for obstetric patients. The Consultants agree that a fasting period for solids of 8 hours or more is preferable for uncomplicated parturients undergoing *elective* cesarean delivery. The Task Force recognizes that in laboring patients the timing of delivery is uncertain; therefore compliance with a predetermined fasting period is not always possible. The Task Force supports a fasting period of at least 6 hours before elective cesarean delivery.

RECOMMENDATIONS: Solid foods should be avoided in laboring patients. The patient undergoing elective cesarean delivery should undergo a fasting period for solids consistent with the hospital's policy for nonobstetric patients undergoing elective surgery. Both the amount and type of food ingested must be considered when determining the timing of surgery.

ANESTHESIA CARE FOR LABOR AND VAGINAL DELIVERY

Overview of Recommendations. Anesthesia care is not necessary for all women for labor and/or delivery. For women who request pain relief for labor and/or delivery, there are many effective analgesic techniques available. Maternal request represents sufficient justification for pain relief, but the selected analgesia technique depends on the medical status of the patient, the progress of the labor, and the resources of the facility. When sufficient resources (e.g., anesthesia and nursing staff) are available, epidural catheter techniques should be one of the analgesic options offered. The primary goal is to provide adequate maternal analgesia with as little motor block as possible when regional analgesia is used for uncomplicated labor and/or vaginal delivery. This can be achieved by the administration of local anesthetic at low concentrations. The concentration of the local anesthetic may be further reduced by the addition of narcotics and still provide adequate analgesia.

Specific Recommendations
Epidural Anesthetics
Epidural Local Anesthetics. The literature supports the use of single-bolus epidural local anesthetics for providing greater quality of analgesia compared to *parenteral opioids*. However, the literature indicates a reduced incidence of spontaneous vaginal delivery associated with single-bolus epidural local anesthetics. The literature is insufficient to indicate causation. Compared to *single-injection spinal opioids* the literature is equivocal regarding the analgesic efficacy of single-bolus epidural local anesthetics. The literature suggests that epidural local anesthetics compared to spinal opioids are associated with a lower incidence of pruritus. The literature is insufficient to compare the incidence of other side effects.

Addition of Opioids to Epidural Local Anesthetics. The literature supports the use of epidural local anesthetics with opioids, when compared with *equal* concentrations of epidural local anesthetics without opioids for providing greater quality and duration of analgesia. The former is associated with reduced motor block and an increased likelihood of spontaneous delivery, possibly as a result of a reduced total dose of local anesthetic administered over time.*

The literature is equivocal regarding the analgesic efficiency of *low* concentrations of epidural local anesthetics with opioids compared to *higher* concentrations of epidural local anesthetics without opioids. The literature indicates that low concentrations of epidural local anesthetics with opioids compared to higher concentrations of epidural local anesthetics are associated with reduced motor block.

No differences in the incidence of nausea, hypotension, duration of labor, or neonatal outcomes are found when epidural local anesthetics with opioids were compared to epidural local anesthetics without opioids. However, the literature indicates that the addition of opioids to epidural local anesthetics results in a higher incidence of pruritus. The literature is insufficient to determine the effects of epidural local anesthetics with opioids on other maternal outcomes (e.g., respiratory depression, urinary retention).

The Task Force and majority of Consultants are supportive of the case-by-case selection of an analgesic technique for labor. The subgroup of Consultants reporting a preferred technique, when all choices are available, selected an epidural local anesthetic technique. When a low concentration of epidural local anesthetic is used, the Consultants and Task Force agree that the addition of an opioid(s) improves analgesia and maternal satisfaction without increasing maternal, fetal or neonatal complications.

---

*No meta-analytic differences in the likelihood of spontaneous delivery were found when studies using morphine or meperidine were added to studies using only fentanyl or sufentanil.

RECOMMENDATIONS: The selected analgesic/anesthetic technique should reflect patient needs and preferences, practitioner preferences or skills, and available resources. When an epidural local anesthetic is selected for labor and delivery, the addition of an opioid may allow the use of a lower concentration of local anesthetic and prolong the duration of analgesia. Appropriate resources for the treatment of complications related to epidural local anesthetics (e.g., hypotension, systemic toxicity, high spinal anesthesia) should be available. If opioids are added, treatments for related complications (e.g., pruritus, nausea, respiratory depression) should be available.

Continuous Infusion Epidural Techniques (CIE). The literature indicates that effective analgesia can be maintained with a low concentration of local anesthetic with an epidural infusion technique. In addition, when an opioid is added to a local anesthetic infusion, an even lower concentration of local anesthetic provides effective analgesia. For example, comparable analgesia is found, with a reduced incidence of motor block, using bupivacaine infusion concentrations of *less than* 0.125% with an opioid compared to bupivacaine concentrations *equal to* 0.125% without an opioid.* No comparative differences are noted for incidence of instrumental delivery.

The literature is equivocal regarding the relationship between different local anesthetic infusion regimens and the incidence of nausea or neonatal outcome. However, the literature suggests that local anesthetic infusions with opioids are associated with a higher incidence of pruritus.

The Task Force and Consultants agree that infusions using low concentrations of local anesthetics with or without opioids provide equivalent analgesia, reduced motor block, and improved maternal satisfaction when compared to higher concentrations of local anesthetic.

RECOMMENDATIONS: Adequate analgesia for uncomplicated labor and delivery should be provided with the secondary goal of producing as little motor block as possible. The lowest concentration of local anesthetic infusion that provides adequate maternal analgesia and satisfaction should be used. For example, an infusion concentration of bupivacaine equal to or greater than 0.25% is unnecessary for labor analgesia for most patients. The addition of an opioid(s) to a low concentration of local anesthetic may improve analgesia and minimize motor block. Resources for the treatment of potential complications should be available.

Spinal Opioids With or Without Local Anesthetics. The literature suggests that spinal opioids with or without

---

*References to bupivacaine are included for illustrative purposes only, and because bupivacaine is the most extensively studied local anesthetic for CIE. The Task Force recognizes that other local anesthetic agents are equally appropriate for CIE.

local anesthetics provide effective labor analgesia without significantly altering the incidence of neonatal complications. There is insufficient literature to compare spinal opioids with parenteral opioids. However, the Consultants and Task Force agree that spinal opioids provide improved maternal analgesia compared to parenteral opioids.

The literature is equivocal regarding analgesic efficacy of spinal opioids compared to epidural local anesthetics. The Consultants and Task Force agree that spinal opioids provide equivalent analgesia compared to epidural local anesthetics. The Task Force agrees that the rapid onset of analgesia provided by single-injection spinal techniques may be advantageous for selected patients (e.g., those in advanced labor).

RECOMMENDATIONS: Spinal opioids with or without local anesthetics may be used to provide effective, although time-limited, analgesia for labor. Resources for the treatment of potential complications (e.g., pruritus, nausea, hypotension, respiratory depression) should be available.

Combined Spinal-Epidural Techniques. Although the literature suggests that combined spinal-epidural techniques (CSE) provide effective analgesia, the literature is insufficient to evaluate the analgesic efficacy of CSE compared to epidural local anesthetics. The literature indicates that use of CSE techniques with opioids when compared to epidural local anesthetics with or without opioids results in a higher incidence of pruritus and nausea. The Task Force and Consultants are equivocal regarding improved analgesia or maternal benefit of CSE versus epidural techniques. Although the literature is insufficient to evaluate fetal and neonatal outcomes of CSE techniques, the Task Force and Consultants agree that CSE does not increase the risk of fetal or neonatal complications.

RECOMMENDATIONS: Combined spinal-epidural techniques may be used to provide rapid and effective analgesia for labor. Resources for the treatment of potential complications (e.g., pruritus, nausea, hypotension, respiratory depression) should be available.

Regional Analgesia and Progress of Labor. There is insufficient literature to indicate whether timing of analgesia related to cervical dilation affects labor and delivery outcomes. Both the Task Force and Consultants agree that cervical dilation at the time of epidural analgesia administration does not impact the outcome of labor.

The literature indicates that epidural analgesia may be used in a triad of labor for previous cesarean section patients without adversely affecting the incidence of vaginal delivery. However, randomized comparisons of epidural versus other specific anesthetic techniques were not found, and comparison groups were often confounded.

RECOMMENDATIONS: Cervical dilation is not a reliable means of determining when regional analgesia should be initiated.

Regional analgesia should be administered on an individualized basis.

Monitored or Stand-by Anesthesia Care for Complicated Vaginal Delivery. Monitored anesthesia care refers to instances in which an anesthesiologist has been called upon to provide specific anesthesia services to a particular patient undergoing a planned procedure.[2] For these Guidelines, stand-by anesthesia care refers to the availability of the anesthesiologist in the facility, in the event of obstetric complications. The literature is silent regarding the subject of monitored or stand-by anesthesia care in obstetrics. However, the Task Force and Consultants agree that monitored or stand-by anesthesia care for complicated vaginal delivery reduces maternal, fetal, and neonatal complications.

RECOMMENDATIONS: Either monitored or stand-by anesthesia care, determined on a case-by-case basis for complicated vaginal delivery (e.g., breech presentation, twins, and trial of instrumental delivery), should be made available when requested by the obstetrician.

REMOVAL OF RETAINED PLACENTA

Anesthetic Choices. The literature is insufficient to indicate whether a particular type of anesthetic is more effective than another for removal of retained placenta. The literature is also insufficient to assess the relationship between a particular type of anesthetic and maternal complications. The Task Force and Consultants agree that spinal or epidural anesthesia (i.e., regional anesthesia) is associated with reduced maternal complications and improved satisfaction when compared to general anesthesia or sedation/analgesia. The Task Force recognizes that circumstances may occur when general anesthesia or sedation/analgesia may be the more appropriate anesthetic choice (e.g., significant hemorrhage).

RECOMMENDATIONS: Regional anesthesia, general endotracheal anesthesia, or sedation/analgesia may be used for removal of retained placenta. Hemodynamic status should be assessed before giving regional anesthesia to a parturient who has experienced significant bleeding. In cases involving significant maternal hemorrhage, a general anesthetic may be preferable to initiating regional anesthesia. Sedation/analgesia should be titrated carefully due to the potential risk of pulmonary aspiration in the recently delivered parturient with an unprotected airway.

Nitroglycerin for Uterine Relaxation. The literature suggests and the Task Force and Consultants agree that the administration of nitroglycerin is effective for uterine relaxation during removal of retained placental tissue.

RECOMMENDATIONS: Nitroglycerin is an alternative to terbutaline sulfate or general endotracheal anesthesia with halogenated agents for uterine relaxation during removal of retained placental tissue. Initiating treatment with a low dose of nitroglycerin may relax the uterus sufficiently while minimizing potential complications (e.g., hypotension).

ANESTHETIC CHOICES FOR CESAREAN DELIVERY

The literature suggests that spinal, epidural or CSE anesthetic techniques can be used effectively for cesarean delivery. When compared to regional techniques, the literature indicates that general anesthetics can be administered with shorter induction-to-delivery times. The literature is insufficient to determine the relative risk of maternal death associated with general anesthesia compared to other anesthetic techniques. However, the literature suggests that a greater number of maternal deaths occur when general anesthesia is administered. The literature indicates that a larger proportion of neonates in the general anesthesia groups, compared to those in the regional anesthesia groups, are assigned Apgar scores of less than 7 at one and five minutes. However, few studies have utilized randomized comparisons of general versus regional anesthesia, resulting in potential selection bias in the reporting of outcomes.

The literature suggests that maternal side effects associated with regional techniques may include hypotension, nausea, vomiting, pruritus and postdural puncture headache. The literature is insufficient to examine the comparative merits of various regional anesthetic techniques.

The Consultants agree that regional anesthesia can be administered with fewer maternal and neonatal complications and improved maternal satisfaction when compared to general anesthesia. The Consultants are equivocal about the possibility of increased maternal complications when comparing spinal or epidural anesthesia with CSE techniques. They agree that neonatal complications are not increased with CSE techniques.

RECOMMENDATIONS: The decision to use a particular anesthetic technique should be individualized based on several factors. These include anesthetic, obstetric and/or fetal risk factors (e.g., elective versus emergency) and the preferences of the patient and anesthesiologist. Resources for the treatment of potential complications (e.g., airway management, inadequate analgesia, hypotension, pruritus, nausea) should be available.

POSTPARTUM TUBAL LIGATION

There is insufficient literature to evaluate the comparative benefits of local, spinal, epidural or general anesthesia for postpartum tubal ligation. Both the Task Force and Consultants agree that epidural, spinal and general anesthesia can be effectively provided without affecting maternal complications. Neither the Task Force nor the Consultants agree that local anesthetic techniques provide effective anesthesia, and they are equivocal regarding the impact of local anesthesia on maternal complications. Although the literature is insufficient, the Task Force and Consultants agree that a postpartum tubal ligation can be performed safely within eight hours of delivery in many patients.

RECOMMENDATIONS: Evaluation of the patient for postpartum tubal ligation should include assessment of hemodynamic status (e.g., blood loss) and consideration of anesthetic risks. The patient planning to have an elective postpartum tubal ligation within 8 hours of delivery should have no oral intake of solid foods during labor, and postpartum until the time of surgery. Both the timing of the procedure and the decision to use a particular anesthetic technique (i.e., regional versus general) should be individualized, based on anesthetic and/or obstetric risk factors and patient preferences. The anesthesiologist should be aware that an epidural catheter placed for labor may be more likely to fail with longer postdelivery time intervals. If a postpartum tubal ligation is to be done before the patient is discharged from the hospital, the procedure should not be attempted at a time when it might compromise other aspects of patient care in the labor and delivery area.

MANAGEMENT OF COMPLICATIONS

Resources for Management of Hemorrhagic Emergencies. The literature suggests that the availability of resources for hemorrhagic emergencies is associated with reduced maternal complications. The Task Force and Consultants agree that the availability of resources for managing hemorrhagic emergencies is associated with reduced maternal, fetal and neonatal complications.

RECOMMENDATIONS: Institutions providing obstetric care should have resources available to manage hemorrhagic emergencies (Table 1). In an emergency, the use of type-specific or O negative blood is acceptable in the parturient.

■ Table 1
SUGGESTED RESOURCES FOR OBSTETRIC HEMORRHAGIC EMERGENCIES*

1. Large bore iv catheters
2. Fluid warmer
3. Forced air body warmer
4. Availability of blood bank resources
5. Equipment for infusing iv fluids and/or blood products rapidly. Examples include (but not limited to) hand squeezed fluid chambers, hand inflated pressure bags, and automatic infusion devices.

*The items listed represent suggestions. The items should be customized to meet the specific needs, preferences, and skills of the practitioner and healthcare facility.

Equipment for Management of Airway Emergencies. The literature suggests, and the Task Force and Consultants agree, that the availability of equipment for the management of airway emergencies is associated with reduced maternal complications.

RECOMMENDATIONS: Labor and delivery units should have equipment and personnel readily available to manage airway emergencies. Basic airway management equipment should be immediately available during the initial provision of regional analgesia (Table 2). In addition, portable equipment for difficult airway management should be readily available in the operative area of labor and delivery units (Table 3)

Central Invasive Hemodynamic Monitoring. There is insufficient literature to indicate whether pulmonary artery catheterization is associated with improved maternal, fetal or neonatal outcomes in patients with pregnancy-related hypertensive disorders. The literature is silent regarding the management of obstetric patients with central venous catheterization alone. The literature suggests that pulmonary artery catheterization has been used safely in obstetric patients; however, the literature is insufficient to examine specific obstetric outcomes. The Task Force and Consultants agree that it is not necessary to use central invasive hemodynamic monitoring routinely for parturients with severe preeclampsia.

RECOMMENDATIONS: The decision to perform invasive hemodynamic monitoring should be individualized and based on clinical indications that include the patient's medical history and cardiovascular risk factors. The Task Force recognizes that not all practitioners have access to resources for utilization of central venous or pulmonary artery catheters in obstetric units.

Cardiopulmonary Resuscitation. The literature is insufficient to evaluate the efficacy of CPR in the obstetric patient during labor and delivery. The Task Force is supportive of

■ Table 2
SUGGESTED RESOURCES FOR AIRWAY MANAGEMENT DURING INITIAL PROVISION OF REGIONAL ANESTHESIA*

1. Laryngoscope and assorted blades
2. Endotracheal tubes, with stylets
3. Oxygen source
4. Suction source with tubing and catheters
5. Self-inflating bag and mask for positive pressure ventilation
6. Medications for blood pressure support, muscle relaxation, and hypnosis

*The items listed represent suggestions. The items should be customized to meet the specific needs, preferences, and skills of the practitioner and healthcare facility.

■ Table 3
SUGGESTED CONTENTS OF A PORTABLE UNIT FOR DIFFICULT AIRWAY MANAGEMENT FOR CESAREAN SECTION ROOMS*

1. Rigid laryngoscope blades and handles of alternate design and size from those routinely used†
2. Endotracheal tubes of assorted size
3. Laryngeal mask airways of assorted sizes
4. At least one device suitable for emergency nonsurgical airway ventilation. Examples include (but are not limited to) retrograde intubation equipment, a hollow jet ventilation stylet or cricothyrotomy kit with or without a transtracheal jet ventilator, and the esophageal-tracheal combitube.
5. Endotracheal tube guides. Examples include (but are not limited to) semirigid stylets with or without a hollow core for jet ventilation, light wands, and forceps designed to manipulate the distal portion of the endotracheal tube.
6. Equipment suitable for emergency surgical airway access
7. Topical anesthetics and vasoconstrictors

*The items listed represent suggestions. The items should be customized to meet the specific needs, preferences, and skills of the practitioner and health-care facility.

†The Task Force believes fiberoptic intubation equipment should be readily available.

Adapted from Practice guidelines for management of the difficult airway: A report by the American Society of Anesthesiologists Task Force on Management of the Difficult Airway. Anesthesiology 1993; 78:599–602.

the immediate availability of basic and advanced life-support equipment in the operative area of labor and delivery units.

RECOMMENDATIONS: Basic and advanced life-support equipment should be immediately available in the operative area of labor and delivery units. If cardiac arrest occurs during labor and delivery, standard resuscitative measures and procedures, including left uterine displacement, should be taken. In cases of cardiac arrest, the American Heart Association has stated the following: "Several authors now recommend that the decision to perform a perimortem cesarean section should be made rapidly, with delivery effected within 4 to 5 minutes of the arrest."[3]

REFERENCES

1. Guidelines for Perinatal Care, 4th ed. American Academy of Pediatrics and American College of Obstetricians and Gynecologists, 1997, pp 100–102
2. American Society of Anesthesiologists: Position on monitored anesthesia care, ASA Standards, Guidelines and Statements. Park Ridge, IL, American Society of Anesthesiologists, October 1997, pp 20–21
3. Guidelines for cardiopulmonary resuscitation and emergency cardiac care: recommendations of the 1992 national conference. JAMA 1992; 268:2249

GUIDELINES FOR REGIONAL ANESTHESIA IN OBSTETRICS

(Approved by House of Delegates on October 12, 1988 and last amended on October 30, 1991)

■■■

These guidelines apply to the use of regional anesthesia or analgesia in which local anesthetics are administered to the parturient during labor and delivery. They are intended to encourage quality patient care but cannot guarantee any specific patient outcome. Because the availability of anesthesia resources may vary, members are responsible for interpreting and establishing the guidelines for their own institutions and practices. These guidelines are subject to revision from time to time as warranted by the evolution of technology and practice.

GUIDELINE I

Regional anesthesia should be initiated and maintained only in locations in which appropriate resuscitation equipment and drugs are immediately available to manage procedurally related problems.

Resuscitation equipment should include, but is not limited to: sources of oxygen and suction, equipment to maintain an airway and perform endotracheal intubation, a means to provide positive pressure ventilation, and drugs and equipment for cardiopulmonary resuscitation.

GUIDELINE II

Regional anesthesia should be initiated by a physician with appropriate privileges and maintained by or under the medical direction[1] of such an individual.

Physicians should be approved through the institutional credentialing process to initiate and direct the maintenance of obstetric anesthesia and to manage procedurally related complications.

GUIDELINE III

Regional anesthesia should not be administered until: 1) the patient has been examined by a qualified individual[2]; and 2) The maternal and fetal status and progress of labor have been evaluated by a physician with privileges in obstetrics who is readily available to supervise the labor and manage any obstetric complications that may arise.

Under circumstances defined by department protocol, qualified personnel may perform the initial pelvic examination. The physician responsible for the patient's obstetrical care should be informed of her status so that a decision can be made regarding present risk and further management.[2]

320

GUIDELINE IV

An intravenous infusion should be established before the initiation of regional anesthesia and maintained throughout the duration of the regional anesthetic.

GUIDELINE V

Regional anesthesia for labor and/or vaginal delivery requires that the parturient's vital signs and the fetal heart rate be monitored and documented by a qualified individual. Additional monitoring appropriate to the clinical condition of the parturient and the fetus should be employed when indicated. When extensive regional blockade is administered for complicated vaginal delivery, the standards for basic anesthetic monitoring[3] should be applied.

GUIDELINE VI

Regional anesthesia for cesarean delivery requires that the standards for basic anesthetic monitoring[3] be applied and that a physician with privileges in obstetrics be immediately available.

GUIDELINE VII

Qualified personnel, other than the anesthesiologist attending the mother, should be immediately available to assume responsibility for resuscitation of the newborn.[3]

The primary responsibility of the anesthesiologist is to provide care to the mother. If the anesthesiologist is also requested to provide brief assistance in the care of the newborn, the benefit to the child must be compared to the risk to the mother.

GUIDELINE VIII

A physician with appropriate privileges should remain readily available during the regional anesthetic to manage anesthetic complications until the patient's postanesthesia condition is satisfactory and stable.

GUIDELINE IX

All patients recovering from regional anesthesia should receive appropriate postanesthesia care. Following cesarean delivery and/or extensive regional blockade, the standards for postanesthesia care[4] should be applied.

1. A postanesthesia care unit (PACU) should be available to receive patients. The design, equipment and staffing should meet requirements of the facility's accrediting and licensing bodies.
2. When a site other than the PACU is used, equivalent postanesthesia care should be provided.

GUIDELINE X

There should be a policy to assure the availability in the facility of a physician to manage complications and to provide cardiopulmonary resuscitation for patients receiving postanesthesia care.

REFERENCES

1. The Anesthesia Care Team (Approved by ASA House of Delegates 10/26/82 and last amended 10/21/92).
2. Guidelines for Perinatal Care (American Academy of Pediatrics and American College of Obstetricians and Gynecologists, 1988).
3. Standards for Basic Anesthetic Monitoring (Approved by ASA House of Delegates 10/21/86 and last amended 10/23/96).
4. Standards for Postanesthesia Care (Approved by ASA House of Delegates 10/12/88 and last amended 10/19/94).

STANDARDS FOR BASIC ANESTHETIC MONITORING

(Approved by House of Delegates on October 21, 1986 and last amended on October 21, 1998)

∎∎∎

These standards apply to all anesthesia care although, in emergency circumstances, appropriate life support measures take precedence. These standards may be exceeded at any time based on the judgment of the responsible anesthesiologist. They are intended to encourage quality patient care, but observing them cannot guarantee any specific patient outcome. They are subject to revision from time to time, as warranted by the evolution of technology and practice. They apply to all general anesthetics, regional anesthetics and monitored anesthesia care. This set of standards addresses only the issue of basic anesthetic monitoring, which is one component of anesthesia care. In certain rare or unusual circumstances, (1) some of these methods of monitoring may be clinically impractical, and (2) appropriate use of the described monitoring methods may fail to detect untoward clinical developments. Brief interruptions of continual† monitoring may be unavoidable. *Under extenuating circumstances, the responsible anesthesiologist may waive the requirements marked with an asterisk (*); it is recommended that when this is done, it should be so stated (including the reasons) in a note in the patient's medical record.* These standards are not intended for application of the care of the obstetrical patient in labor or in the conduct of pain management.

STANDARD I

Qualified anesthesia personnel shall be present in the room throughout the conduct of all general anesthetics, regional anesthetics and monitored anesthesia care.

OBJECTIVE

Because of the rapid changes in patient status during anesthesia, qualified anesthesia personnel shall be continuously present to monitor the patient and provide anesthesia care. In the event there is a direct known hazard, e.g., radiation, to the anesthesia personnel which might require intermittent remote observation of the patient, some provision for monitoring the patient must be made. In the event that an emergency requires the temporary absence of the person primarily responsible for the anesthetic, the best judgment of the anesthesiologist will be exercised in comparing the emergency with the anesthetized patient's condition and in the selection of the person

---

†Note that "continual" is defined as "repeated regularly and frequently in steady rapid succession" whereas "continuous" means "prolonged without any interruption at any time."

left responsible for the anesthetic during the temporary absence.

STANDARD II

During all anesthetics, the patient's oxygenation, ventilation, circulation and temperature shall be continually evaluated.

OXYGENATION

Objective

To ensure adequate oxygen concentration in the inspired gas and the blood during all anesthetics.

Methods

1. Inspired gas: During every administration of general anesthesia using an anesthesia machine, the concentration of oxygen in the patient breathing system shall be measured by an oxygen analyzer with a low oxygen concentration limit alarm in use.*
2. Blood oxygenation: During all anesthetics, a quantitative method of assessing oxygenation such as pulse oximetry shall be employed.* Adequate illumination and exposure of the patient are necessary to assess color.*

VENTILATION

Objective

To ensure adequate ventilation of the patient during all anesthetics.

Methods

1. Every patient receiving general anesthesia shall have the adequacy of ventilation continually evaluated. Qualitative clinical signs such as chest excursion, observation of the reservoir breathing bag and auscultation of breath sounds are useful. Continual monitoring for the presence of expired carbon dioxide shall be performed unless invalidated by the nature of the patient, procedure or equipment. Quantitative monitoring of the volume of expired gas is strongly encouraged.*
2. When an endotracheal tube or laryngeal mask is inserted, its correct positioning must be verified by clinical assessment and by identification of carbon dioxide in the expired gas. Continual end-tidal carbon dioxide analysis, in use from the time of endotracheal tube/laryngeal mask placement, until extubation/removal or transfer to a postoperative care location, shall be performed using a quantitative method such as capnography, capnometry or mass spectroscopy.*
3. When ventilation is controlled by a mechanical ventilator, there shall be in continuous use a device that is capable of

detecting disconnection of components of the breathing system. The device must give an audible signal when its alarm threshold is exceeded.

4. During regional anesthesia and monitored anesthesia care, the adequacy of ventilation shall be evaluated, at least, by continual observation of qualitative clinical signs.

CIRCULATION

Objective

To ensure the adequacy of the patient's circulatory function during all anesthetics.

Methods

1. Every patient receiving anesthesia shall have the electrocardiogram continuously displayed from the beginning of anesthesia until preparing to leave the anesthetizing location.*

2. Every patient receiving anesthesia shall have arterial blood pressure and heart rate determined and evaluated at least every five minutes.*

3. Every patient receiving general anesthesia shall have, in addition to the above, circulatory function continually evaluated by at least one of the following: palpation of a pulse, auscultation of heart sounds, monitoring of a tracing of intra-arterial pressure, ultrasound peripheral pulse monitoring, or pulse plethysmography or oximetry.

BODY TEMPERATURE

Objective

To aid in the maintenance of appropriate body temperature during all anesthetics.

Methods

Every patient receiving anesthesia shall have temperature monitored when clinically significant changes in body temperature are intended, anticipated or suspected.

STANDARDS FOR POSTANESTHESIA CARE

(Approved by House of Delegates on October 12, 1988 and last amended on October 19, 1994)

■ ■ ■

These standards apply to postanesthesia care in all locations. These standards may be exceeded based on the judgment of the responsible anesthesiologist. They are intended to encourage quality patient care, but cannot guarantee any specific patient outcome. They are subject to revision from time to time as warranted by the evolution of technology and practice. Under extenuating circumstances, the responsible anesthesiologist may waive the requirements marked with an asterisk (*); it is recommended that when this is done, it should be so stated (including the reasons) in a note in the patient's medical record.

STANDARD I

All patients who have received general anesthesia, regional anesthesia or monitored anesthesia care shall receive appropriate postanesthesia management.[1]

1. A Postanesthesia Care Unit (PACU) or an area which provides equivalent postanesthesia care shall be available to receive patients after anesthesia care. All patients who receive anesthesia care shall be admitted to the PACU or its equivalent except by specific order of the anesthesiologist responsible for the patient's care.
2. The medical aspects of care in the PACU shall be governed by policies and procedures which have been reviewed and approved by the Department of Anesthesiology.
3. The design, equipment and staffing of the PACU shall meet requirements of the facility's accrediting and licensing bodies.

STANDARD II

A patient transported to the PACU shall be accompanied by a member of the anesthesia care team who is knowledgeable about the patient's condition. The patient shall be continually evaluated and treated during transport with monitoring and support appropriate to the patient's condition.

STANDARD III

Upon arrival in the PACU, the patient shall be re-evaluated and a verbal report provided to the responsible PACU nurse by the member of the anesthesia care team who accompanies the patient.

1. The patient's status on arrival in the PACU shall be documented.
2. Information concerning the preoperative condition and the surgical/anesthetic course shall be transmitted to the PACU nurse.

3. The member of the Anesthesia Care Team shall remain in the PACU until the PACU nurse accepts responsibility for the nursing care of the patient.

STANDARD IV
The patient's condition shall be evaluated continually in the PACU.

1. The patient shall be observed and monitored by methods appropriate to the patient's medical condition. Particular attention should be given to monitoring oxygenation, ventilation, circulation and temperature. During recovery from all anesthetics, a quantitative method of assessing oxygenation such as pulse oximetry shall be employed in the initial phase of recovery.* This is not intended for application during the recovery of the obstetrical patient in whom regional anesthesia was used for labor and vaginal delivery.
2. An accurate written report of the PACU period shall be maintained. Use of an appropriate PACU scoring system is encouraged for each patient on admission, at appropriate intervals prior to discharge and at the time of discharge.
3. General medical supervision and coordination of patient care in the PACU should be the responsibility of an anesthesiologist.
4. There shall be a policy to assure the availability in the facility of a physician capable of managing complications and providing cardiopulmonary resuscitation for patients in the PACU.

STANDARD V
A physician is responsible for the discharge of the patient from the postanesthesia care unit.

1. When discharge criteria are used, they must be approved by the Department of Anesthesiology and the medical staff. They may vary depending upon whether the patient is discharged to a hospital room, to the Intensive Care Unit, to a short stay unit or home.
2. In the absence of the physician responsible for the discharge, the PACU nurse shall determine that the patient meets the discharge criteria. The name of the physician accepting responsibility for discharge shall be noted on the record.

REFERENCE

1. Refer to Standards of Post Anesthesia Nursing Practice 1992 published by ASPAN, for issues of nursing care.

INDEX

Note: Page numbers in italics refer to illustrations; page numbers followed by t refer to tables.